Seen and Heard

Seen and Heard:

Exploring Participation, Engagement and Voice for Children with Disabilities

Miriam Twomey and Clare Carroll (Eds)

PETER LANG

Oxford · Bern · Berlin · Bruxelles · New York · Wien

Bibliographic information published by Die Deutsche Nationalbibliothek.
Die Deutsche Nationalbibliothek lists this publication in the Deutsche
National-bibliografie; detailed bibliographic data is available on the
Internet at http://dnb.d-nb.de.

A catalogue record for this book is available from the British Library.

Library of Congress Cataloging-in-Publication Data:

Names: Twomey, Miriam, 1963- editor. | Carroll, Clare, 1975- editor.
Title: Seen and heard : researching with children with disabilities:
    engagement, participation and voice/Miriam Twomey and Clare Carroll
    (eds).
Description: First edition. | Oxford; New York: Peter Lang, [2018] |
    Includes bibliographical references and index.
Identifiers: LCCN 2018023023 | ISBN 9781787075160 (alk. paper)
Subjects: LCSH: Children with disabilities.
Classification: LCC HV888 .S44 2018 | DDC 305.9/08072—dc23 LC record
available at https://lccn.loc.gov/2018023023

Cover design by Peter Lang Ltd.

Cover image: Detail from Raffael's *Madonna Sixtina*, reproduced under
a Creative Commons Attribution 2.0 Generic license (source: Wikimedia
Commons).

ISBN 978-1-78707-516-0 (print) • ISBN 978-1-78707-517-7 (ePDF)
ISBN 978-1-78707-518-4 (ePub) • ISBN 978-1-78707-519-1 (mobi)

© Peter Lang AG 2018

Published by Peter Lang Ltd, International Academic Publishers,
52 St Giles, Oxford, OX1 3LU, United Kingdom
oxford@peterlang.com, www.peterlang.com

Miriam Twomey and Clare Carroll have asserted their right under the
Copyright, Designs and Patents Act, 1988, to be identified as Editors of this
Work.

This publication has been peer reviewed.

Printed in Germany

Contents

Foreword

The movement towards establishing inclusive learning environments has been a long and convoluted journey. Everyone appears to agree that inclusion is a good idea, however, agreement about how inclusive education is to be understood and implemented is elusive. If something such as inclusion appears to be indisputably a good to be strived for why has it taken so long to become embedded in ordinary classroom practice. There is no shortage of international and national policies advocating inclusive education, many of these policies have been mandated through enabling legislation and yet resistance to inclusion is apparent.

Gary Thomas (2013) observes that the movements advocating inclusion originated in the social and political spheres rather than within education. He argues very cogently that inclusive education was not based on egalitarian perspectives but had emerged from special education. As a result, it can be argued that in many school environments inclusive education is special education dressed up in new clothes more appropriate for a twenty-first-century audience. Inclusive education is still shackled to the notions of difference and disability that characterized special educational thinking and practice. As educators, our understanding of what constitutes learning has evolved to realize that all learning is social and that failure in learning is attributable to many factors including school culture, pedagogical practice and understanding of difference. As a society, there is a growing awareness that failure in learning has immediate and long-term consequences for the individual concerned, their families and communities and society itself. Young people considered to be failures are likely to be 'excluded from the expectations, the activities, the resources, the worlds of their peers' (Thomas 2013: 480).

Establishing inclusive school environments is multi-faceted, involving the development of a responsive school culture, principled leadership, informed and knowledgeable educators and a willingness to reshape how support for all learners is conceptualized. However, it is also critical that the voice of children and young people is respected and acted upon. In recent years there has been a growing recognition of the importance of the voice of children and young people, particularly those from traditionally marginalized communities, in decision making processes that affect their lives. Children and young people identified as having special educational needs are well able to articulate their opinions on educational provision, as demonstrated in Rose and Shevlin's (2015) report. These children and young people particularly appreciated a supportive school ethos characterized by positive relationships with their teachers and the availability of personalized support to address their specific learning and social needs. Children and young people identified how a non-judgemental, encouraging approach by teachers enabled them to tackle the challenges they experienced in learning.

Early childhood education encounters many of the challenges experienced by primary and post-primary schools in establishing inclusive learning environments. Inclusive early childhood education needs to enable all children, including those who are vulnerable to exclusion, to belong, to become active participants and to learn alongside each other in their local community (European Agency for Special Needs and Inclusive Education (EASNIE) 2017). Inclusive early childhood environments are characterized by how they value each child within a supportive learning community where positive relationships are the norm and everyone is focused on the individual child's progress in stark contrast to a slavish adherence to attaining national standards of competence (EASNIE 2017).

This book, edited by Miriam Twomey and Clare Carroll, offers a unique opportunity to access the voice of children within early childhood settings who are receiving early intervention supports. These children are often the most marginalized and vulnerable within our society and many are voiceless in shaping their lives. The international interdisciplinary perspectives presented in this book are focused on enabling these children to begin to have agency in their lives. Current support mechanisms for these children are usually characterized by an emphasis on eligibility and identification which often obscures the need to develop innovative interventions designed to enable these children to become active participants in their learning, belong within their peer group and become recognized within their local communities. The insights developed through the interdisciplinary perspective presented in this book will be essential in establishing viable, sustainable inclusive early education environments that welcome and value every child.

We all need to interrogate our own assumptions and beliefs about how we as educators, health professionals and researchers value and support our most vulnerable children in their early years. Prepare to be challenged and energized through engaging with the ideas and innovative practices documented in this book and we can begin together to implement these insights in establishing the inclusive learning environments in early childhood education that will benefit all children including our most vulnerable.

Michael Shevlin
(Professor in Inclusive Education, Trinity College Dublin)

References

European Agency for Special Needs and Inclusive Education (EASNIE) (2017). *Inclusive Early Childhood Education: New Insights and Tools*. Brussels: EASNIE.

Rose, R., and Shevlin, M. (2015). This is what works for me: students reflect on their experiences of special needs provision in Irish mainstream schools. In E. West (ed.), *Including Learners with Low-Incidence Disabilities*, pp. 183–202. Bingley: Emerald Group Publishing Ltd.

Thomas, G. (2013). A review of the thinking and research about inclusive education policy, with suggestions for a new kind of inclusive thinking. *British Educational Research Journal*, 39(3), 473–490.

MIRIAM TWOMEY AND CLARE CARROLL

Introduction: Why voice and why now?

This book endeavours to explore new thinking around children's participation, engagement and voice in initiating collaborations with national and international authors from a range of disciplines committed to this field of research. This book emerged following the editors' doctoral and postdoctoral work on listening to young children's voices. The editors recognized the need to share and understand how researchers are currently exploring children's voice from hard-to-reach groups in an authentic manner. The editors also sought to disentangle myths associated with participation, engagement and impairment and to legitimize voice in all its forms. This book will explore innovative approaches to researching with children who previously may have not been listened to, sharing various interpretations of 'voice' and what is known about voice. It explores children's voice from a number of philosophical, methodological and interpretive orientations (including but not limited to psychological, sociological, anthropological, medical, legal, therapeutic, and educational). This book aims to engage with a community that are particularly interested in researching with children who have a disability (or are at risk of a disability) and who may be eligible for Early Intervention or education services. The editors are committed to a rights-based approach and hope to support and extend the increasing view that we need to learn and understand through children's eyes (using environmental, visual, tactile, movement-based supports), or other innovative ways of encouraging their participation and engagement. This highlights children's participation and engagement as pre-requisites to voice, or possibly manifesting voice itself, and also draws on a culture of listening, encouraging research with children who would historically have been without voice or agency. We are mindful of Charles Dickens' representations of childhood and the much-used aphorism 'children should be seen and not heard'. Children were identified as lesser human beings and experienced a long history of not being seen or heard. Having a voice may be integral to a process of becoming more human or as a means towards self-actualization. Accessing the worlds of children with disabilities will explore critical questions framing this dialogue. It will appraise the use of innovative approaches to voice other than spoken language and how we can address the challenges to our perceptions of competence when researching with children with disabilities.

The importance of researching with children with disabilities has received considerable attention, but little has been written about the particular challenges of researching with children with disabilities from a range of disciplinary perspectives. International policy frameworks orchestrate a policy agenda for this book and have vehemently encouraged children's rights. A vast range of sociological, developmental, anthropological, economic and political research underpins modern definitions of the child. Theorizing about childhood in this book reflects childhood not wholly as a biological state but in terms of who the child is, or will be, as a state of being that is self-determining, legitimate and influenced by rights. This book will draw on theories that are child first, understanding that a person is not defined by their disability, but will also include such descriptions as the disabled child in the sense of being disabled by society. The United Nations Convention on the Rights of the Child (1989) states that the best interests of the child must be the primary consideration and that the child's views must be given due weight in accordance with the child's age and maturity. In Ireland the National Children's Strategy (2000: 6), states that 'children will have a voice in matters which affect them and their views will be given due weight in accordance with their age and maturity'. Drawing on international and national policy, this book focuses on an area worthy of deep exploration. Representing a range of countries, cultures and contexts, adopting a rights-based approach, contributing authors will explore participation, engagement, and voice from hard to reach groups using a range of innovative methods. We want this book to move 'beyond voice', as in the search for children's voice or giving them a voice, to acknowledging the changing and different positions from which children speak. We believe that this newer discourse is a central feature and a common thread underpinning this book. This collection of chapters adds to this newer paradigm and will contribute significantly to this area of research.

The UNCRC (1989) has promoted the rights of children guiding the central tenets of this book: participation, engagement and voice. This Convention contains fifty-two standards setting out the Rights of a Child. Most countries are signatories to the Convention. Many countries adopt the use of the standards wholly or in part to promote children and young people's participation. Deemed specifically to promote children's participation are the following articles: Article 12: Children and young people have the right to say what they think should happen, when adults are making decisions that affect them, and to have their opinions taken into account; Article 13: Children and young people have the right to get and to share information, as long as the information is not damaging to them or others; and Article 23: Children and young people who have any kind of disability have to receive care and support as well as all the rights in the Convention so that they can live full and independent lives. Acknowledging these rights, this book will address the contested issues of participation, engagement and voice for children with disabilities, where challenges exist due to the nature or degree of disability or impairment and the impact of the environment. The benefits of the UNCRC (1989) are now represented as the explicit presence of the child's voice. While present, this voice is understated and occasionally silent (Lewis 2010). In the absence of voice, a different form of expression is required. A child's ability to communicate, grow, develop and learn should not be confined to normative expectations. It is important as Kelly (2005) reminds us to consider the child as experiencing agent – a site of meaning and knowledge in the world (2005: 182). More recently, there is evidence of shifts in thinking about childhood and disability. Childhood and disability are now increasingly reconceptualized in terms of voice, agency, competency and rights. We need to extend a discourse that recognizes the child as an experiencing agent, listening to their voice as a source of understanding. We are hoping to explore innovative and creative methods of accessing the voice of the child, who may have a range of difficulties, looking at research 'with' rather than 'on' children as a priority and enabling children with cognitive, communication, social, physical or medical difficulties to have a voice, in whatever way that may be represented. McLeod (2018: 4) stresses that 'the importance of communication rights goes beyond just enabling freedom of opinion, expression and language. Once these rights are realized, people are more readily able to realize other human rights'.

A notable shift has taken place when considering research on the participation and engagement of the child with a disability, where the impact of context, environment and the challenges in everyday life are prioritized. To this end, regarded as an international benchmark in documenting children and young person's participation and wellbeing, The International Classification of Functioning, Disability and Health for Children and Youth (ICF-CY) (WHO 2007) which is derived from the International Classification of Functioning, Disability and Health (ICF) (WHO 2001) is significant in terms of a move away from the binary and dualist presentation of a medical or social model to its emphasis on the person's functioning in terms of body structures, activity, participation and the environment. This framework is designed to record the characteristics of the developing child and the influence of the environment. The ICF (WHO 2001) and ICF-CY (WHO 2007) provide a framework to document functions and structures of the body, activity limitations and participation restrictions manifested in infancy, childhood and adolescence. They provide a holistic presentation accounting for the biopsychosocial perspectives that may contribute to overall health and well-being. Bjorck-Akesson et al. (2010) confirm that the ICF model and ICF-CY may provide a common language and framework which are feasible for use in early childhood intervention. Their findings are based on several studies including those involving young children. Importantly, the children's findings indicate that a child's perception of engagement and motivation needs to be considered in the participation component. Bjorck-Akesson et al. (2010) indicate that the ICF-CY could also effectively support interdisciplinary profiling of a child's functioning across culturally diverse contexts. Researchers contend that capturing the multidimensional nature of participation in everyday activities is challenging and highlight that the subjective experience of involvement of the child in activities and participation is important (Granlund et al. 2012; Hammel et al. 2008; Lyons, Brennan and Carroll 2016).

This book contends that perspectives of the child need to be facilitated when considering the factors that support and hinder research and practice. While participation has received intense attention as an outcome based on the ICF-CY, participation of children with disabilities is generally inconsistent and lacks clarity (Imms et al. 2016). The authors argue that while participation appears to comprise a family of constructs [including engagement] it includes attendance and involvement, preferences, activity competence and sense of self. A restriction or failure to participate can be observed as low engagement. While engagement is considered an essential component in a child's participation, there is no clear definition of child engagement. Definitions vary according to their use and are dependent on the context or field of enquiry. Drawing on research from an Early Childhood Care and Education [ECCE] perspective, research on the quality of Swedish preschool interventions and children's longitudinal outcomes in terms of engagement was conducted by Castro et al. (2015). Notably a strong correlation between quality preschool environments and engagement was observed in ECEC settings in Swedish preschools over time. In a scoping review of articles on predictors of engagement, the effectiveness of engagement interventions, and interpersonal aspects of care within mental health interventions, authors King, Currie, and Petersen (2014) highlight some of the complexities and considerations. For example, in their review, articles varied on how engagement was conceptualized and whether it was an outcome, an event, or a process.

Imms et al. (2016) also see a strong association between these approaches and how the concepts associated with 'quality of life' (QOL) have been developed by Ronen and colleagues over the past decade or more. The degree to which the child pays attention, is involved, or is motivated has been referred to as engagement. Engagement has been defined by Maxwell et al. (2012) and Ronen and Rosenbaum (2013) for children with neurological and developmental conditions. Ronen and Rosenbaum's (2013) conceptualization builds on the World Health Organization's concepts of 'health', 'functioning' and 'quality of life' for young people with neurodisabilities by emphasizing the importance of engaging with patients in the identification of both treatment goals and their evaluation. Therefore, participation is necessary for an intervention to have a positive effect on a child. According to Maxwell (2012: iii), proposed relationships exist between the participation construct and five central dimensions of the environment described as: 'availability, accessibility, affordability, accommodability and acceptability'. Di Marino et al. (2018) emphasize the effect of the child's family and environmental factors on the participation of the child and the role of the environment in supporting children with disabilities. The authors note that participation includes frequency, involvement and desire for change in activities and may be strongly influenced or dependent on practitioners' ability to modify the environment to help children participate.

The construct of participation within an activity and whether the environment is accommodated to the child and accepted by the child is also important. Kemp, Kishido, Carter and Sweller (2013) found that children with disabilities engaged more in free-play and meal-routine activities. These activities provided better opportunities for active engagement than did group activities. The authors also found that children were more actively engaged during meal-routine activities than during free play. However, children with Autism Spectrum Disorders [ASD] did not actively engage in free play activities. Bearing this in mind there are a range of children with disabilities who experience difficulties in terms of participation and engagement. In short, many children with disabilities have not had their experiences documented nor voices heard. This demonstrates the need for researchers to be innovative within and sensitive to the complex challenges of researching with children with disabilities and accessing their meaning. Bjorck-Akesson et al. (2010) highlight that when considering a child's participation, motivation and engagement also need to be considered. Furthermore, participation of a heterogeneous group of young children with neurodevelopmental disabilities requires the researcher to be creative and to use an open and flexible approach in the development of research tools to facilitate communication (Carroll and Sixsmith 2016; Franklin and Sloper 2009; Kelly 2007; Mitchell and Sloper 2011; Paige-Smith and Rix 2011). Juxtaposition of the subjective experiences of families and children themselves (WHO 2007) with professionals' views is necessary when positioning individual child factors alongside environmental factors, such as opportunities for participation in intervention planning for children with disabilities (Lyons et al. 2016).

International and national perspectives on voice will interrogate Fielding's (2007) contention that previously silenced voices have yet to be heard. This book is also mindful of the complex power imbalances that shape the ideological contexts of research on children's voice and its representation. Komulainen (2007) claims that the concept of children's voice is socially constructed. Spyrou (2011) suggests that as critical, reflective researchers we need to move beyond claims of authenticity and account for the complexity involved in children's voice research by exploring its messy, multi-layered and non-normative character. For children who communicate differently and challenge our assumptions about voice, allowing their voices to remain unheard may be easier. Implications drawn from this collection of voices will be used to inform us about the experiences of children in Early Intervention or school settings. In the search for identity, the voices of these children will be foregrounded. Due to their explicit difficulties engaging with the world around them and inherent difficulties differentiating and authoring self and other, children with multiple and complex difficulties may experience obstructions in expressing their voice. The need to listen to children's voices has been echoed by researchers (Kellet 2006; Kelly 2005; Lewis 2002). Increasingly the participation of disabled children has been prioritized through the following:

- Lundy's (2007) argument that enabling voice is not enough; space, influence and audience are necessary components to make it meaningful.
- If voice exists is it socially constructed?
- Is it authentic?
- How do we know this?
- Are certain voices privileged and others silenced?
- Are there other ways of expressing voice?

Organization and description of this book

This book presents empirically based international research representing the lives of children with additional needs or disabilities, including children with neurodevelopmental disorders or at risk of developing them. We have endeavoured to reflect a diverse group of children with differing needs; however, we have considered their need to be heard as an overarching need, something all children have in common, from infancy to later childhood. While children with disabilities are a significant focus of this book, we are also cognisant of new initiatives in Ireland and internationally which prioritize inclusion and which prompt us to consider that the diversity of need may be present in all childhood environments, where children need to have a voice. Reflecting the diversity of interest in research with children, this book contains a broad range of contributions reflecting a wide range of research and practice internationally focusing on themes of participation, engagement, agency and voice. This book includes:

- A multi-disciplinary approach to eliciting voice acknowledging the significance of drawing on expertise from speech and language therapy, psychology, occupational therapy and education, to mention a few. This diversity of disciplines also draws on health, education, Early Childhood Studies, and medical anthropology.
- A range of creative methods and innovative suggestions for eliciting the voice of children.
- Insights from researchers working with children using participatory methods aimed at eliciting the voice of the child.

Throughout this book there is discussion on ethics, data collection, case studies and theoretical standpoints. These contributions have been divided into three parts:

- Part I: Legislation, policy and theories
- Part II: Innovative explorations of different forms of voice
- Part III: Disciplinary illustrations and explorations around voice

Part I: Legislation, policy and theories

The first part of this book sets the context with both national and international examples guiding us through the legislative aspects, policy orientation and the sociology of childhood associated with children's voice. It is foregrounded by Professor Kay M. Tisdall's chapter which provides a wonderful introduction to this book in that it demonstrates how ideas and concepts from human rights inform and challenge ways of undertaking research with children. In particular, it considers how the United Nations Convention on the Rights of the Child [UNCRC] and the United Nations Convention on the Rights of Persons with Disabilities can challenge conceptualizations of capacity and competence, communication and voice, and research ethics. Dr Mary Wickenden's chapter draws on her background as a Speech and Language Therapist as well as her training as a Medical Anthropologist and challenges the concepts of voice, inclusion and participation drawing on multiple research studies involving children who communicate in unconventional ways. She presents the challenges of participatory research and encourages readers to consider that all children having the right to be consulted and contributing to society is not a universal view. The chapter by Ms Elena Jenkin and colleagues reflects on theoretical constructs of childhood, disability and postcolonialism and interrogates why it is imperative to listen to children with a disability, particularly in developing countries. Ms Jenkins and her colleagues present methodological considerations with research design through the use of a case study including children with a disability from developing countries. Their chapter shares the diversity in experiences and priorities for children in developing countries through the use of a range of methods to 'restore' the rights of young children with disabilities to share their voice. Finally, Dr Karen Watson presents her research in Australia using a poststructural framework and drawing on data produced as part of a larger ethnographic study. This chapter explores the idea of researching among children in three 'inclusive' early childhood classrooms. This research-oriented chapter explores theoretical and methodological implications of participation – moving beyond adult definitions of participatory or 'adult centric' perspectives on participation.

This part of the book highlights that children's participation is on the human rights agenda across the world, emphasizing the importance of recognizing human dignity and valuing all children as paramount.

Part II: Innovative explorations of different forms of voice

The second part of the book presents innovative explorations of different forms of voice from a number of authors. Professor Melanie Nind leads with a research and methodologically oriented chapter, clearly and explicitly leading thinking relative to the educative value of listening. This provides an excellent theoretical base for understanding how children's voices are accessed and interpreted. Practical examples from the authors research and other important studies are used to illustrate exploring and accessing different forms of voice with children experiencing profound disability using a multimodal lens. Professor Nind's chapter pays tribute to the work of others in extending our thinking on the concept of attendance. Her evaluation of this concept moves beyond empathy and she stresses the selflessness which appeals to her in the work of others. Dr Ben Simmons engaging chapter draws us into the phenomenology of intersubjectivity and research with profoundly disabled children as a novel, distinct and innovative approach to developing an experiential framework for exploring and analysing the lived social experiences of children with Profound and Multiple Disability (PMLD). This chapter will present engaging, ground-breaking work in terms of voice and the child with PMLD. This original exploration will ignite researchers and practitioners to consider alternate ways of embodying voice through new methodologies, finding alternatives to verbal means. Dr Miriam Twomey shares the importance of a phenomenological frame to overcome deficit theorizing when researching with young nonverbal children with ASD. Dr Twomey urges researchers, practitioners and families to be creative, inventive and open-minded in considering movement as a means of engagement. Dr Twomey challenges readers to view a child's development as a trajectory rather than a destination and to focus on timing, tuning in, and being responsive to children who may not communicate verbally. Movement and being moved are brought to the foreground with the purpose of encouraging readers to be open to engagement at a bodily level. The need to hear and understand the voices of children with ASD and neurodevelopmental disabilities who are nonverbal is illustrated through the use of puppetry. Developing innovative and alternative modes of communication for children with severe speech impairments, Dr Martine M. Smith extends points raised in the first part of this book and encourages readers to consider the individuality and uniqueness of voice and communication style. This chapter illustrates how the co-construction of interactions is imperative for successful communication between children who use Augmentative and Alternative Communication (AAC) systems and their communication partners. Dr Smith raises the need to understand more from the perspectives of children who use communication devices. Dr Clare Carroll illustrates the impact of policy and context on the child and family in Early Intervention in Ireland with the positioning of the child within a multi-layered approach to Bronfenbrenner's ecological systems. This chapter offers a nuanced approach to participation through the use of innovative methodological approaches reaching young children with Down syndrome.

Part III: Disciplinary illustrations and explorations around voice

The third part of the book includes chapters from the fields of Occupational Therapy/Science, Speech and Language Therapy, Psychology and Early Years education. Dr Helen Lynch situates the UNCRC, UNCRPD and ICF-CY from an Occupational Science perspective. She shares strategies and challenges to support research with children with disabilities from an Occupational Science perspective. She prompts the reader to consider agency, purposefulness and participation through 'doing' and challenges researchers to explore the use of multiple methods, in particular the use of video as a qualitative method. Dr Lynch shares how considering the research questions and purpose of the study will determine the method of analysis. Dr Maria Prellwitz and Dr Helen Lynch propose that while often restricted by physical barriers and social exclusion, children with disabilities have a right to play and participate in play with other children in community playspaces and playgrounds. Frequently, spaces and structures set up for children's outdoor play are not accessible to children with disabilities. This may result in a lack of interaction between children with and without disabilities reinforcing attitudinal barriers and stigmatization. The authors aim to remediate this by presenting a background to designing for play, based on empirical research with children with disabilities, landscape architects and other disciplines. Dr Rena Lyons extends concepts from the first part of this book with particular reference to children with speech and developmental language disorders. She challenges readers to

listen to children with speech and developmental language disorders as we
need to understand how we as practitioners and researchers can support
them to develop. Dr Lyons reiterates how the voice of children has been
neglected in research and acknowledges that it is only recently that children
with speech and developmental language disorders have been included in
research, thus being respected. Dr Line Caes and Dr Siobhan O'Higgins
situate the evidence related to young children and children with cognitive
impairments' experiences of pain. The authors propose that all children
need to share their pain experiences. This will require creativity and an
exploration of existing self-report and proxy tools used by researchers and
practitioners when exploring pain. The authors illustrate this through a
participatory research example of innovative and creative techniques to
explore pain with young children and children with cognitive impairment.

The chapter by Dr Carolyn Blackburn illustrates the use of a time-
sequenced observation of children in early childhood settings with a focus
on private speech of young children and children with speech, language
and communication needs. Her findings support the use of episodes of
solitary play for all children, thus challenging Kincheloe's notion of education as commodification. Dr Blackburn considers the use of non-directive
approaches in Early Childhood Education. Children engage more in private speech during unstructured child-led activities. In the final chapter,
Professor Nóirín Hayes theorizes the need for a dynamic approach to inclusion and acknowledgement of the child in context. Professor Hayes provides
the reader with a universal view of inclusion as the context for participation
where children are not defined by their differences. Attention is paid to the
significant gap between recognizing young children as active participants
in their own learning and development, with rights to being meaningfully
included in day-to-day practice, and actually including them as partners in
the creation and realization of an inclusive curriculum in practice.

This book aims to consider the significant contribution of an interdisciplinary exploration of voice. An interdisciplinary exploration challenges
us to think differently, to move out of our 'comfort zone' in order to con-
ceptualize alternatively and divergently, adopting views and belief systems
that characterize voice differently. In particular, it invites us to look critically
at our own and others' conceptualizations of researching with children;

acknowledging that our views and opinions of voice impact how we go about researching voice. As editors, we also share a desire to shine a light on innovative research which accesses and engages with children who are considered hard to reach, while respecting the views and opinions of those children whose voice has not always been heard. We include a notion that voice can be 'seen' and 'heard' which challenges the researcher to interrogate their own assumptions about what voice is. Acknowledging that voice, in whatever form it takes, may be a means of representation for a child and that it may present differently will affect our practice; influencing the questions we ask, the way we carry out our research and subsequently our approach to participants. It is also worth noting that children's languages may be part of a larger inclusive collective involving Mihkail Bakhtin's (1986) notions of dialogical landscape and collective voices, where the origins of language and thought are products of human interaction, where in finding ourselves we are found by the other, and where we are inescapably influenced by the other and the other's engagement with us. To this end we hope that this book answers our current question – why voice and why now?

References

Bakhtin, M. (1986). *Speech Genres and Other Late Essays*. Edited by Caryl Emerson and Michael Holquist. Translated by Vern W. McGee. Austin, TX: University of Texas Press.

Bjorck-Akesson, E., Wilder, J., Granlund, M., Pless, M., Simeonsson, R. J., Adolfsson, M., and Lillvist, A. (2010). The International Classification of Functioning, Disability and Health and the version for Children and Youth as a tool in child habilitation/early childhood intervention – feasibility and usefulness as a common language and frame of reference for practice. *Disability and Society*, 32 (S1), S125–S138.

Carroll, C., and Sixsmith, J. (2016). Exploring the facilitation of young children with disabilities in research about their early intervention service. *Child Language Teaching and Therapy*, 32(3), 313–325.

Castro, S. Granlund, M and Almqvist, L. (2015). The relationship between classroom quality-related variables and engagement levels in Swedish preschool classrooms:

a longitudinal study. *European Early Childhood Education Research Journal*, 25 (1), 122–135. DOI: 10.1080/1350293X.2015.1102413.

Fielding, M. (2007). Beyond 'Voice': New roles, relations, and contexts in research-ing with young people. *Discourse: Studies in the Cultural Politics of Education*, 28 (3), 301–310.

Granlund, M., Arvidsson, P., Björck-Åkesson, E., Simeonsson, R. J., Maxwell, G., Adolfson, M., et al. (2012). Differentiating activity and participation of chil-dren and youth with disability in Sweden. *American Journal of Physical Medical Rehabilitation*. 91 (2S), S84–S96.

Hammel, J., Magasi, S., Heinmann, A., Whiteneck, G., Bogner, J., and Rodriguez, E. (2008). What does participation mean? An insider perspective from people with disabilities. *Disability and Rehabilitation*, 30, 1145–1460.

Lyons, R., Brennan, S. and Carroll, C. (2016). Exploring parental perspectives of participation in children with Down Syndrome. *Child Language Teaching and Therapy*, 32, 79–93.

Kemp, C., Kishida, Y., Carter, M., and Sweller, N. (2013). The effect of activity type on the engagement and interaction of young children with disabilities in inclusive childcare settings. *Early Childhood Research Quarterly*, 28 (1), 134–143.

King, G., Currie, M., and Petersen, P. (2014). Review: Child and parent engagement in the mental health intervention process: A motivational framework. *Child and Adolescent Mental Health*, 19 (1), 2–8.

McLeod, S. (2018). Communication rights: Fundamental human rights for all. *International Journal of Speech-Language Pathology*, 20(1), 3–11. DOI: 10.1080/17549507.2018.1428687.

Ronen, G. M., and Rosenbaum, P. L. (2013). Concepts and perspectives of 'health' and life quality 'outcomes' in children and young people with neurological and developmental conditions. In G. M. Ronen and P. L. Rosenbaum (eds), *Life quality outcomes in children and young people with neurological and developmen-tal conditions: Concepts, evidence and practice clinics in developmental medicine*, pp. 329–343. London: Mac Keith Press.

Simeonsson, R. J. (9 June 2016). *UNCRC & ICF-CY: Defining and documenting universal rights of children.* Paper presented at the International Society on Early Intervention Conference: Children's Rights and Early Intervention, University of Stockholm, Sweden.

World Health Organization. (2001). International Classification of Functioning, Disability and Health. Geneva: World Health Organization.

World Health Organization. (2007). International Classification of Functioning, Disability and Health – Children and Youth Version. Geneva: World Health Organization.

PART I

Legislation, policy and theories

KAY M. TISDALL

1   Applying human rights to children's[1] participation in research

Introduction

Over the last twenty years, there has been a significant 'turn' in the social sciences and related disciplines, to undertaking research *with* rather than *on* children. Whereas in the past adults were often treated as informants on behalf of children, researchers increasingly recognize that children can respond and participate on their own behalf and provide meaningful contributions to address the research questions. Whereas formerly children were the objects of research ethics, childhood researchers firmly assert that children should be able to agree in their own right to their research participation. Research itself is no longer the sole preserve of adults; children themselves are increasingly taking on different roles within research processes, from advising research studies as consultants, to peer researchers collecting and analysing data, to co-producing projects with adults (Bradbury-Jones and Taylor 2015; Davis 2009). This change to research with children, rather than on children, has thus created new opportunities and challenges for research methods, governance, procedures and ethics.

At least one inspiration for this change is the international recognition of children's human rights. In 1989, the UN General Assembly ratified the United Nations Convention on the Rights of the Child (CRC). It is now

---

1   This chapter uses the 'term' children, as the book overall is focusing on younger children. The CRC itself defines a child as 'every human being below the age of eighteen years unless, under the law applicable to the child, majority is obtained earlier' (Article 1).

the most ratified international human rights treaty ever (all States Parties have ratified it except the USA). With ratification, States Parties have a duty to implement the CRC provisions. The CRC is an extensive document of 54 articles, covering all types of human rights from civil to economic to cultural, and has three additional Optional Protocols.[2] CRC's participation rights have been particularly influential because they challenge traditional conceptualizations of childhood as merely passive recipients of services and solely vulnerable dependents on their parents, families and communities. Children have the right to have their views duly considered in all matters affected the child. More recently, this right to participation was re-articulated in the United Nations Convention on the Rights of Persons with Disabilities (CRPD) (2006), in Article 7. Children's participation is firmly on the human rights agenda internationally.

This chapter will explore the implications of human rights, and particularly of the CRC and CRPD, for research with children. First, it provides an overview of the human rights framework and its potential applications to research. Then the chapter explores three themes, which are particularly enhanced and/or challenged by human rights: a reconsideration of communication and 'voice'; pervasive concepts of capacity and competence; and research ethics. The chapter concludes by outlining how a human rights approach continues to challenge research with children.

Human rights framework: potential applications to research

Human rights are recognized for all people, simply on the basis of their being human. These rights are inalienable – they cannot be given away or abrogated; they are universal – they apply to all people in all countries in

2   Optional Protocol to the Convention on the Rights of the Child on the sale of children, child prostitution and child pornography; Optional Protocol to the Convention on the Rights of the Child on the involvement of children in armed conflict; Optional Protocol to the Convention on the Rights of the Child on a communications procedure.

all contexts; and human rights must be addressed holistically – the range of human rights must be realized, rather than prioritizing one and not addressing others. Such ideas are both powerful and controversial. Rights can be variously defined and conceptualized but core to virtually all human rights theories are requirements for duty-bearers to recognize and realize the rights of the rights-holders (e.g. see Jones 1994; Mahoney 2007). There are requirements therefore both for duty bearers' accountability and for rights holders' access to redress if their rights were not upheld. It is these elements that distinguish a rights framework from other popular ones, such as wellbeing (Bradshaw 2014; Camfield et al. 2009) or vulnerability (Fineman 2013; Herring 2012). Rights fundamentally respect a person's dignity. They are important 'moral coinage' (Freeman 1983: 2) as well as having political and legal power. Rights are described as political 'trump cards' by Dworkin (1997: xi), as so fundamental they cannot be politically compromised (although in practice they may well be). Human rights basis in international law gives them political 'stickiness': while laws can be changed, this typically takes time and a certain amount of consensual agreement. Thus rights recognized in law are less quickly and easily changed than other areas of policy, such as the definitions of 'wellbeing' or a charitable concern for vulnerable children. Applying a human rights framework to children, disabled[3] people and disabled children, thus powerfully asserts their human dignity and value, shines a light on discrimination against them, and thus can change how individuals and society perceive them.

Human rights are not without their critics, however, both conceptually and in practice. Conceptually, rights have been roundly criticized for being based on a false premise of the autonomous rational individual. Instead, critics (e.g. Arneil 2002; Sandel 1992) suggest that people are inherently social, no one is autonomous and rationality is not a necessary criterion to have rights. King (1997) is provocative, in suggesting that a

---

3   As I am currently working in the UK, this chapter will largely use the phrases 'disabled children' or 'disabled people' (rather than children with disabilities or people with disabilities) as this is generally the preferred phrasing of the disability movement and its advocates here. When quoting or citing other documents, however, the chapter keeps to their use of terminology (e.g. the CRPD uses the phrases 'persons with disabilities' and 'children with disabilities').

rights framework for children narrows the focus, away from fundamental issues of war, national disasters and global capitalism, which are not or inadequately addressed by human rights yet have the greatest impacts on children's lives worldwide. In practice, human rights face a strong critique about their universal application, as being culturally inappropriate in many parts of the world and merely the latest version of colonialism and the Global North's imposition on the Global South (e.g. Valentin and Meinert 2009). States Parties may ratify the conventions but implementation remains varied and accountability procedures at an international level are relatively weak (Alston and Crawford 2000). Thus, there are potential drawbacks of a human rights approach, in recognizing relationships, cultures, and addressing wider social issues.

All human rights treaties apply to disabled children. This chapter considers the ones particular to disabled children and to people more generally. The creation of both the CRC and CRPD were contentious in themselves – why is a separate convention required for children, or for disabled people, when they are already included within other human rights treaties? But the arguments were made that specific attention needed to be focused on these groups, to ensure their particular rights were articulated and recognized (see Hanson 2014; Kanter 2015).

The CRC has four general principles (UN Committee on the Rights of the Child 2003): Article 2 (non-discrimination); Article 3(1) (a child's best interests must be a primary consideration in all actions concerning children); Article 4 (inherent right to life, survival and development) and Article 12(1) on children's views. Article 12 is but one of the participation rights within the CRC, which includes Article 13 (freedom of expression), Article 14 (freedom of thought, conscience and religion), Article 15 (freedom of association and peaceful assembly) and Article 17 (access to information). But it is Article 12(1) that is the most cited for encouraging children's participation, and the one often viewed as transformative and radical for children and childhood (Holzscheiter 2010; Reid 1994). Article 12(1)'s precise wording is:

> States Parties shall assure to the child who is capable of forming his or her own views the right to express those views freely in all matters affecting the child, the views of the child being given due weight in accordance with the age and maturity of the child.

Article 12 must be applied widely, with a broad understanding of 'all matters affecting the child' (UN Committee on the Rights of the Child 2009: para 26–27). This is elaborated upon for young children, as needing to be:

> ... anchored in the child's daily life at home (including, when applicable, the extended family) and in his or her community; within the full range of early childhood health, care and education facilities, as well as in legal proceedings; and in the development of policies and services, including through research and consultations. (2005: para 14)

Children's views must also be considered seriously (UN Committee on the Rights of the Child 2009: para 28). In summary, then, the UN Committee on the Rights of the Child underlines the considerable responsibility of families, professionals and others to support young children in their rights to participate. Participation must be part of young children's daily lives.

Article 23 of the CRC particularly addresses the rights of disabled children. The Article is lengthy, starting with the recognition that a disabled child 'should enjoy a full and decent life, in conditions which ensure dignity, promote self-reliance and facilitate the child's active participation in the community' (Article 23[1]). Subsequent sub-sections address disabled children's right to special care, resources and affordable assistance across a range of services, and international exchange of information.

The CRPD is composed of 50 articles.[4] Article 7 is dedicated to children with disabilities:

1. States Parties shall take all necessary measures to ensure the full enjoyment by children with disabilities of all human rights and fundamental freedoms on an equal basis with other children.
2. In all actions concerning children with disabilities, the best interests of the child shall be a primary consideration.
3. States Parties shall ensure that children with disabilities have the right to express their views freely on all matters affecting them, their views being given due weight in accordance with their age and maturity, on

---

4 The CRPD also has an Optional Protocol on communications.

an equal basis with other children, and to be provided with disability and age-appropriate assistance to realize that right.

These provisions echo three of the CRC's general principles, in terms of non-discrimination (Article 2), children's best interests (Article 3) and children's views (Article 12).

Given the above, the implications for research are considerable. Numerous authors have articulated what a rights-based approach could be for childhood research (e.g. Bessell 2016; Collins 2012; Lundy and McEvoy 2012; special issue of Children's Geographies 2009 7(4)). Beazley and colleagues (2009) write of children's right to be researched properly, which they summarize into four elements based on certain CRC articles: children should be research participants; methods should make it easy for children to express their experiences, views and opinions; children should be protected from harms that could result from research participation; and the quality of research should be ensured, in terms of methods, analysis, management and supervision. Others go further, such as Lundy and colleagues. Rights-based research requires stepping back from conventional research approaches, across the disciplines, to ensure human rights standards are applied to all aspects of research – from design, to fieldwork, to ethics. Lundy and McEvoy (2012) elaborate on changes that must be made. Research questions must be framed in the language of rights. The research itself must build rights-holders' capacity to claim their rights and duty-bearers to fulfil their obligations. The former requires support for children to form their views, so they can have informed and formed views when they are involved in research. Children need to participate in the various elements of research fieldwork, analysis and dissemination. Just as human rights must be considered holistically, so must their application to research. As suggested in the introduction, a particular emphasis of such rights-based approaches – and the biggest challenge perceived to conventional research – is the participation of children.[5]

5   For example, see <https://www.qub.ac.uk/research-centres/Centrefor ChildrensRights/ChildrensRights-BasedResearch/ARights-BasedApproachto ChildrensParticipationinResearch> (accessed 4.5.17)

The sections below pick up three issues related to participation, of particular salience to research with disabled children.

Communication and 'voice'

The Conventions give strong grounding for children's participation in research and particularly for respect for children's own views on matters that affect them. This has precipitated an enthusiasm for children to be participants in research, as important contributors to answering research questions about their lives, experiences, attitudes and views. It has encouraged researchers to develop and use a variety of 'participative' or 'creative' methods. While largely but not solely qualitative, such methods range from photo tours, where children are encouraged to take pictures with cameras or other devices, to story-telling and puppets, to drawing and other arts-based activities (e.g. see Aldridge 2015; Johnson et al. 2014; Lyons and Roulstone 2017; Tisdall et al. 2009). Such methods are argued as more effectively and ethically involving children in research, in comparison to relying solely on 'traditional' research methods such as filling in tickboxes on a quantitative self-report survey or face-to-face interviews. Kesby, for example, argues that such methods create better knowledge: they will 'access and valorize previously neglected knowledge and provide more nuanced understandings of complex, social phenomena' (2000: 423). Better knowledge in turn will create better data, better decision-making and best results. These methods create better knowledge, because they are 'in tune with children's ways of seeing and relating to the world' (Thomas and O'Kane 1998: 337). This also makes them more ethical, argue Thomas and O'Kane (1998), as they give children more control over the research process. Participatory methods are characterized as inclusive, in at least two ways. First, often children have choice in methods, so that if one method were not preferred or suitable, another one is used (e.g. see Clark and Moss 2001). Thus a wider range of children can be involved, who have different communication preferences. Second, the participatory methods can recognize communication in addition to or instead of words, the latter of which are so often relied upon within social science research methods (Komulainen 2007). Such participatory methods have been widely used in childhood research and have been specifically used in research with disabled children (e.g. Brady et al. 2012; Raibee et al. 2005).

This inclusivity fits well with the interpretation of children's participation rights by the UN Committee on the Rights of the Child. The Committee's General Comment on Early Childhood, for example, emphasizes that adults need to demonstrate patience and creativity, adapting to the interests, understanding levels and preferred ways of communication with young children (2005: para 14). It fits with a disability rights paradigm, which recognizes impairments but argues that society creates the disability through oppression, discrimination and barriers (Tisdall 2012; Watson 2012). It is for the research to change, rather than the individual with the impairment. The emphasis then becomes the researcher's responsibility to find ways for children to participate, rather than excluding children because they do not neatly fit into the researcher's set protocols. Children's involvement as research participants has often been celebrated as giving 'voice' to children and thus recognizing their rights to participate. It has resulted in numerous publications that contain lists of quotations from children and other productions of and from children such as podcasts, videos and artistic creations. Projects abound that are 'child-led', which typically means that children work on all research stages – from research questions to fieldwork to analysis and subsequent dissemination (Michail and Kellett 2015; Spalding 2011). There is an enthusiasm, therefore, amongst committed adult researchers to expanding traditional methods to facilitate children's participation and to ensure their voices are heard.

While maintaining the commitment, there is a growing recognition in the literature that the emancipatory claims for participatory methods and presenting the 'voice' of the child are not inevitably met. Simply using an art-based method, such as drawing, or taking a photo tour with a child, does not necessarily mean that the child has more control over the research process that the child enjoys participating, or that participatory methods will meet different children's communication needs. For example, children can feel pressured about drawing, particularly as they get older and if they are in a school setting; they can feel their drawing is judged by external standards, that they are not a 'good' at drawing, or that they must follow conventions on how they should depict something (Einarsdóttir et al. 2009; Tisdall 2015). Participatory methods are often reduced to text for the analysis, as children are encouraged to talk or write about what pictures they took or what art they created. This helps check the researcher's understanding of the data and thus interpretation. But it privileges text and crowds out the other communication methods. The claims to present children's 'voice' have also been recognized as problematic. First, the use of a singular voice belies the diversity of children, who may not have a homogenous view or experience but instead considerable heterogeneity. Second, Komulainen (2007) points out that voice privileges certain forms of communication, which may not be available for particular disabled children. While voice can be put into inverted commas, to indicate it is not to be understood narrowly but widely, such phrases feed into discourses that exclude disabled children. Third, 'voice' presumes that there is a fixed perspective, which a researcher can access and present. Whether we take a modernist or post-modern view, this expectation is unrealistic. We can expect any person's view to change over time, by context, and by how it is elicited (for discussion, see Gallacher and Gallagher 2008; James 2007). Lastly, research can be presented as the voice of the child or children without acknowledging the researcher's role. For example, reports abound that have been written by adult researchers, who have selected the quotations as excerpts from transcripts, arranged the quotations within a narrative, and presented both analysis and recommendations. The adult's role can be equally pervasive, in editing of videos or art exhibitions. Children may have limited to no involvement in any of these analytical and presentational processes.[6] The researcher's role may well have considerable merit, in terms of technical expertise, paid time and dedication. What is more problematic is that the co-production, the contribution of both the researcher and the children in different or similar ways, is not acknowledged reflectively and reflexively (see Gallagher 2008).

6　To note that there are a growing number of research projects that do involve children more deeply in research production, including analysis and presentation.

Thus, the CRC gave considerable impetus to recognizing the rights of children to participate and has been picked up with enthusiasm by numerous researchers. As practice and experiences accumulate, more critical perspectives are emerging that can hone how such research is designed and carried out. For example, we can recognize that many research participants can enjoy 'participatory' methods and that they may be very good methods to answer particular research questions but such methods do not inevitably create better knowledge nor are they inherently more ethical and more inclusive. Any method, whether labelled participatory or not, will include and exclude certain people. The question then becomes about making considered decisions in light of this. The emancipatory claims of such research can be more thoughtfully tested, to consider the different possibilities for children's involvement in research. Arguably, we need far more research that is based on children's own priorities and is undertaken to their own design. But research can also be productive that is not 'child-led' but respectfully engages children as participants and advisers, and recognizes the respective roles of those involved. A more critical appraisal and judicious consideration of robust research will only strengthen its quality – and be more respectful of children's rights to participate.

Competence and capacity

The CRC and CRPD have established a place for children's participation, where it may not have existed before in legislation nor in practice. Whereas previously children may not have been judged as competent enough to be involved in making a decision, and thus lacking the capacity to participate, Article 12(1) of the CRC and Article 7(3) of the CRPD assert that they have the right to express their views freely in all matters affecting them.

This right is to be interpreted generously, according to the CRC Committee: a child should be presumed to have the capacity to form his or her own view and 'it is not up to the child to first prove his or her capacity' (UNCRC 2009: para 20); a child need not have comprehensive knowledge to be considered capable of having a view (UNCRC 2009: para 21); there is no age limit on the rights of the child to express his or her views (UNCRC 2009: para 21); and the right should be applied to younger as well as older children (UNCRC 2005). Thus a child's capacity is relevant to their participation rights but should be defined generously. Further, children's capacity should be supported: information is a precondition to a child's 'clarified view' (UNCRC 2009: para 25) and an identified right of the CRC. Age-appropriate assistance should be provided for children, to facilitate their participation (Article 7, CRPD and Article 23, CRC). Thus children's capacity is recognized as not necessarily set but something that can develop and change with further skills, experience and knowledge – and children have the right to be supported in this way. The development of children's capacities is explicitly addressed in Article 5 of the CRC, which recognizes the 'evolving capacities of the child' as balancing parental rights and responsibilities to direct and guide children with the increasing autonomy of children (see Lansdown 2005 for analysis).

This 'place' for children's participation, where it may not have been respected before, has numerous implications for research. First, it has encouraged a host of research studies to be funded, from non-governmental organizations seeking to present research of children's views to influence services or policy, to statutory bodies needing children's views in order to evaluate or change their services or policy. Second, it has increased children's inclusion as research participants, as well as other research roles. Third, it asks questions about the informational as well as other support and assistance to participate in research. As Lundy and McEvoy (2012) point out, this can be challenging to certain research designs and expectations, where providing information before research participation can be considered leading and thus biasing the research. A rights-based approach has widened the depth and breadth of children's participation.

However, there are caveats to this progressive depiction. As more extensively discussed in Tisdall (forthcoming), capacity and competency are terms frequently used in the literature and policy around children's participation but rarely with definition. Children are assumed to have 'evolving capacities' while adults do not; the result is children having less responsibilities than adults but more protection (Lansdown 2005: xiii).

While the General Comment on Article 12 does advocate a wide interpretation of children's capacity, Article 12 and thus the General Comment
allows for some children to be considered *insufficiently* mature and *not*
capable of having an informed view and thus not able to exercise Article 12
(CRC) or Article 7(3) (CRPD).

This can play out problematically in research, in at least three ways.
First, children and particularly disabled children can still be excluded from
research. While participation rights have encouraged researchers to look to
their own competence to facilitate children's research participation, rather
than excluding children as incompetent, this only goes so far. Children
are casually discriminated against by age, which would be unacceptable
for other equalities issues such as race, gender or religion. Consider, for
example, the amount of public investment in surveys that only include
those aged sixteen or eighteen and above, despite the surveys addressing
issues of considerable import to children – such as crime, poverty, and
quality of life. If this is true for children generally, it is even more true for
younger children. Some research methods literature, for example, continues to assert that questionnaires are best not used with children under
the age of 8 (e.g. Bell 2007). Yet other studies show that, with the appropriate information and methods, children at much younger ages can contribute
meaningfully to such questions and issues (e.g. see Greig et al. 2007). The
details of the original studies are not always considered and such references
are regularly used as a quick way to explain why younger children are not
included. Disabled children risk exclusion as well. The support to ensure
their participation can be considered too expensive or time-consuming and
this can justify their exclusion (to recognize that a research team may well
do this reluctantly but the fact is that the justification is accepted). Thus,
the 'place' for children in research has arguably expanded due to recognizing participation rights but certain exclusions are still easily justified, on
the basis of the children not being competent or not having the capacity to
participate, without extensive evidence nor consideration of alternatives.

Second, because such exclusion is recognized by a host of committed
researchers, specialist projects are developed, where researchers ensure
the resources and methods are there to include disabled children. While
immensely worthwhile in themselves, there remains the risks that research

with young disabled children is not mainstreamed into research with children more generally, just as research with children is not necessarily mainstreamed into research with adults. It also can lead to projects focusing on issues related to disability, rather than the myriad of issues that may be important to children who have a disability. This has been raised by disabled children themselves (Barnardo's Scotland et al. 2011; McMellon and Morton 2014), who do not always want the focus to be on their disability and who want to have their views considered on other issues of relevance to them.

Third, ethical practices remain unsettled about children's capacity to agree to participate in their own right within research. It would be conventional within childhood research that children's agreement to participate is paramount, if the child were the one taking part. Thus if a child did not want to participate, or withdrew their participation during the research, this must be respected by the researchers. What is less decided is parents' (or other legal guardians') role in agreeing or not to the child participating. In some arenas, a parent's consent is required; thus leading to the potential that a competent child wants to participate in a project but the parent does not agree. Typically the parent's view prevails.

Part of this problem lies with the construction of 'informed consent'. The practical problems of achieving informed consent are well-rehearsed in the literature (e.g. see Alderson and Morrow 2011). It is also more conceptual, as informed consent is set in a contractual framework[7] – as exemplified by the request for signatures to demonstrate agreement. A contract presumes sufficient information on both sides, to make a contract valid. Yet certain types of research such as ethnographies or action research can begin with very open agendas and lead to unexpected findings and outputs; whether information can be sufficiently explained to meet the above criteria is difficult. Should contract terms not be met, the injured party should have legal redress; the articulation of this within research governance is still in its infancy. A contractual framework is based on legal capacity to agree and sufficient competence to do so. Given the above problems, other

---

7   This section draws on Scottish contract law (e.g. MacQueen and Thomson 2016).

frames may in fact be more ethical – such as trust, professionalism and professional accountability – and indeed human rights.

Overall, then, children's participation rights have expanded their place in research: to be involved as participants as well as other roles and to decide on their own behalf if they want to participate and to continue to do so. However, the participation rights are highly qualified. Article 12(1) and Article 7(3) are far from 'self-determination'. Capacity and competency are loosely defined concepts within the field, which are easily used to exclude as well as include children in research. It is questionable whether they are useful concepts to guide children's participation. It is increasingly realized that all people have evolving capacities and that competence is situational and relational rather than intrinsic and individual (Tisdall forthcoming).

Research ethics

If informed consent remains a major discussion point in the literature, it is not the only one that childhood research considers. For those located within 'childhood studies' and 'children's rights studies', research ethics have long been an obsession and the subject of considerable attention, debate and concern. Trends can be picked out in terms of the discussions. First, research ethics should permeate all aspects of the research, from its original design to its fieldwork and analysis, to its dissemination. Second, research ethics are more than meeting regulatory requirements; they require a deep consideration of principles and ongoing reflective practice. Third, research ethics are still largely what adults think are good for children, rather than having extensive involvement from children in deciding ethical practice, judging it or holding researchers to account. The first two trends are in line with a human rights approach, in taking a holistic view and respecting the human dignity of those involved in research. The third remains an outstanding issue, given children's participation rights as internationally agreed.

Research ethics for children's involvement as research participants have become increasingly established on certain issues: what can be considered 'default' positions such as caveats on confidentiality (typically, a researcher is required to have a process for reporting any concerns about child abuse) and protecting anonymity (typically, a researcher would not use a child's name when reporting on the research). As children become involved as more than participants in research projects, some of these positions are being questioned or raising new issues.

One is the ownership of research and who benefits thereof. As more research projects are involving children in roles such as advisers, researchers and more, issues arise about due recognition. Frequently, adults are paid to undertake research studies. Should children be paid if they take on similar roles? Replacement costs for lost wages is commonplace, for children, but that is not the same as paid employment as researchers. In Europe, law prohibits most paid employment for children under the age of 15.[8] Interpretations of health and safety requirements can preclude children being in certain institutional environments, such as Universities. Questions arise about the position, respect and power relationships of such involvement. Who owns the data and the rights of authorship? Research is frequently published with the names of the adult researchers as authors or due recognition of the researchers. This public naming can be problematic given the default positions of anonymizing children who are involved in research. A convention is growing that children's first names will be used, following mutual agreement, if they have been involved in such co-production. But does this fully and long-term recognize their intellectual property? Such issues extend into the 'knowledge exchange' elements of the research, where the research engages with other stakeholders, typically to maximize research impact. Again, if there are widespread concerns about using children's photographs and children's digital footprints more generally, the ethical sensitivities of involving children in knowledge exchange – and balancing their participation rights with concerns about protection – grow. There are outstanding issues, of continued debate in the literature and in practice, about how to balance agreements now – which children

---

8   Council Directive 94/33/EC of 22 June 1994 on the protection of young people at work, <http://eur-lex.europa.eu/legal-content/EN/ALL/?uri=CELEX:31994L0033> (accessed 25.8.17).

may have been well informed about and given their agreement – with the longevity, searchability and replicability now possible in digital technology. Will they be as content to have their outputs at age 5 readily seen by others when they are in their teens or older?

The literature on childhood research, generally and specifically with younger children and with disabled children, has much to contribute to ethics discussions more widely. Its holistic and questioning approach is well aligned with the breadth of human rights and its value base in human dignity and respect. Increased involvement of children has raised new challenges, particularly in balancing the protective assumptions of research ethics with children's participation rights – and, further, ownership and intellectual property.

Conclusion

The increased recognition of children's human rights, and particularly their participation rights, has influenced certain research arenas. More projects are involving children as research participants, as well as other roles as advisers, consultants, peer researchers and projects that are 'child-led'. There have been leading projects in this regard of disabled children and young children – and combinations thereof. There has been accompanying interest in methods to involve children in these ways, with the proliferation of methods labelled 'participative' and 'creative' that seek to tap into ways that children do and want to communicate, sensitively and ethically. There has been a widening of who is considerable capable and competent enough to participate in various methods, on particular topics, and in various ways (McNamee and Seymour 2012).

This progressive depiction is heartening, for those committed to children's human rights. It is not necessarily so embedded that its continuation will be guaranteed; certainly, with the 'innovation' of children's participation now past, funding may well not prioritize such projects in times of financial austerity and enhanced research competition. It is not necessarily mainstreamed into research more generally: while studies might be queried about why gender has not been considered and incorporated into the research design, the involvement in children would rarely be expected (despite children being a notable proportion of any country's population).[9] Just as human rights more generally can feel threatened by other worldwide priorities and pressures, so can children's participation in research.

As experiences of children's participation in research have broadened and deepened, so has an 'insiders' critique that seeks to interrogate some of the practices and their underlining assumptions. This book's focus – young disabled children – provides a very productive lens to do so. It leads to questioning the emancipatory claims of children's participation. It, for example, allows us to question the inclusivity and exclusivity of research methods (whether participatory, creative or traditional), the continued preoccupations with children's competency and capacity, and ethical issues that arise when we are involved in forms of co-production and child-led research in terms of anonymity, authorship and ownership.

Despite the revolutionary claims for children's participation rights within the CRC, and repeated in the CRPD, this chapter demonstrates that they are highly qualified rights, with adult judgements of children's capacity and competency still determining children's inclusion or exclusion. Best interest concerns can further trump children's participation, particularly when only children are seen as having evolving capacities and requiring protection. It is timely to recognize that the CRC and CRPD are minimum thresholds, subject to the political consensus at the time. There are opportunities to extend children's participation rights. What if we decided that ideas of children's competency and capacity were not the relevant criteria to determine research participation and research ethics, and particularly not ones that saw competence and capacity as individually set characteristics but relational and situational? If we take co-production seriously, how does this challenge certain established ideas of how to do and judge research, about protective aspects of research ethics in light of ownership and contribution?

9   Ranging from 14 per cent to 48 per cent of a country's population, aged 0–14 estimated as of 2017. <http://data.worldbank.org/indicator/SP.POP.0014.TO.ZS> (accessed 4.5.17).

If we recognize that the exclusion of young disabled children from most research, and its treatment as a niche specialism, as a form of discrimination, how would that change research investments from funders – to influence not only children's research but research more generally? Human rights remains a radical framework that continues to challenge research practice, asking us to go further in truly recognizing and respecting children's human dignity in research governance, practice and ethics.

References

Alderson, P., and Morrow, V. (2011). *The Ethics of Research with Children and Young People*. London: Sage.

Aldridge, J. (2015). *Participatory Research*. Bristol: Policy Press.

Alston, P., and Crawford, J. (eds) (2000). *The Future of UN Human Rights Treaty Monitoring*. Cambridge: Cambridge University Press.

Arneil, B. (2002). Becoming versus Being: A Critical Analysis of the Child in Liberal Theory. In D. Archard and C. M. Macleod (eds), *The Moral and Political Status of Children*, pp. 70–96. Oxford: Oxford University Press.

Barnardo's Scotland, Children in Scotland, and the Centre for Research on Families and Relationships (2011). *Children and Young People's Participation in Policy-Making*. Retrieved from: <http://www.research.ed.ac.uk/portal/files/14094815/Participation_briefing_2_FINAL.pdf>.

Beazley, H., Bessell, S., Ennew, J., and Waterson, R. (2009). The right to be properly researched: research with children in a messy, real world. *Children's Geographies*, 7 (4), 365–378.

Bell, A. (2007). Designing and testing questionnaires for children. *Journal of Research in Nursing*, 12 (5), 461–469.

Bessell, S. (2016). Rights-based research with children: Principles and practice. In: R. Evans, L. Holt, and T. Skelton (eds), *Methodological Approaches*, pp. 1–18. Singapore: Springer Singapore.

Bradbury-Jones, C., and Taylor, J. (2015). Engaging with children as co-researchers. *International Journal of Social Research Methodology*, 18 (2), 161–173.

Bradshaw, J. (2014). Overview: Social Policies and Child Well-Being. In A. Ben-Arieh, F. Casas, I. Frønes and J. Korbin (eds), *Handbook of Child Well-Being*, pp. 2921–2943. Dordrecht: Springer.

Brady, L., Shaw, C., Davey, C., and Blades, R. (2012). Involving children and young people in research – principles into practice. In P. Beresford and S. Carr (eds), *Social Care, Service users and User Involvement: building on research*, pp. 226–242. London: Jessica Kingsley.

Camfield, L., Streuli, N., and Woodhead, M. (2009). What's the Use of 'Well-Being' in Contexts of Child Poverty? Approaches to Research, Monitoring and Children's Participation. *International Journal of Children's Rights*, 17 (1), 65–109.

Clark, A., and Moss, P. (2001). *Listening to young children: the Mosaic approach*. London: National Children's Bureau and Joseph Rowntree Foundation.

Collins, T. M. (2012). Improving Research of Children Using a Rights-Based Approach: A Case Study of Some Psychological Research about Socioeconomic Status. *Frontiers in Psychology*, 3, 293.

Davis, J. M. (2009). Involving Children. In E. K. M. Tisdall, J. M. Davis and M. Gallagher (eds), *Research with Children and Young People: Research design, methods and analysis*, pp. 154–167. London: Sage.

Dworkin, R. (1977). *Taking Rights Seriously*. Boston, MA: Harvard University Press.

Einarsdóttir, J., Dockett, S., and Perry, B. (2009). Making meaning: children's perspectives expressed through drawings. *Early Child Development and Care*, 179 (2), 217–232.

Fineman, M. A. (2013). Equality, autonomy and the vulnerable subject in law and politics. In M. A. Fineman and A. Grear (eds), Vulnerability: Reflections on a new ethical foundation for law and politics, pp. 13–17. Farnham: Ashgate.

Freeman, M. D. A. (1983). *The Rights and Wrongs of Children*. London: Francis Pinter.

Gallacher, L., and Gallagher, M. (2008). Methodological Immaturity in Childhood Research? *Childhood*, 15 (4), 499–516.

Gallagher, M. (2008). Power is not an evil: Rethinking Power in Participatory Methods. *Children's Geographies*, 6 (2), 137–150.

Greig, A., Taylor, J., and Mackay, T. (2007). *Doing research with children* (2nd ed). London: Sage.

Hanson, K. (2014). Separate childhood laws and the future of society. *Law, Culture and the Humanities*, 12 (2), 195–205.

Herring, J. (2012). Vulnerability, Children and the Law. In Freeman, M. (ed.), *Law and Childhood Studies*, pp. 243–263. Oxford: Oxford University Press.

Holzscheiter, A. (2010). *Children's Rights in International Politics: The Transformative Power of Discourse*. Basingstoke: Palgrave Macmillan.

James, A. (2007). Giving Voice to Children's Voices: Practices and Problems, Pitfalls and Potentials. *American Anthropologist*, 109 (2), 261–272.

Johnson, V., Hart, R., and Colwell, J. (2014). *Steps to engaging young children in research*. Retrieved from: <https://bernardvanleer.org/publications-reports/steps-engaging-young children-research-volume-1-guide/>.

Jones, P. (1994). *Rights*. Basingstoke: Palgrave.

Kanter, A. (2015). *The development disability rights under international law: from charity to human rights*. London: Routledge.

Kesby, M. (2000). Participatory Diagramming: Deploying Qualitative Methods through an Action Research Epistemology. *Area*, 32 (4), 423–435.

King, M. (1997). *A Better World for Children? Explorations in Morality and Authority*. Abingdon: Routledge.

Komulainen, S. (2007). The ambiguity of the child's 'voice' in social research. *Childhood*, 14 (1), 11–28.

Lansdown, G. (2005). *The Evolving Capacities of the Child*. Florence: UNICEF Innocenti Research Centre.

Lundy, L., and McEvoy, L. (2012). Vulnerability, Children and the Law. In Freeman, M. (ed.), *Law and Childhood Studies*, pp. 75–91. Oxford: Oxford University Press.

Lyons, R., and Roulstone, S. (2017). Labels, identity and narratives in children with primary speech and language impairments. *International Journal of Speech-Language Pathology*, 19 (5), 503–518.

McMellon, C., and Morton, S. (2014). *Disabled children and young people: making choices and participating in everyday decisions*. Retrieved from: <http://www.capability scotland.org.uk/media/404784/making_choices_and_participation_literature_review_839755 pdf>.

McNamee, S., and Seymour, J. (2012). Towards a sociology of 10–12 year olds? Emerging methodological issues in the 'new' social studies of childhood. *Childhood*, 20 (2), 156– 168.

MacQueen, H., and Thompson, J. (2016). *Contract Law in Scotland*. Haywards Heath: Bloomsbury Professional.

Mahoney, J. (2007). *The Challenge of Human Rights*. Oxford: Blackwell.

Michail, S., and Kellett, M. (2015). Child-led research in the context of Australian social welfare practice. *Child & Family Social Work*, 20 (4), 387–395.

Rabiee, P., Sloper, P., and Beresford, B. (2005). Doing research with children and young people who do not use speech for communication. *Children & Society*, 19 (5), 385–396.

Reid, R. (1994). Children's Rights: Radical Remedies for Critical Needs. In S. Asquith and M. Hill (eds), *Justice for Children*. London: Martinus Nijhoff Publishers.

Sandel, M. (1982). *Liberalism and the Limits of Justice*. Cambridge: Cambridge University Press.

Spalding, V. (2011). *We are researchers – child-led research: children's voice and educational value*. Retrieved from: <https://cerp.aqa.org.uk/research-library/we-are-researchers-child-led-research-childrens voice-and-educational-value>.

Thomas, N., and O'Kane, C. (1998). The ethics of participatory research with children. *Children and Society*, 12 (5), 336–348.

Tisdall, E. K. M. (2012). The Challenge and Challenging of Childhood Studies? Lessons from disability studies and research with disabled children. *Children & Society*, 26 (3), 181–191.

Tisdall, E. K. M. (2015). Participation, Rights and 'Participatory' Methods. In A. Farrell, S. L. Kagan, and E. K. M. Tisdall (eds), *The SAGE Handbook of Early Childhood Research*, pp. 73–88. London: Sage.

Tisdall, E. K. M. (forthcoming). Challenging competency and capacity? Due weight to children's views in family law proceedings. *International Journal of Children's Rights*.

Tisdall, E. K. M, Davis, J. M., and Gallagher, M. (2009). *Research with Children and Young People: Research design, methods and analysis*. London: Sage.

United Nations Committee on the Rights of the Child (2003). *General Comment No. 5 General measures of implementation of the Convention on the Rights of the Child*. Retrieved from: <http://tbinternet.ohchr.org/_layouts/treatybodyexternal/Download.aspx?symbolno=CRC%2fC%2f2003%2f5&Lang=en>.

United Nations Committee on the Rights of the Child (2005). *General Comment No. 7 Implementing Child Rights in Early Childhood*. Retrieved from: <http://www2.ohchr.org/english/bodies/crc/docs/AdvanceVersions/GeneralComment7Rev1.pdf>.

United Nations Committee on the Rights of the Child (2009). *General Comment No. 12 The right of the child to be heard*. Retrieved from: <http://www2.ohchr.org/english/bodies/crc/docs/AdvanceVersions/CRC-C-GC-12.pdf>.

Valentin, K., and Meinert, L. (2009). The Adult North and the Young South. *Anthropology Today*, 25 (3), 23–28.

Watson, N. (2012). Theorising the Lives of Disabled Children: How Can Disability Theory Help?, *Children and Society*, 26 (3), 192–202.

MARY WICKENDEN

2 'I have a lot to say!': A human rights perspective on recognizing the voices of disabled children globally

Introduction

The rights and perspectives of disabled children[1],[2] are slowly but surely rising up global, national and local agendas. This is as a result of a number of coalescing movements and agendas, which now show encouraging signs of uniting for the benefit of disabled children, a previously neglected and 'silenced' group.

In the last 3 decades or so, understanding about the importance of the perspectives of children and young people generally have changed radically, in the wake of the development of 'Childhood Studies', as a multidisciplinary arena of practice, reflection and investigation (James and James 2004). The 'new' or now not so new 'sociology of childhood' proposed that children are social actors, who have important things to say about their lives, and that importantly these are very different from the views of

---

1 I am using the term children to mean anyone under eighteen. Where I refer to 'young people', I mean broadly those aged between fourteen and twenty-four.

2 In relation to the debate about the use of the terms disabled children vs children with disabilities, I prefer the former as I choose to align myself with the terminology used in the UK. This recognize that disability is constructed by society, not an inherent part of the person. However, I recognize that internationally the terms 'people with disabilities' or 'children with disabilities' are more commonly used, as these are in line with the practice adapted by the United Nations Convention on the Rights of People with Disabilities [UNCRPD] (United Nations [UN] 2006) and related documents. I have used the two terms interchangeably in this chapter.

adults such as parents or teachers who might previously have been asked
to speak for them (Ansell 2009; Beazley et al. 2009; Ennew et al. 2009).
This recognition of children as citizens in their own right, has resulted in
acceptance that they should be consulted about many aspects of their lives
and communities. Their perspectives are important in understanding them,
in informing policy and practice and in making these relevant, as well as in
projects with purely research rather than applied objectives (Hart 2008).

Participatory research with children gives us unique insights into
their lifeworlds and the communities they live in (Crivello et al. 2008).
However there remain contested areas within this movement, for instance
about power dynamics around consulting children (Hunleth 2011), the
role of culture and context in children's lives, about child development
(Rogoff 2003) and about motivations and methodologies in childhoods
research (Tisdall and Punch 2012). There are diverse views about what
can be expected of children and young people in relation to their skills
and types of participation, as well as their possible motivations and interests in participating in consultations (Alderson 1995; Hill 2008). There
have also been concerns about whether seeking children's views can be
tokenistic (James 2007) and about whether they are perhaps patronize
or exoticized in certain contexts. Another critique is that children are
easily homogenized by purely developmental approaches (Burman 2008;
Rogoff 2003), that 'ordinary' children not living in so-called 'difficult circumstances' are overlooked, and that artificial binaries between children
in different contexts (e.g. the 'Global North and South' or middle versus
working class) are too firmly drawn (Twum-Danso 2016). A culture of
seeking out and valuing children's and young people's perspectives is now
established, although this varies in its reach, dynamism and application
across contexts globally (Kirby et al. 2003; Kellett 2005; Skelton 2008).
This view of children as competent people who contribute to society and
have a right to be consulted is of course embodied in and supported by the
UN Convention on the Rights of the Child (1989). However, this view
of children is by no means universal and in some contexts the idea that
children can have their own ideas or indeed should be asked about them
is still novel or seen as inappropriate. Local understandings of the status,
value, expected roles and capacities of children and young people vary

enormously across cultures and contexts (Woodhead and Montgomery 2002; Lansdown 2005).

In parallel and over a similar period of about the last twenty to thirty years, major changes in thinking have taken place in the disability world. Thus 'Disability Studies' has become established as an arena for cross-disciplinary exploration of the lives and concerns of disabled people (Shakespeare 2013). Alongside this academic flowering has come the evolution of the disability advocacy and rights movements within civil society. These developments both contributed to and are the result of the emergence of the 'social model' of disability, which conceptualizes disabled people's often devalued and excluded position as being the result of societal barriers, as opposed to directly resulting from individuals' differences, so called impairments (Shakespeare 1994; Thomas 2004; Barnes and Mercer 2010; Oliver and Barnes 2012). These ideas although originating in various forms in the UK, US and Scandinavia, have spread to other contexts globally to a greater or lesser extent. So in nearly every country, disabled people have gradually acquired more power and are using louder voices to express their particular concerns and perspectives (International Disability Alliance [IDA] 2016). Again echoing changes in the childhood arena, although nearly thirty years later, the United Nations Convention on the Rights of People with Disabilities [UNCRPD] (UN 2006) underlines their right to an equal life and is used by them to illuminate where these rights are denied and to lobby for their increased recognition as citizens. Although many countries including the UK have lead the way in this movement and in changing attitudes to disability, at the global level and in many low and middle income countries, levels of discrimination and exclusion have yet to change substantially (WHO 2011). Exploring attitudes and practices in relation to disabled people cross-culturally reveals many layers of complexity when we take into account the intersecting influences of culture, faith and beliefs, socio-economic circumstances, structural, legal and policy environments (Ghai 2001; Ferri and Connor 2006; Grech and Soldatic 2016).

Largely as a result of very effective lobbying by the global and national disability movements (Disabled People International (DPI); IDA), the rights and wellbeing of disabled people is now rising fast up international and local policy and practice agendas. An affirmative approach sees diversity as something to be appreciated and celebrated (Swain and French 2000). The success of this is epitomized in the recognition of the need for an 'inclusive approach' in the new global goals for international development: The Sustainable Development goals (SDGs), which aim that 'no one is left behind' (UN 2015; IDA 2016). Importantly this means that policy, and lawmakers and service providers, whether government or non-government need to think about how to gather the perspectives of disabled people, in order to respond to their needs and see them as equal citizens alongside others. If truly inclusive participation takes place, those whose voices have previously been very quiet or unheard will be amplified for the first time.

In these two advocacy and academic arenas outlined above: about children and about disability, new conceptualizations are bringing about radical changes. Both groups are being consulted more than ever before and so their voices are beginning to be heard. In this chapter, I will discuss whether the benefits of these two movements are effectively being combined to benefit the group who fall into both categories: disabled children, to give them a voice? They are historically one of the most silenced groups, being members of two traditionally disempowered and devalued sections of society. If both children and disabled people now have their rights recognized, is this happening or can it happen for disabled children? Further, for those with the most excluded types of impairments, those having unusual modes of thinking, behaviour and communication, can they be recognized as having voices which should be listened to, albeit unusual ones and how can their participation and inclusion be ensured?

Disabled children – Bringing childhoods and disability arenas together

Until very recently disabled children have not generally been included in or benefitted from the two movements described above, which have influenced thinking about nondisabled children and disabled adults so radically. Although they are members of both these structurally disadvantaged minority groups, they have been somewhat forgotten by both. This is however now beginning to change and ideas from the two arenas are being productively combined (Tisdall 2012). Lansdown (2012) has interrogated the ways in which disabled children are or are not protected and served by the two UN Conventions (UNCRC and UNCRPD). The former treaty having been written three decades earlier now looks outdated in its wording about disabled children, the UNCRPD sounding more positive and less segregationist. However even in the decade since the launch of the latter treaty, ideas and terminology have evolved and now the emphasis is more firmly on the inclusion of disabled people, whether adults or children in mainstream activities, on rights to participation, to appropriate accommodations and accessibility. Changes in the wording and the vocabulary used precipitates people to think proactively about inclusive approaches across sectors. Funding also needs to change to ensure that there are resources to ensure that disabled adults and children can join in with a whole range of activities in their communities alongside their peers. These changes often focus first on physical access, but those are the easy wins, there also need to be changes in attitudes, information and expectations so that all feel welcomed into a full range of societal roles and contexts. Thus as well as 'inclusive education', there is now increasingly talk of 'inclusive health', 'inclusive leisure' and 'inclusive research'.

These new ideas lead naturally to recognition of the necessity of hearing disabled children's voices, but are still perhaps not well understood. Many authors still report the devalued status of disabled children and the negative assumptions that are made about them in policy and in practice, both in the UK (Goodley and Runswick-Cole 2011) and internationally (UNICEF 2013; Curran Runswick-Cole 2013; Burman et al. 2015). Often there is an observable gap between legal instruments and policy intentions and implementation in reality. This is particularly true in low income settings, where many disabled children are still shockingly disadvantaged and silenced compared with their nondisabled peers (UNICEF 2011, 2013). These reports highlight the lack of basics such access to education and healthcare, as well as higher rates of malnutrition, mortality and abuse of disabled children. However, they have not yet really resulted in consultation directly with them or amplification of their voices.

All children may at times be unfairly regarded as incompetent and incapable of forming or expressing their own views, but this is even more so for disabled children. Although their impairments may affect what and how they can think and communicate, this is hugely variable and dependent on their ages, the type and severity of impairment they have and all importantly on the availability of appropriate assistive devices and personal support. There has so far been a tendency to assume low competency in all disabled children (Davis and Watson 2000). This kind of thinking then limits consideration of whether and how they might be asked for their opinions. It is often just assumed that this is not possible (Wickenden and Kembhavi-Tam 2014). Disabled children are then for the most part invisible in society, before the law, in research and in consultations (Corker and Davis 2000; Sabatello 2013; Feldman et al. 2013).

In the light of the two UN conventions and in recognition of disabled children as citizens with rights, it could be argued that it is unethical and a denial of their rights not to do inclusive research or other consultations with them (Allan 2005). There is a need to find ways actively to include them, rather than assuming that they cannot join in. Although there has been some increase in the amount of targeted disability-focused research undertaken, some of it avowedly participatory, this has been almost exclusively with adults. There is still a serious lack of inclusion of a disability lens, or disabled people as participants in mainstream research or consultation activities. Thus projects which set out to explore the perceptions of children in a community, about universal topics of relevance to all, such as: their school, transport, the environment or whatever, are still very unlikely to plan to include disabled children alongside their peers. This is despite the fact that is likely that 5–10 per cent of the children in a community will have a disability (UNICEF 2013). This inclusion in mainstream consultations, would necessitate firstly, recognition of their right and probable desire to join in and secondly consideration of the accommodations needed to support them at the design, resourcing and practical stages (Wickenden and Elphick 2016).

Different voices

Voice as a concept conjures up powerful and emotive images. It can represent personal power and autonomy as well as opportunities for self-expression and important aspects of identity. Thus 'having a voice' or hearing people's voices' is a powerful trope. Often the idea of previously hidden or neglected minority groups being revealed and given a chance to tell others about their lives is described as 'giving them a voice' or hearing their voices (HelpAge 2015). However, it is interesting to consider what kinds of voices these are. Voice can of course be considered from either the physical or the meta-phorical perspective. Opportunities to have 'a voice' maybe facilitated or denied in a number of ways, either at the individual or the structural level. Being given a chance to have a say, is then a metaphorical way to describe having agency and being empowered. People have different kinds of voices and these, depending on what they are like, may be more or less acknowl-edged and recognized.

A person's physical voice is a very individual aspect of them, each speaker having their own unique and instantly recognisable features which are linked to aspects of their physical body, so someone might have a deep or high voice, a gravelly or smooth voice and so on. Additionally, the way the person uses their voice and their style of communication more gen-erally are very individual and characteristic of them. This develops from early in life, and it evolves as a child grows and matures. Furthermore, this becomes a 'social voice' through being overlaid with the individual's life experiences, much as Shilling (1994) argues that the unfinished natural body is 'completed' through social action. Used philosophically or anthropologi-cally the 'voice' is the expression of both internal and external dialogues, a representation of the person. Thus, the ways in which a person talks and moves are like a 'fingerprint' of selfhood, simultaneously unconscious and conscious. The kind of voice a person has is 'read' by others as part of understanding them. It can however be misleading. Disabled children or adults may have voices that are unconventional in various ways. They may not be able to speak physically at all and use nonverbal, augmentative or alternative communication (AAC) (e.g. symbols, pictures, and gestures), have slow, indistinct or an unusual quality of speech or be deaf and so use sign language. Thus their 'voice' is of a different kind.

Conventional verbal communication using natural speech is a powerful medium and because it is fast, efficient and very flexible, will always dominate over other types of voices. Paterson and Hughes argue that this is what happens in a disablist world, where the most usual types of voices prevail. They suggest that 'norms of communication and norms of intercorporeal interaction reflect the carnal needs of non-disabled actors' (1999: 604). Thus the verbal world and 'vocal bodies' are exclusionary because they powerfully structure society. Some disabled people have very unusual voices, talking through multi-modal methods, which are often a complex dance combining body movement, speech, signs, gestures, alternative and augmentative systems used together. People who know them well such as family members are able to interpret and translate their 'voices', but unfamiliar people may not recognize that the person is talking and has things to say. Human beings use communication for many purposes, with many types of voice. It is easy to see then how certain types of voice will be particularly muted for some individuals if their form of talking is not recognized and adapted to. For example, it might be possible for them to express everyday needs at home, but they might never be asked about their inner thoughts, not able to be a gossip at school or a human rights advocate!

Someone who has an unusual physical voice is then easily silenced because others do not see them as having a metaphorical voice that is a right to say things, although in a different way. They are then disempowered. For people with unconventional communication in a vocal world, it is difficult to have a metaphorical voice without being problematized. Their unusual physical voices negatively overshadow their right to metaphorical voices. Disabled children with unusual communication may if they are not given opportunities to have their metaphorical voice heard, learn to be passive and will grow used to being excluded. This then can be the start of a lifetime of internalized oppression (Mason 1992). We can see how the usual 'hierarchy of exclusion' across impairment groups (Deal 2007), which commonly leaves those with cognitive, communication and behavioural difficulties the most left out might be promulgated, because of the lack of recognition of these unusual voices. Thus in setting out to hear the voices of disabled children there is a need to proceed with caution and to develop methods of research and consultation which rather than exacerbating this hierarchy, actively recognize and encourage those whose physical and or metaphorical voice is weak. Disabled children may then have particular and unusual types of physical voices. They may also be able to talk using speech but still have a weak metaphorical voice because of the response of society to them and the ways that they are different.

If researchers set out with all good intentions to collect the perspectives of disabled children, they need to be wary of being too aligned to concepts around normative child development. General guidelines about what children can be expected to do at different ages do not take into account huge individual and cultural variation. These child development norms can easily lead to expectations of some kind of 'typical' child and possibly to making assumptions about the competencies (or more likely lack of them) of disabled children (Skelton 2008). Children anyway are very diverse in what they can do and what they want to say, and those with disabilities even more so. James (2007) points out that in the rush to hear 'children's voices' there is a risk of cliché and tokenism and that as a powerful rhetorical device, there is a danger that adults in simplifying, clarifying or mediating may 'reinforce established prejudices' about them (2007: 267). This is a particular risk for disabled children. It is essential that many different types of voice are recognized, heard and valued. The way that unusual voices are interpreted, mediated and reported is also a matter for important consideration (Wickenden 2011).

The way disabled children see themselves

The way that disability and disabled children are understood in any particular cultural context will affect the type of citizens they can be and the ways in which they will or will not be included in society (Thomas 2004; Hughes 2007). I have heard disabled children in multiple contexts insisting that they have more in common with their nondisabled peers than they have differences. They just want to be treated as a 'normal kid'. The reverse assumption, that they are essentially different will lead to further othering of them, a process that often begins with the acquiring of the label disabled. Once perceived as a separate category of person, or in extreme cases as nonhuman or a 'non-person', it is somehow easier to justify their exclusion and denial of their human rights. Sadly, extreme ill treatment, neglect, abuse and other disadvantages are not uncommonly experienced by disabled children globally (UNICEF 2013).

There is plenty of evidence from disabled adults and now an increasing amount from disabled children that they do not see themselves as different from others. When asked to describe themselves and what their priorities are, their responses are very markedly similar to those of their nondisabled peers. Thus their impairment or disabled status is not usually the first thing they mention. In examples taken from UK disabled teenagers who use AAC, we can see that they are more likely to mention their role within their family:

> I am helpful.
> I am the joker.
> I am a chatterbox.

Or things they like or are positive characteristics:

> I love chocolate.
> I support Chelsea.
> I am a sporty girl.
> I am competitive like my dad.
> I love the Kaiser Chiefs

These kinds of self-descriptions show that given an opportunity to describe and demonstrate who they are, these young people focus more on things which accentuate their 'normality' to use a contested concept, or their ordinariness. Thus disabled children often demonstrate a different set of interests and priorities from those they are assumed to have. Their main identity then is not a disabled one (Watson 2002). The data quoted above is from disabled teenagers in the UK, but rather similar responses are also found from studies I have done with disabled children in South Asia and in East Africa (Wickenden 2016, 2017). Noticeably then, despite huge differences in culture and context, and disparities in available resources, disabled children given an opportunity to express themselves say that they want to be known for what they can contribute to their families and communities and for aspects of themselves that accentuate their competence, their age-related interests and their aspirations for the future. E.g. a disabled teenage boy in India said:

> I want to work to help my family.

And a girl in Uganda said:

> I want to be someone who can be someone.

The evidence from these studies clearly supports the work of both Albrecht and Devleiger (1999) and Mackenzie and Leach Scully (2007) who all argue that nondisabled people regularly underestimate the positive aspects of disabled people's lives. Others assume that they cannot be having a good quality of life, if they are living lives that nondisabled people cannot imagine. In order to counter these ableist preconceptions we need to seek out the perspectives of disabled children themselves. If we do not facilitate and enable disabled children to 'have a voice', then we will not understand how they see themselves and how they can be enabled to resist infantilizing, homogenizing and pathologizing assumptions about them.

Understandings and expectations of disabled children's participation

Closely related to the idea of 'hearing' disabled children's voices are the concepts of inclusion and participation. These are common buzzwords and aspirations of our times. Children's participation in particular has received increased attention latterly (Percy-Smith and Thomas 2009), although sadly inclusive approaches to this less so. Both inclusive approaches and participatory research are routes to the amplification of disabled children's physical and metaphorical voices. An inclusive approach which includes everybody, whatever kind of voice they have demands especially good and adapted listening from others. Ways of consulting and doing research that use multi-modal, communication methods using pictures, symbols and signs and which do not automatically privilege talking are needed. This demands a considerable switch in mind-set and flexibility by the adults designing such projects. They need to start with a 'can do' attitude, where all children are assumed to be able to participate, not that some can't. Often judgements are made too quickly about children's competence without trying out a range of modes and methods of engaging them. Their evolving capacities and the need for adaptations and for them to get familiar with a new situation are all often overlooked (Lansdown 2005; Skelton 2008). So a child who appears not to be following or contributing, may be recognized later as doing so in their own way, given time and appropriate support. Styles of and expectations of participation can sometimes be too conventional and narrow and therefore unaccepting of diversity. So traditionally a 'participating child' might be seen as one who is attentive, responsive and active. A child like this clearly understands and responds conventionally as and when expected. This makes adults' jobs easy. However, a child who has severe physical impairments or intellectual/behaviour impairments may be more difficult to recognize as participating, because his or her participation looks different. Additionally, styles of participation and expectations of disabled children vary cross-culturally (Nelson et al. 2016). Whatever the context, the way someone appears and behaves can have dramatic and negative effects on how they are seen as a person (Garland-Thomson 2006). Thus someone who appears different is easily essentialized as unable to participate or as not having a voice (Fuss 1989). In order to hear these unusual voices there is a need to accept a diversity of ways to participate and of being. Twum-Danso (2016) argues for recognition of diversity amongst children generally, rather than a homogenizing tendency. Disability is then just one kind of diversity, which needs to be accommodated to and indeed celebrated.

I have argued that disabled children's voices are often silenced or muted. So it is good to reflect on what they might want to tell us about, given the opportunity. Albrecht and Devlieger (1999) argue that if we seek disabled people's perspective this will 'humanize' them and surprise us. They will not necessarily say what people expect! If we are considering disabled children's perspectives, we need to make sure that we don't just pursue adult led agendas, as we may miss hearing what they really want to tell us about. It is tempting to ask them about practical aspects such as service provision: their experiences of school, health or social care (Franklin and Sloper 2009). These are of course important and they can reveal important information if we ask them directly (Garth and Aroni 2003). However, they may prioritize other things to tell us about. Research which explores their lives more broadly and follows their lead is also important. From this we can learn about their lived realities in a more nuanced way and set these perspectives alongside those of adults such as their parents and teachers (Singh and Ghai 2009; Witchger et al. 2014).

Conclusion

In this chapter, I have discussed changes in conceptions of children and of disability in the last few decades. However, sadly, in this era of rights, and the implementation of UN conventions (UNCRC and UNCRPD) for both groups, disabled children's voices are still silenced and need to be heard. An inclusive approach to consultations with children and to research would necessarily mean that their physical, information, communication and attitudinal access needs should be met to enable them to have a voice. Their skills and abilities may be diverse and sometimes different from other children but they are not incompetent. They have ideas and experiences to share and they may do this with unusual communication modes, such as signing, pictures, symbols, communication devices and natural gestures alongside or rather than with conventional speech. Thus they may not have 'a physical voice' in the way that nondisabled children do, but they can be given the chance to have a metaphorical voice. This would allow them to realize for example article 12 of the UNCRC- the right of the child to form and express his own ideas. All children whatever their skills and support needs can participate in one way or another, and the concept of participation needs to be broadened in the discourse, to recognize different forms of joining in. A truly inclusive approach, would be affirmative and celebratory, seeing all children's contributions, however unconventional as important and valuable and providing insights into their worlds which cannot be gathered in any other way. The onus is on adults around them and society at large to enable and recognize their potential contribution. Disabled children resist conceptions of them as incompetent, as devalued, as destined to be eternally childlike and as unworthy to have a voice. Given a voice they say that they are ordinary children with important things to tell us.

References

Albrecht, G. L., and Devleiger, P. J. (1999). The disability paradox: high quality of life against all odds. *Social Science and Medicine*, 48, 977–988.

Allan, J. (2005). Inclusion as an ethical project. In S. Tremain (ed.), *Foucault and the government of disability*, pp. 281–297. Ann Arbor: The University of Michigan Press.

Barnes, C., and Mercer, G. (2010). *Exploring Disability*. Cambridge: Polity.

Beazley, H., Bessel, S., Ennew, J., and Waterson, R. (2009). Editorial: The Right to Be Properly Researched – Research with Children in A Messy Real World. *Children's Geographies*, 7 (4), 365–378.

Burman, E. (2008). *Deconstructing developmental psychology*. London: Routledge.

Burman, E., Greenstein, A., and Kumar, M. (2015). Editorial: Frames and debates for disability, childhood and the global South: Introducing the special issue. *Disability and the Global South* 2 (2), 563–569.

Corker, M., and Davis, J. M. (2000). Children with disabilities – invisible under the law. In J. Cooper and S. Vernon (eds), *Disability and the law*. London: Jessica Kingsley.

Crivello, G., Camfield, L. and Woodhead, M. (2009). How can children tell us about their wellbeing? Exploring the potential of participatory research approaches within Young Lives. *Social Indicators Research*, 90, 51–72.

Curran, T., and Runswick-Cole, K. (eds) (2013). *Disabled Children's Childhood Studies: Critical approaches in a global context.* Basingstoke: Palgrave Macmillan.

Davis, J. M., and Watson, N. (2000). Disabled Children's rights in everyday life: problematising notions of competency and promotion self-empowerment. *International Journal of Children's Rights,* 8, 211–228.

Deal, M. (2007). Aversive Disablism: subtle prejudice toward disabled people. *Disability and Society,* 22 (1), 93–107.

Disabled People's International (DPI) (2016). Retrieved from: <http://www.dpi.org>.

Ennew, J., et al. (2009). *The right to be properly researched: how to do rights-based, scientific research with children.* Bangkok: Black on White Publications.

Feldman, M. A., Battin, S, M., Shaw, O. A., and Luckasson, R. (2013). Inclusion of children with disabilities in mainstream child development research. *Disability and Society,* 28 (7), 997–1011.

Ferri, B. A., and Connor D. J. (2006). *Reading resistance: Discourses of exclusion in desegregation and inclusion debates.* New York: Peter Lang.

Franklin, A., and Sloper, P. (2009). Supporting the participation of children with disabilities and young people in decision-making. *Children and Society,* 23, 3–15.

Fuss, D. (1989). *Essentially Speaking.* New York: Routledge.

Garland-Thompson, R. (2006). Ways of Staring. *Journal of Visual Culture,* 5 (2), 173–192.

Garth, B., and Aroni, R. (2003), 'I value what you have to say': Seeking the perspective of children with a disability, not just their parents. *Disability and Society,* 18, 561–576.

Goodley, D., and Runswick-Cole, K. (2011). Problematising policy: Conceptions of 'child', 'disabled 'and 'parents' in social policy in England. *International Journal of Inclusive Education,* 15(1), 71–85.

Grech, S., and Soldatic, K. (eds) (2016). *Disability in the Global South: A Critical Handbook.* Switzerland: Springer International Publishing.

Hart, J. (2008). Children's Participation and International Development: Attending to the Political. *International Journal of Children's Rights,* 16, 407–418.

HelpAge International (2015). *'We can also make change':* Voices of the marginalised. Retrieved from: <http://www.refworld.org/docid/55c9e46b4.html>.

Hill, M. (2006). Children's Voices on ways of having a voice: Children's and young people's perspectives on methods used in research and consultation. *Childhood,* 13, 69–89.

Hughes, B. (2007). Being disabled: towards a critical social ontology for disability. *Disability and Society,* 22(7), 673–683.

Hunleth, J. (2011). Beyond on or with: Questioning power dynamics and knowledge production in 'child-orientated' research methodology. *Childhood,* 18(1), 81–93.

International Disability Alliance (IDA) (2016). *High Level Political Forum. Ensuring that no one is left behind Position paper by Persons with Disabilities.* Retrieved from: <http://www.internationaldisabilityalliance.org/blog/day-one-high-level-political-forum-2016>.

James, A. (2007), Giving voice to children's voices: Practices and problems, pitfalls and potentials. *American Anthropologist,* 109, 261–272.

James, A., and James, A. L. (2004). *Constructing Childhood.* London: Palgrave.

Kellett, M. (2005). *Children as active researchers: a new research paradigm for the 21st century?* ESRC, UK.

Kirby, P., et al. (2003). *Building a culture of participation: involving children and young people in policy, service planning, delivery and evaluation.* London: Department for Education and Skills.

Lansdown, G. (2012), *Using the human rights framework to promote the rights of children with disabilities.* New York: UNICEF.

Lansdown, G. (2005). *The evolving capacities of the child.* Florence: Save the Children, UNICEF Innocenti Research Centre.

Leonard Cheshire International (LCI). (2014). *Young Voices – speak out.* Retrieved from: <http://www.LCDisability.org/youngvoices>.

Mason, M. (1992). Internalised oppression. In R. Rieser and M. Mason (eds), *Disability Equality in the Classroom: A Human Rights Issue* (2nd ed.), pp. 27–28. London: Disability Equality in Education.

Nelson, F., Masulani-Mwale, C., Richards, E., Theobald, S., and Gladstone, M. (2016.) The meaning of participation for children in Malawi: insights from children and caregivers. *Child: Care, Health and Development,* 43 (1), 133–143.

Oliver, M., and Barnes, C. (2012). *The New Politics of Disablement.* Basingstoke: Palgrave.

Paterson, K., and Hughes, B. (1999). Disability Studies and Phenomenology: the carnal politics of everyday life. *Disability and Society,* 14 (5), 597–610.

Percy-Smith, B., and Thomas, N. (2010). *A Handbook of Children and Young People's Participation Perspectives from theory and practice.* London: Routledge.

Rogoff, B. (2003). *The cultural nature of human development.* Oxford: Oxford University Press.

Sabatello, M. (2013). Children with disabilities: A critical appraisal. *International Journal of Children's Rights,* 21 (3), 464–487.

Shakespeare, T. (1994). Cultural representation of disabled people: dustbins of disavowal? *Disability and Society,* 9, 283–299.

Shakespeare, T. (2013). *Disability Rights and Wrongs Revisited.* London: Palgrave.

Shilling, C. (1994). *The body and social theory.* London: Sage.

Singh, V., and Ghai, A. (2009). Notions of self: lived realities of children with disabilities. *Disability and Society,* 24 (2), 129–145.

Skelton, T. (2008). Research with children and young people: exploring the tensions between ethics, competence and participation. *Children's Geographies*, 6 (1), 21–36.

Swain, J., and French, S. (2000). Towards an affirmative model of disability. *Disability and Society*, 15, 569–582.

Thomas, C. (2004). How is disability understood? An examination of sociological approaches. *Disability and Society*, 19 (6), 569–583.

Tisdall, E. K. M. (2012). The challenge and challenging of childhood studies? Learning from disability studies and research with disabled children. *Children and Society*, 26 (3), 181–191.

Tisdall, E. K. M., and Punch, S. (2012.) Not so 'new'? Looking critically at childhood studies. *Children's Geographies*, 10 (3), 249–264.

Twum-Danso, A. (2016). From the singular to the plural: Exploring diversities in contemporary childhoods in sub-Saharan Africa. *Childhood*, 23 (3), 455–468.

UNICEF (2011). Calls for Children with Disabilities to Be Included in All Development (3 December). Retrieved from: <http://www.unicef.org/media/media_60790.html>.

UNICEF (2013). *State of the World's Children: Children with Disabilities*. UNICEF: New York. Retrieved from: <http://www.unicef.org/sowc2013>.

UNICEF (2013). *Engaging Children with disabilities in decisions that affect their lives*. Retrieved from: <https://www.unicef.org/disabilities/files/Take_Us_Seriously.pdf>.

United Nations. (2006). *UN convention on the rights of persons with disabilities*. New York: United Nations.

United Nations (2015). *Sustainable development Goals* (SDGs). Retrieved from: <http://www.un.org/sustainabledevelopment>.

Watson, N. (2002). Well I know this is Going to Sound Very Strange to You but I Don't see Myself as a Disabled Person: identity and disability. *Disability and Society*, 17 (5), 509–527.

Wickenden, M. (2011). Whose voice is that? Issues of identity, voice and representation arising in an ethnographic study of the lives of disabled teenagers who use Augmentative and Alternative Communication (AAC). *Disability Studies Quarterly*, 31(4). DOI: doi.org/10.18061/dsq.v31i4.1724.

Wickenden, M. (in press 2018). 'Disabled' versus 'nondisabled': another redundant binary. In A. Twum-Danso Imoh, M. Bourdillon, S. Meichsner and F. Wanderley (eds), *Global Childhoods Beyond the North South Divide*. London: Palgrave Macmillan.

Wickenden, M., and Elphick, J. (2016). Don't forget us, we are here too! Listening to the perspectives and priorities of children with disabilities and their families living in contexts of poverty. In S. Grech and K. Soldatic (eds). *Disability in the*

Global South: A Critical Handbook, Chapter 24. Switzerland: Springer International Publishing.

Wickenden, M., and Kembhavi, G. (2014). Ask us too! Doing participatory research with children with disabilities in the Global South. *Childhood,* 21(3), 400–417.

Witchger Hansen, M., Siame, M., and Van der Veen, J. (2014). A qualitative study: Barriers and support for participation for children with disabilities. *African Journal of Disability,* 3(1) 112.

Woodhead, M., and Montgomery, H. (eds) (2002). *Understanding childhood: an interdisciplinary approach.* Milton Keynes: Open University and Wiley.

World Health Organization and World Bank (2011). *World Report on Disability.* Geneva: WHO Press. Retrieved from: <http://www.who.int/disabilities/world_report/2011/report.pdf>.

ELENA JENKIN, ERIN WILSON, ROBERT CAMPAIN AND
MATTHEW CLARKE

3 Beyond childhood, disability and postcolonial theory: young children with disability in developing countries can tell their own stories

Introduction

There are at least ninety-five million children with disability[1] globally
(World Health Organization [WHO] 2011) and it is estimated that
80 per cent of the disability population reside in developing countries (Grech
2012). Despite this, we have very little human rights data pertaining to children with disability (Office of the United Nations High Commissioner for
Human Rights [OHCHR] 2012), particularly data that are self-reported by
children themselves and situated in developing countries (Wickenden and
Elphick 2016). The lack of information about this group poses substantial
problems as 'the information about children generated and used by both
governments and civil society determines the policies and programmes that
directly affect children's experiences of childhood and the extent to which
their rights are fulfilled' (Miljeteig and Ennew 2017: 25). A lack of data,
therefore, leads to policies that do not necessarily include or support children
with disability to access their human rights entitlements or, worse, further
discriminate against them (Johnson 2017; Liebel and Invernizzi 2016).

 Children with disability have been frequently excluded from research
and where data are collected it is often via the use of adult proxies as data

---

1   In this chapter, person first language – children with disability – will be used as per the
    Convention on the Rights of Persons with Disabilities (United Nations [UN] 2006).

sources about children. This is despite proxy information being found to be inaccurate, particularly for children with disability living in poverty (Huus et al. 2015; Invernizzi and Williams 2011). Exclusion from research occurs for multiple reasons. Children with disability are often viewed by researchers through a deficit or charity lens, where they are perceived to be incapable to consent or speak for themselves and their impairments are seen as preventing them from participation. Ignorance on the researchers' behalf can lead them to develop inaccessible research methods which inadvertently or explicitly exclude children with disability. This can extend to an overly literal focus on the 'voice' of children resulting in the exclusion of children with communication and/or cognitive impairments who do not use speech to communicate. Such practices lie in contrast to a human rights lens that views children with disability as having emerging capacities, a 'voice' and a right to express their opinion as declared in the United Nations Conventions on the Rights of the Child (CRC) (UN 1989) and the Rights of Persons with Disabilities (CRPD) (UN 2006).

This chapter explores the theoretical legacy that has led to these constructions of childhood and disability, particularly considering the implications of this for children with disability in developing countries. Theories of childhood, disability, and postcolonialism, and the potentially disrupting ideas of human rights and postcolonialism, engender a range of methodological issues for researching children with disability in developing countries. One methodological approach, adopted for the Voices of Pacific Children with Disability project conducted in Vanuatu and Papua New Guinea (PNG), is presented as an example that attempts to address these issues. Within this methodology, an inclusive method of data collection and dissemination was utilized. This method enabled children aged five to eighteen with diverse disabilities to identify life priorities and aspirations, which were analysed in relation to the CRPD (UN 2006) as a means to present data on the human rights priorities of this group. A brief snapshot of data provided by the five to six-year-old cohort is presented in this chapter.[2] The children's views that were captured via this process were later

---

2   Results for the entire cohort have been presented elsewhere (Jenkin et al., 2017a). The focus here is on the younger cohort to demonstrate that young children can

disseminated via a range of strategies, to inform (and hopefully transform) community attitudes towards children with disability, as well as policy and programme development.[3] Overall, this case study represents an exploration of the link between theoretical issues and research design towards unlocking the utility of children with disability's voices as a mechanism for change in developing countries.

Theoretical lenses constructing children with disability in developing countries

Research about children with disability in the developing world are shaped and influenced directly, or indirectly, by Western dominant theories of childhood, disability, and postcolonisation. Each of these, separately and combined, act to silence and marginalize the voices of children with disability in the developing world. Each theory is briefly presented and critiqued below with the aim of foregrounding issues to inform a more transformative (or 'critical postcolonial disability') research methodology (Chataika 2012).

The theoretical lens of early childhood

Western conceptualizations of childhood have been dominated by developmental stage theory that positions the early years as foundational, laying the pathways for learning, relationships and functioning, and identifying the dependency upon others for care during these early years (Ezell 1983–1984;

---

self-report on their lives in a meaningful way that can then inform a range of positive supports and interventions.

3   A range of resources were produced from the project including: policy briefs and commentary (see for example Wilson et al. 2016); three films for community awareness (see <http://www.voicesofchildrenwithdisability.com/films>) and a guide to the inclusive methods used (see Jenkin et al. 2015).

Platz and Arellano 2011; Woodhead 2006). In this view, the child is seen as incomplete (Davis 2013; Liebel 2012) or 'becoming', rather than 'being' already competent and active (Vogler et al. 2008). The approach is also a normative one, where children have been pathologized 'who failed to meet the standardized developmental targets' (Davis 2013: 415). However, critics have argued that the notion of the normative universal child fails to capture the diversity of children's lives that are impacted by gender, culture, socio-economic situation, class and other aspects (Curran and Runswick-Cole 2014; Priestly 1998), though disability is rarely mentioned as a factor of this diversity and is largely missing from the field of childhood studies (Curran and Runswick-Cole 2014).

A further critique of the universalizing norm of the developmental paradigm has been that of the exclusion of the experiences of children in developing countries (Woodhead 2006). To address this, a social and cultural critique emphasizes that child development occurs in relation to social relationships and is embedded in specific cultural contexts (Woodhead 2006). To some extent, this liberates concepts of early childhood from Western individualized goals of autonomy and independence, previously taken as standard global key concepts of early childhood development, and allows these to be replaced with collectively driven concepts such as interdependence and respect of parents/elders that align with cultural values held in many developing countries and indigenous cultures (Woodhead 2006).

Childhood theory and research have now shifted to recognize the agency of children and the situations that shape and influence their social and cultural constructions (Davis 2013). This 'rights' shift enshrines the importance of children participating in decisions that affect their lives. The CRC (UN 1989) has advanced this perspective of childhood and an acknowledgement of children's emerging capacities and 'voice'. However, while the CRC has assisted to bring about reforms in policy in many countries across the world, Woodhead (2006) reports that it has little focus on young children, and very few states are discussing or reporting on this group. So too, has the CRC been critiqued for its overly universalizing conception of children's rights (Liebel 2012). Paying attention to the diverse experiences and priorities of young children in developing countries and the context within which they live, is a vital aspect to not only respecting but understanding and advancing their human rights.

The theoretical lens of disability

As with early childhood, Western academics have progressed a range of theoretical disability paradigms that shape views, services and attitudes towards children with disability and, in turn, impact on the life experiences of children with disability (Kenny 2006). The medical model of disability emphasizes impairment as a deficit or a deformity requiring medical treatment and rehabilitation (Davis 2013; Priestley 1998). Children who could not overcome their impairment have been deemed as abnormal, inferior, deviant and backward (Priestley 1998; Trani et al. 2011) and children with disability have been 'rarely viewed in a way that appreciated what they were in the present' (Cosaro in Davis 2013: 415). The medical model has often been accompanied by a segregated approach that ghettoized children with disability from their peers, school, community and, often, from their family (Davis 2013). This deficit focus is also evident in the charity model of disability which pities children for their impairments (Kenny 2006) and views them as helpless and in need of help from others (Kenny 2006; Priestley 1998). Capacities held by children with disability are not recognized within either construct (Davis 2013; Harpur 2012). Both the medical and charity models differentiate between the abled and disabled, and involve 'asymmetrical power relations whereby the professional expert (such as doctor or social worker) ... or family member speaks and decides for them' (Kenny 2006: 294).

The social model of disability responds to the previous deficit focused models (Harpur 2012; Marks 1997) and views impairment as a normal part of the human condition. In this model, disability is constructed by a society or environment that fails to consider differences (Marks 1997) or remove barriers (Oliver 2013; Watson 2012), such as attitudes, natural or built structures, communication and legislation (Marks 1997). Dismantling barriers that construct disability is viewed as everyone's role rather than an individual's problem (Llewellyn and Hogan 2000; Marks 1997). However, a focus solely on difference or barriers tends to overly frame children with disability as victims of these factors and reinforce the 'powerless nature of childhood' (Davis 2013: 417). Lacking is a focus on children's ideas, capacities or skills and what strategies they, along with their families, utilized to overcome adversity (Davis 2013). The human rights model of disability expands the social model definition (Harpur 2012) and addresses these concerns whereby the rights, evolving capacities, agency and views of children and adults with disability are enshrined and respected (Kenny 2006; UN 2006).

As with theories of childhood, Western theories of disability have been transposed in many situations to developing countries, and have achieved 'hegemonic status' (Grech 2012: 59). Missing from the literature are models, beliefs and practices that are local to developing countries, and the universal definition of disability within the CRPD has been critiqued as failing to capture the real experiences felt by a diverse range of children (and adults) with disability in these contexts (Grech 2012). Critical postcolonial understandings of disability, discussed below, offer a potential way to address these concerns.

The theoretical lens of postcolonialism

As discussed above, dominant Western ideology has imposed specific approaches upon developing countries to attend to 'problems experienced by children in the Global South, which ... poorly account for the social, economic, political and cultural realities' of these nations (Bessell et al. 2017: 237). Similarly, Grech (2012) reports that the 'colonial constructions of, and approaches to, disability seep into and make up the contemporary landscape (including the transmission/imposition of knowledge and practices)' (p. 53–53) in developing country contexts. This includes Western expertise in the form of development (Chataika 2012), compounded by policies and practices that either decide what is best for children with disability or ignore their existence altogether, reinforcing oppressive practices (Barker and Murray 2010). Holt and Holloway (2006) warn that there is a tendency to dichotomize children according to whether they live in developed or developing countries, with no diversity within either of these parallel worlds. Such oversimplified categorizations can imply that children and adults with disability in the developing world are perpetually oppressed (Grech 2012: 59), making invisible the strengths and emerging capacities of children with disability along with the 'agency, resilience, love and care of families who continue to ensure the survival of their own disabled members' (Grech 2012: 60).

Postcolonial theory offers a way to challenge and re-make colonialist dominance, both materially and epistemologically (Liebel 2017). Until recently, postcolonial theory has not considered the role of children or notions of childhood, but now focuses attention on how 'children's way of life and constructions of childhood are interwoven with postcolonial power relations' (Liebel 2017: 86) and the disparities brought about via colonization and globalization. Despite this, disability has been 'absent from the postcolonial theory discourse' (Barker and Murray in Chataika 2012: 264), potentially relegating children and adults with disability into the shadows (Chataika 2012), adding yet another layer of oppression. However, moves to embrace a critical postcolonial view of disability identify the potential to liberate or de-colonize the notion of 'disability', recognizing it as 'fluid, dynamic and shifting, constantly (re)negotiated' (Grech 2012: 58). Disability needs to be acknowledged as a 'highly complex variable, ... [cutting] across the range of political, social and cultural experiences' (Watson 2012: 194) and defined and understood through a complexity of layers such as gender (CRPD 2015; Don et al. 2015; Nguyen et al. 2015), age, impairment type, power, poverty (Emerson and Hatton in Watson 2012), race (Stienstra and Nyerere 2016), ethnicity (Stienstra and Nyerere 2016; Watson 2012), class (Priestley 1998), rurality (Gartrell and Hoban 2016), cultural beliefs, colonization (Ghai 2012; Grech 2012), and a 'myriad of other social identities that converge, articulate and shift to shape how individuals experience life' (Acker-Verney 2016: 1). Finally, postcolonialism offers a direction for research 'decolonization', proposing a transformative shift in the power relations and purpose of research (Chataika 2012), one that focuses on a deep learning of each context, and making marginalized knowledges, such as those of children with disability in developing countries, 'present and credible' (Grech 2012: 66).

Methodological implications for conducting research about children with disability in developing countries

The above discussion outlines three theoretical lenses (childhood, disability and postcolonialism) that shape both how children with disability are viewed and how research about them is constructed. Taken together, these three lenses construct young children with disability in developing country contexts as underdeveloped, deficient, and incompetent. For researchers seeking to conduct research with young children with disability in developing country contexts, critiques of these three theoretical lenses offer a range of methodological issues to be addressed and strategies to implement. The Voices of Pacific Children with Disability research project was conducted in Vanuatu and PNG between 2013 and 2015, through a partnership with Deakin University, Save the Children, the Vanuatu Disability Promotion and Advocacy Association and the PNG Assembly of Disabled Persons.[4] Specifically, the project aimed to address the research question, 'What are the human rights needs and priorities of children with disability in Vanuatu and Papua New Guinea?' Data were collected from eighty-nine children with disability (aged five to eighteen), including fifteen children aged five and six, across both countries.

Partnership approach

The first hurdle of research design was the negotiation of power between partners in the project. As Chataika (2012) identifies, project funding in international development is commonly allocated to a lead agency in the Global North, who later seeks 'downstream' partners in the Global South to support a 'pre-set research agenda' (p. 254). In the case of the 'Voices' project, academic researchers based in Australia (the authors),

---

4   The research was funded through the Australian Development Research Award scheme (Department of Foreign Affairs and Trade [DFAT]).

commenced discussions through pre-existing relationships with Disabled Peoples Organizations (DPOs) in both countries prior to application for grant funds, which focused on a discussion of their priorities in relation to children with disability. However, in recognition of the need to best connect with children in each country, a partnership with a child rights and service delivery agency (operating in both countries) was also established and included in the discussions. The research design was heavily based on this partnership with local agencies which facilitated a mutual sharing of expertise in research (from the authors), disability (from local disability leaders, DPO members and local researchers with disability) and children (from the local child rights organization).

A further aspect of power sharing and mutual capacity building was the employment of local researchers, most of whom were adults with disability. Recognizing the tension many people with disability have in their availability for employment, positions were open to full time, part time or consultant work to provide flexibility. Support was provided to ensure researchers' work environment was as accessible as possible given the contexts and remote locations. Local researchers had cultural knowledge and resources that external researchers did not: they were sensitive to and worked within cultural norms and expectations; they were already well known and connected with their local communities; they adhered to cultural protocols and spoke local dialects; and they had an in-depth understanding of the multiple factors within each context that affected participation and meaning making. Their deployment in the project grounded it in, and translated it for, the multiple local contexts within each country.

Decolonizing of concepts: Localizing meaning of disability and childhood

Given the dominance of Western theories of childhood and disability, the methodology needed to overtly seek to counteract these discourses and practices that externally construct and subordinate young children (Acker-Verney 2016). A method for enabling the privileging of local understandings of disability and childhood was required. The partnership approach discussed above was critical to explicating meanings related to disability and childhood. As part of this process, members from local DPOs attended all research workshops held in each country to develop methods. This included the DPOs providing training to all partners on a contextual understanding of disability, facilitating discussion of disability (and terminology re disability) in local languages and critiquing oppressive constructions of disability. Similarly, local child protection workers (from the child rights agency) provided training in relation to child safety and reporting of concerns. Overall, this process resonates with that described by Mutua and Swadener (2004) as the 'process of valuing, reclaiming, and foregrounding indigenous voices and epistemologies' (p.186) and is consistent with community development theory outlined by Ife (2013) in relation to the importance of valuing local language, knowledge, and process. This process provided important dialogue about understandings of disability, and also engendered considerable discussion of the interpretation of maltreatment of children with disability in some contexts.

Privileging context

Critiques of theories discussed above have all emphasized the importance of diversity and context to exploring meanings related to the lives of children with disability in developing countries. This project set out to include a wide diversity of children, located in both rural and urban environments, across a span of ages between five and eighteen years, with diverse disabilities, and who communicated through different modes.

The project sought to apply a human rights lens as an integral focus to respecting the emerging capacities and strengths of diverse children with disability, and to valuing what they have to say in an attempt to understand and advance their human rights priorities. Liebel (2012) calls for a move away from the legislative and technical focus of human rights, to a more in-depth understanding of how human rights are experienced by children themselves within their diverse contexts. In line with this, we sought to engage children in identifying their human rights and life priorities, but recognized that these would be diverse and differently constructed across the cohort. Therefore, we designed three questions to ask children that were deliberately open ended and that could encompass a diversity of responses. Children were asked:

I. What is important to you in your life?
II. What are your hopes and dreams?
III. What would make your life better or happier?

Researchers developed a variety of ways these questions could be asked depending on the age of the child and capacity to understand the question.[5] The questions, along with informed consent processes, were translated by local researchers into Bislama, Tok Pisin or the local language, and the conversation with children and families was conducted in the language of choice or via other modes (sign language, gesture, body language etc.). When gaining assent from the child, and consent from the parent or care-giver, we used a variety of materials to provide child-friendly and accessible information. This included pictures, plain-language English, local translation and photos. We continually re-visited the issue of assent and consent at all stages of the research when engaging with children as well as reminding each child and their parents or care-givers that they could withdraw at any time.[6]

Central to the privileging of context was the time spent by researchers with each child and each community. Rarely adequately provided for in research, time (and appreciation for a different pace that is more aligned with Pacific culture) is essential for children with disability who may not be used to speaking to previously unknown adults and safely expressing their views. Time was built in for researchers to visit children many times

---

5   Researchers customized their communication approaches and modes to suit the needs and preferences of children. This involved trialling different inclusive data collection tools, observation of the child's responses and interests and, when appropriate, drawing on support from the child's parents or carers to assist with communication and interpretation. For the five to six-year-old age group, most children received five or more visits. See Jenkin et al. 2015 for further details of methods and case study examples.

6   For further discussion on ethical issues of assent and consent when researching with children with disability see Jenkin et al. 2015.

(between two and six visits) in order to understand each child's context (including the factors influencing the experience of disability), build a rapport, collect data and then check that the researchers had recorded the children's priorities correctly (see Jenkin et al. 2017a).

Enabling children to self-report: young children as 'present and credible'

Curran and Runswick-Cole (2014) and Davis (2013) call for more research that enables children with disability to voice their own diverse experiences and agendas so that researchers can support them with the changes they wish to pursue. The research team worked to identify and anticipate both the barriers to communication experienced by children with diverse disabilities, as well as the strengths and interests children and their families might bring to engagement with the research. Local researchers worked with Deakin University researchers to develop a method of data collection that enabled the communication of participating children through aural, oral, visual and tactile means using such techniques or 'tools' as story-telling, story in a bag (filled with locally identifiable items as conversation starters), an audio-library of sounds, drawing, the use of dolls (for role play and story-telling), taking or selecting photographs, and guided tours by children around their environment (Jenkin et al. 2017a; Jenkin et al. 2015). In addition, the use of sign language interpreters was important, particularly in PNG where PNG Sign Language is used. The approach successfully enabled a wide diversity of children with disability to participate. Of eighty-nine participants (aged five to eighteen years), 54 per cent had a cognitive disability, 48 per cent of children had a communication disability, 48 per cent had a physical disability, 30 per cent had a hearing disability and 27 per cent had a vision disability.[7]

---

7   All disability categories were based on extended discussions with parents and not
     formal diagnoses which were frequently absent. Given the lack of formal diagnoses,
     impairment was ascertained using an amended version of the Washington Group
     'Short Set of Questions on Disability' (Washington Group 2010) to identify func-
     tional impairments and level of difficulty as per the parent's information. For the

The approach required an understanding that children's 'voice' is diverse, is not equated with speech alone, and that methods to enable children to communicate through a variety of means beyond speech and text, needed to be adopted and valued as legitimate and rigorous (Sorin 2009; Tisdall 2012). Researchers were supported to observe children's attention levels, tone of voice, restlessness, eye contact and energy in order to capture everything that the child communicated, and to ensure that the child was expressing assent. An important element of this method was the involvement of a child's carer or communication partner to assist in interpreting the child's communication and views where the child used a communication mode that was not understandable to researchers who did not know the child well. Rather than this being considered a mechanism of proxy report, researchers sought to enable the child to utilize their communication partners as key supports to their communication. Family members also sometimes provided additional information, which was noted separately and, as Irwin and Johnson (in Sorin 2009) found in their research, 'parents scaffolding of stories added a richness and completeness that might not have been accessible on first or even subsequent meetings' (p.134).

Commitment to change

Child participants are often denied access to the final phases of the research including findings and dissemination (McLeod 2008, and Porter and Lacey 2005, both in Gray and Winter 2011). Traditional research outputs are frequently inaccessible to the child audience and the communities in which they reside (Jenkin et al. 2016). By contrast, Chataika (2012) asserts that 'research "decolonization" means that the processes and outputs should be

---

purposes of data analysis, researchers aligned impairments with broad disability categories – intellectual, communication, physical, hearing and vision. These labels should be understood as broad and indicative of only some features associated with each formal disability category. They are used for the purpose of analysis only (in the absence of diagnosis or population level prevalence data) and we do not suggest that they would meet the strict criteria of formal diagnoses.

communicated to and used to benefit the researched communities' (p. 266). Consistent with this, the research process, outcomes and dissemination strategies of the project, aimed to generate awareness of the priorities as identified by children with disability, in order to disrupt power inequalities and bring about social change within children's family, community and via policy change. Following PNG and Vanuatu's strong tradition of oral and visual story telling as a source of knowledge dissemination, and calls to make child research results accessible to children and their communities (Graham et al. 2013; Harcourt and Sargeant 2009), key findings were reported by child participants, in their language, through film (with additional accessibility features). These films were screened locally and then regionally[8].

The priorities of young children with disability in Vanuatu and Papua New Guinea

The approach used above generated substantial interest and participation in the research project in both urban and rural communities in Vanuatu and PNG. While a total of eighty-nine children took part in the research, for the purpose of this chapter, the focus will be on priorities reported by children aged five to six years, which included five children in Vanuatu (four male, one female) and ten children in PNG (six male, four female). These young children self-reported information about seven of twenty-six Articles of the CRPD (across Articles 5–30). The data evidence that young children with disability in developing countries can speak about their social, cultural and economic realities in a way that can inform human rights actions, community attitude change, and policy and programme development.

---

8   For more information see Jenkin et al. (2016). Films can be viewed at <http://www. voicesofchildrenwithdisability.com/films>.

Employment and livelihood

Over half of the children (nine boys and girls) from Vanuatu and PNG, identified work, employment and livelihoods (Article 27) as their main aspiration for the future (as did their older peers aged seven to eighteen). Young children with diverse disabilities (hearing, vision, physical and intellectual) aspired to an equally diverse range of jobs, indicating a desire to one day work so that they could help support their families and themselves, and to contribute to their communities. This theme of interdependence and mutual support between child, family and wider community was strong in both countries (and across all age cohorts). Employment and livelihood was a major focus for children across the three discussion questions, highlighting this as a significant human right priority for children with disability in both countries.

The following quotes provide both researcher descriptions of the research tools in use and details of the child's viewpoint (using pseudonyms).

> Norbert was provided with toys and photos and we asked him which photos he liked and which toy he liked. Norbert chose the car and the photo of the policeman. We asked him why he chose the car and the photo of the policeman. He replied, *I want to be a policeman and drive a car to chase the criminals.* (Norbert is five years old, lives in rural PNG and has a physical disability).

> Olima was very shy when we first met him – so we go slowly, slowly. He liked using the camera and was happy to go walkabout [a data collection technique]. He took photos of trees and the environment around him. Olima wants to become a carpenter in the future so the timber from the trees is important. He told us he will use the timber to build a house and build houses for other people. (Olima is six and lives in Vanuatu. He has developmental delay and physical impairment).

Cultural life, recreation and leisure

Recreation, leisure and cultural life (Article 30 of the CRPD) was also a key priority for children with disability in both countries. Young children with diverse and multiple disabilities talked about the importance of being included in recreational activities (music, singing, sports), custom and church ceremonies, as well as playing with friends. This priority was echoed by older children.

> I asked Inisi what is the important thing in her life using the photos and she picked the photo of the ball. She said she likes playing basketball. She has her own ball and enjoys playing around with small kids. (Inisi is five and lives in PNG. She has a developmental delay).

Education

Education (Article 24) was also an important priority for children with disability in both Vanuatu and PNG. Children talked about how school was also a place to meet, spend time with and 'do the same things as' other children. School was frequently seen as important to getting a job later in life. Some children and families talked about how this aspiration was at risk, with no resources (such as teacher's aides or assistive technology) to support the child's needs in a school setting.

> We asked Mawi to look at the photos on the lap top. She pointed to the photo of the three children walking to school and using sign language said, *I would like to complete my school and work in a store. I have seen a young girl with a hearing aid working in a store serving ice cream.* (Mawi is six years old, lives in PNG and is deaf).

> Isa chose the pictures of reading books. She said, *I want to go to school and read books. I will become a teacher and earn money for my parents.* (Isa is five years old, lives in PNG and has a hearing impairment and developmental delay).

Adequate standard of living and poverty

Poverty and standard of living (Article 28) were also key priorities and concerns for children with disability, particularly for children in PNG. Discussion focused on having adequate food, housing and warmth, with some children talking about being hungry.

> During the discussion, I used the photo tool. Naiho said food is the very important thing in his life. He picked a photo of a plate of food (Naiho is five and lives in rural PNG. He has a physical impairment).

Family

Children also discussed the importance of home and family life (Article 23), recognizing the importance of family to their current and future security. Family members reported providing personal care (e.g. helping the child toilet, bathe and eat), as well as teaching language and other skills, including those useful for work.

Summary

The research method enabled us to engage with a wide range of children, including young children, with diverse disabilities in both countries, contributing to a wider understanding of what it means to be a child. Overall, young children were able to highlight things of importance in their lives and, despite the localize descriptors, these were able to be related to more universally framed human rights entitlements within the CRPD. This suggests that a postcolonial, context-specific approach to meaning making can be used in tandem with a more universal human rights model.

In all cases, sometimes despite significant limitations on their lives, young children with disability viewed themselves as having agency in both their present and future lives, with a strong focus on future employment and livelihood activities, with even young children aligning future employment or livelihood with a desire to reciprocate to their communities and families. Children frequently acknowledged the importance of family, explicating how their own agency was supported rather than compromized by the interdependence between families, communities and individuals. Both 'agency' and 'disability' are potentially re-interpreted in this context, where interdependency is normalized.

Finally, the experiences and viewpoints of children with disability, reflecting both the current 'being' of childhood (Vogler et al. 2008) as well as future aspirations, have utility to influence change in a range of ways. For example, data about the anticipated employment and livelihood strategies of children should be used to inform vocational education provision (currently very limited for young people with disability in the

Pacific), as well as relevant livelihood support strategies. Similarly, data about the important role of families, poor standards of living additional costs of related to meeting children's disability specific needs feed into calls for financial and social protection programmes in these countries. In this project, the broader findings have been presented to communities and governments through the varied dissemination strategies of the project including accessible film, policy briefs, resources for inclusive research and other publications (see Jenkin et al. 2016; Jenkin et al. 2017b). The role of film (where children report their own views and aspirations) has been a key medium for addressing attitudes about children with disability (both locally and internationally).

Conclusion

The process of listening to young children with disability restores their right to express their 'voice' and their views, and have these inform the development of policy and programmes to meet their needs. However, researching with children with disability in developing countries cannot be undertaken without engaging with a critical examination of the theories that construct, and also those that disrupt, how we understand childhood, disability and developing countries. The Voices of Pacific Children with Disability project aimed to overcome the hegemony of Western views of childhood, disability and development contexts, by using an approach that privileged local knowledge, and enabled self-report of diverse children with disability about their experiences as they prioritize them in their own contexts. In particular, this approach evidenced that five and six year olds with disability, and their older peers, are able to explain the realities of their lives in ways that provide meaningful information for human rights and other analyses. As a result, the project sought a range of ways to utilize children's voices for social change activities via the integration of research data into policy and programmes and community education. The involvement of children with disability in research of this kind, and its visibility in their communities, has contributed to attitude change that affirms and makes visible children's agency, competency and rights.

Acknowledgements

We wish to thank all of the children and their families in PNG and Vanuatu who shared their personal stories with the researchers. We are grateful to our partners (mentioned in the chapter above) and the dedicated researchers from PNG and Vanuatu who carried out the research, namely Ishmael Leanave, Louisah Nohan Neras, Zeena McSivvi, Peter Wasape, Kalo James, Marguerite Goulding and Leitare Joel.

References

Acker-Verney, J. M. (2016). Embedding intersectionality and reflexivity in research: doing accessible and inclusive research with persons with disabilities. *Third World Thematics: A TWQ Journal*, 1 (3), 411–424.

Australian Research Alliance for Children and Youth and the New South Wales Commission for Children and Young People (2009). Executive Summary. In Australian Research Alliance for Children and Youth and the New South Wales Commission for Children and Young People, *Involving children and young people in research: a compendium of papers and reflections from a think tank co-hosted by the Australian Research Alliance for Children and Youth and the NSW Commission for Children and Young People on 11 November 2008*, pp. V–VI. Retrieved from: <https://www.aracy.org.au/publication-sresources/command/download_file/id/108/filename/Involving_children_and_young_people_in_research.pdf>.

Barker, C., and Murray, S. (2010). Disabling postcolonialism: global disability cultures and democratic criticism. *Journal of Literary and Cultural Disability Studies*, 4 (3), 219–236.

Bessell, S., Beazley, H., and Waterson, R. (2017). The Methodology and Ethics of Rights-Based Research with Children. In A. Invernizzi, B. Milne, M. Liebel and K. Soldatic (eds), *Children Out of Place and Human Rights*, pp. 211–231. Switzerland: Springer International Publishing.

Chataika, T. (2012). Disability, Development and Postcolonialism. In D. Goodley, B. Hughes and L. Davis (eds), *Disability and Social Theory: New Developments and Directions*, pp. 252–269. Basingstoke: Palgrave Mcmillan.

Curran, T., and Runswick-Cole, K. (2014). Disabled children's childhood studies: a distinct approach?. *Disability and Society*, 29 (10), 1617–1630.

Davis, J. (2013). Conceptual issues in childhood and disability: integrating theories from childhood and disability studies. In N. Watson, A. Roulstone and C. Thomas (eds), *Routledge Handbook of Disability Studies*, pp. 415–425. Oxon: Routledge.

Don, Z., Salami, A., and Ghajarieh, A. (2015). Voices of girls with disabilities in rural Iran. *Disability and Society*, 30 (6), 805–819.

Ezell, M. J. M. (1983–1984). John Locke's Images of Childhood: Early Eighteenth Century Response to *Some Thoughts Concerning Education*. *Eighteenth-Century Studies*, 17 (2), 139–155.

Gartrell, A., and Hoban, E. (2016). 'Locked in Space': Rurality and the Politics of Location. In S. Grech and K. Soldatic (eds), *Disability in the Global South: The Critical Handbook*, pp. 337–350. Switzerland: Springer International Publishing.

Ghai, A. (2012). Engaging with Disability with Postcolonial Theory. In D. Goodley, B. Hughes and L. Davis (eds), *Disability and Social Theory: New Developments and Directions*, pp. 270–286. Basingstoke: Palgrave Mcmillan.

Graham, A., Powell, M., Taylor, N., Anderson, D., and Fitzgerald, R. (2013). Ethical Research Involving Children. Florence: UNICEF Office of Research – Innocenti. Retrieved from: <http://childethics.com/wp-content/uploads/2013/10/ERIC-compendium-Getting-Started-section-only.pdf>.

Gray, C., and Winter, E. (2011). Hearing voices: participatory research with preschool children with and without disabilities. *European Early Childhood Education Research Journal*, 19 (3), 309–320.

Grech, S. (2012). Disability and the majority world: A neocolonial approach. In D. Goodley, B. Hughes and L. Davis (eds), *Disability and Social Theory: New Developments and Directions*, pp 52–69. Basingstoke: Palgrave Mcmillan.

Harpur, P. (2012). Embracing the new disability rights paradigm: the importance of the Convention on the Rights of Persons with Disabilities. *Disability & Society*, 27 (1), 1–14.

Holt, L., and Holloway, S. L. (2006). Editorial: Theorising other childhoods in a globalised world. *Children's Geographies*, 4 (2), 135–142.

Huus, K., Granlund, M., Bornman, J., and Lyngegård, F. (2015). Human rights of children with intellectual disabilities: comparing self-ratings and proxy ratings. *Child: care, health and development*, 41 (6), 1010–1017.

Ife, J. (2013). *Community Development in an Uncertain World*. Melbourne: Cambridge University Press.

Invernizzi, A., and Williams, J. (2011). *The Human Rights of Children: From Visions to Implementation*. London: Routledge.

Jenkin, E., Wilson, E., Murfitt, K., Clarke, M., Campain, R., and Stockman, L. (2015). *Inclusive Practice for Research with Children with Disability: A Guide*. Melbourne: Deakin University. Retrieved from: <http://www.voicesofchildrenwithdisability. com/wp-content/uploads/2015/03/DEA-Inclusive-Practice-Research_ACCES-SIBLE.pdf>.

Jenkin, E., Wilson, E., Clarke, M., Campain, R., and Murfitt, K. (2016). Spreading the word: using film to share research findings and knowledge about children with disabilities in Vanuatu and Papua New Guinea. *Knowledge Management for Development Journal*, 11 (1), 69–84.

Jenkin, E., Wilson, E., Clarke, M., Campain, R., and Murfitt, K. (2017a). Listening to the voices of children: understanding the human rights priorities of children with disability in Vanuatu and Papua New Guinea. *Disability and Society*, 32 (3), 358–380.

Jenkin, E., Wilson, E., Clarke, M., Murfitt, K., and Campain, R. (2017b). Children with disability: human rights case study. In S. Kenny, B. McGrath and R. Phillips (eds), *The Routledge Handbook of Community Development: Perspectives From Around the Globe*, pp. 370–381. New York: Routledge.

Johnson, V. (2017). Moving beyond voice in children and young people's participation. *Action Research*, 15 (1), 104–124.

Kenny, S. (2007). *Developing Communities for the Future* (3rd edn.). South Melbourne: Thomson.

Liebel, M. (2012). Framing the issue: Rethinking children's rights. In M. Liebel (ed.), *Children's Rights from Below: Cross-cultural perspectives*, pp. 9–28. Basingstoke: Palgrave Macmillan.

Liebel, M. (2017). Children Without Childhood? Against the Postcolonial Capture of Childhoods in the Global South. In A. Invernizzi, M. Liebel, B. Milne and R. Budde (eds), *Children Out of Place' and Human Rights: In Memory of Judith Ennew*, pp. 79–97. Switzerland: Springer International Publishing.

Liebel, M., and Invernizzi, A. (2017). Introduction. Children Out of Place: Their Written and Unwritten Rights. In A. Invernizzi, M. Liebel, B. Milne and R. Budde (eds), *'Children Out of Place' and Human Rights: In Memory of Judith Ennew*, pp. 1–5. Switzerland: Springer International Publishing.

Llewellyn, A., and Hogan, K. (2000). The Use and Abuse of Models of Disability. *Disability & Society*, 15 (1), 157–165.

Marks, D. (1997). Models of disability. *Disability and Rehabilitation*, 19 (3), 85–91.

Miljeteig, P., and Ennew, J. (2017). The Greatest Violation of Children's Rights Is That We Do Not Know Enough About Their Lives or Care Enough to Find Out More. In A. Invernizzi, M. Liebel, B. Milne and R. Budde (eds), *'Children Out of Place' and Human Rights: In Memory of Judith Ennew,* pp. 23–49. Switzerland: Springer International Publishing.

Mutua, K., and Swadener, B. B. (2007). Decolonizing Research in Cross-Cultural Contexts. In J. A. Hatch (ed.), *Early Childhood Qualitative Research*, pp. 185–206. New York: Routledge.

Nguyen, X. T., Mitchell, C., de Lange, N., and Fritsch, K. (2015). Engaging girls with disabilities in Vietnam: making their voices count. *Disability and Society,* 30 (5), 773–787.

Office of the High Commissioner for Human Rights Regional Office for the Pacific (2012). *Human Rights in the Pacific – Country Outlines 2012.* Fiji: United Nations.

Oliver, M. (2013). The social model of disability: thirty years on. *Disability and Society*, 28 (7), 1024–1026.

Platz, D., and Arellano, J. (2011). Time Tested Early Childhood Theories and Practices. *Education,* 132 (1), 54–63.

Priestley, M. (1998). Childhood Disability and Disabled Childhoods: Agendas for research. *Childhood,* 5 (2), 207–223.

Sorin, R. (2009). Learning from Learners – Early Childhood Voices in Research. In Australian Research Alliance for Children and Youth and the New South Wales Commission for Children and Young People, *Involving children and young people in research: a compendium of papers and reflections from a think tank co-hosted by the Australian Research Alliance for Children and Youth and the NSW Commission for Children and Young People on 11 November 2008*, pp. 131–144. Retrieved from: <https://www.aracy.org.au/publications-resources/command/download_file/id/108/filename/Involving_children_and_young_people_in_research.pdf>.

Stienstra, D., and Nyerere, L. (2016). Race, Ethnicity and Disability: Charting Complex and Intersectional Terrain. In S. Grech and K. Soldatic (eds), *Disability in the Global South: The Critical Handbook*, pp. 255–268. Switzerland: Springer International Publishing.

Tisdall, E. (2012). The challenge and challenging of childhood studies? Learning from disability studies and research with disabled children. *Children and Society,* 26 (3), 181–191.

Trani, J., Bakhshi, P. and Biggeri, M. (2011). Re-thinking Children's Disabilities Through the Capability Lens: A Framework for Analysis and Policy Implications. In M. Biggeri, J. Ballet and F. Comim (eds), *Children and the Capability Approach*, pp. 245–270. Basingstoke: Palgrave Mcmillan.

United Nations (1989). *Convention on the Rights of the Child*. New York: United Nations. Retrieved from: <http://www.ohchr.org/EN/ProfessionalInterest/Pages/CRC.aspx>.

United Nations (2006). *Convention on the Rights of Persons with Disabilities*. New York: United Nations. Retrieved from: <https://www.un.org/development/desa/disabilities/resources/general-assembly/convention-on-the-rights-of-persons-with-disabilities-ares61106.html>.

United Nations (2015). *Addressing the vulnerability and exclusion of persons with disabilities: the situation of women and girls, children's right to education, disasters and humanitarian crises*. New York: Conference of States Parties to the Convention on the Rights of Persons with Disabilities Eighth session, 9–11 June 2015. Retrieved from: <https://digitallibrary.un.org/record/844726/files/CRPD_CSP_2015_4-EN.pdf>.

Vogler, P., Crivello, G., and Woodhead, M. (2008). *Early childhood transitions research: A review of concepts, theory, and practice. Working Paper No. 48*. The Hague, The Netherlands: Bernard van Leer Foundation. Retrieved from: <http://library.bsl.org.au/jspui/bitstream/1/4282/1/Early_childhood_transitions_research_A_review_of_concepts_theory_and_practice.pdf>.

Washington Group (2010). *Short Set of Questions on Disability*. Retrieved from: <http://www.cdc.gov/nchs/washington_group/wg_questions.htm>.

Watson, N. (2012). Theorising the lives of disabled children: How can disability theory help?. *Children and Society*, 26 (3), 192–202.

World Health Organization and World Bank (2011). *World Report on Disability*. Geneva: WHO Press.

Wickenden, M., and Elphick, J. (2016). Don't forget us, we are here too! Listening to disabled children and their families living in poverty. In S. Grech and K. Soldatic (eds), *Disability in the Global South: The Critical Handbook*, pp. 167–185. Switzerland: Springer International Publishing.

Wilson, E., Campain, R., Jenkin, E., Murfitt, K., and Clarke, M. (2016). Legitimizing children's evidence: Inclusive participatory research with children with disability. *Development Bulletin*, 77, 20–24.

Woodhead, M. (2006). Changing perspectives on early childhood: theory, research and policy. *International Journal of Equity and Innovation in Early Childhood*, 4 (2), 5–48.

KAREN WATSON

4 Researching *among* children: Exploring discourses and power in the 'inclusive' early childhood classroom

Introduction

In early childhood research, over the past decade or more, there has been a rethinking of the way we examine the lives of young children. There has been a critique of research *on* or *about* children, and a movement toward researching *with* or *for* children (Christensen and James 2008; Christensen and Prout 2002; Mayall 2002; Punch 2002). Researchers have deliberated over improving methods of including children, by offering them a participatory role, by addressing the issue of power imbalances and by considering the importance of rapport building with child participants (Gallacher and Gallagher 2008; O'Kane 2008; Sumsion 2003). Including children's voices in research, and recognizing their subjective agency, reflects a wider acknowledgement of children's rights produced in the United Nations Convention on the Rights of the Child (UNICEF 1989) and the sociology of childhood (James and Prout 1997).

This chapter offers another way of examining how researchers can come to know more about young children, and how they come to know themselves and others, and understand their world. While recognizing the value of researching *with* children, some reassessment of previous research methodology arose, during a six-month long poststructural ethnography in three 'inclusive' early childhood classrooms (Watson 2017). The classrooms, all located within early childhood centres, are situated in two regional urban centres of New South Wales, Australia. While each preschool classroom is unique in its own way, they all provided for the most part, a 'standard' child-centred program. The 75 children in this research, aged between two and six years, are viewed from a contemporary perspective, where children are positioned as competent beings, capable of negotiating their world and their growing understandings of it. Each inclusive classroom, at the time had several children with a diagnosis enrolled. The terms 'child with a diagnosis' 'diagnosed child', 'marked child' or the 'not normal' child, and the binary opposites of 'undiagnosed', 'unmarked' and 'normal' child, are used to avoid other labels that locate the problem within the child. The word 'diagnosis' best describes how the child is marked by medical and psychological discourses. Marked by a diagnosis bestowed on them by a medical professional. Using the term child with a diagnosis underscores the way a diagnosis positions the child in the classroom setting and goes some way in disrupting business-as-usual. There is intentionally no commentary on children's diagnostic labels From a poststructural perspective, the discursively produced labels, and associated homogenizing characteristics of a diagnosis, that define and prescribe the diagnosed child and their behaviours, are vigorously challenged (Watson 2017).

As an early intervention teacher, troubled by classroom practices and taken for granted assumptions about inclusion, the study set out to investigate inclusive and exclusive processes from *inside* the classroom. Attention was afforded to how the already included group of children, the taken for granted 'normal', produced and reproduced themselves within normative classroom discourse, and how they positioned those viewed as different; the diagnosed child, considered in need of including. How do young children negotiate difference in their early years classroom? How do they make decisions about who is included and who is excluded?

In the first part of the chapter, an appreciation of the notion of researching *among* children is explored. This emerged, as my experiences in the classroom stirred a questioning of current research literature. In the second half I discuss the research tools used while researching *among* children, with an analysis and discussion of the children's understandings of each other and their inclusionary and exclusionary practices.

Questioning the notion of researching *with* children

A substantial body of the research literature regarding researching with and/or for children highlights the issue of adult-child power relations. The child research paradigm gives much consideration to the importance of redressing notable power imbalances. In addition, the imperative to build rapport with children is often deliberated, as a way to procure children's participation and realization of their voice in research. 'Child friendly' participatory techniques have also been on offer within the field (Gallacher and Gallagher 2008).

Researching with children, as opposed to researching on or about children (Alderson 2008; O'Kane 2008), endeavours to re-position adults in an attempt to 'empower' children. The literature considers a variety of ways that a researcher could 'act' or 'be' when attempting to alter power differentials. Christensen (2004) proposes that a researcher could position themselves as an 'unusual type of adult', who displays a different and deeper level of interest in the children's social world and their perspectives. Corsaro (1985) and Mayall (2008), promote the notion of the 'least-adult role', where the researcher makes an effort to get involved in the children's everyday lives, while renouncing any adult privilege and authority (Warming 2005). These proposals assume that the adult researcher has a degree of control or choice in their research relationship with children. Offering children a participatory role, using prescribed participatory techniques, is advocated as a way of ensuring children's involvement, but this has been critiqued, as it is often found that children are quite capable of performing 'beyond the limits of prescribed participatory techniques' (Gallacher and Gallagher 2008: 507).

Complex power relations

The possibility of adults empowering children in the research process, is challenged by poststructural theory as power is not a commodity that can be acquired or relinquished (Gallacher and Gallagher 2008). A poststructural perspective challenges the impression that one can give power to another, as power exists in actions and in relations (Foucault 1982). In this study power relations were regularly manoeuvred by the children, as they actively negotiated and re-negotiated my position as a researcher. It was in our interactions and relations that power was produced and reproduced in the classroom context. Ailwood's research experience, as a 'visiting adult of obscure status' (Ailwood 2010: 24) characterizes in some ways my experience, where relations remained unfixed and continuously challenged.

Mayall (2008) suggests trying to downplay the hierarchical power in adult-child interactions. Taking up this advice I positioned myself as a 'researcher'. For the children, this was perhaps a less familiar or recognisable adult role. As a researcher, I was not a teacher. In the classroom hierarchy, the teacher is positioned as the 'boss' (Watson 2017) and at the top of the chain of command. My attempts to 'unfix' this adult-child relation met with mixed success. Most of the time power relations fluctuated, as the children slowly came to see me as 'less than a teacher'. The following conversation underlines my 'less than a teacher' status. Pseudonyms have been used for all participants.

> As Amelia arrived at preschool she walked up to me sitting on a platform in the middle of the yard. I was taking notes at the time.
> AMELIA: 'You're really getting to be a teacher now' (she said as she patted me on the back).
> ME: 'Why do you say that?'
> AMELIA: 'Because you write stuff and take pictures.' (Watson 2017: 26)

Amelia seems to be praising my efforts in trying to 'become' a teacher. In patting me on the back, she expressed her authority over me, showing me that she positioned me as not quite the same as other adults in the classroom. On many occasions, as the children tried to reposition me as a teacher, I explained that I was a researcher, not a teacher. When they requested my interference in managing their conflicts or asked for my support in reinforcing rules, I referred to my lack of authority in the classroom context. Amelia however had diligently observed my teacher-like performances, such as writing stuff and taking photographs, and so she positioned me as a practising teacher: 'You're really getting to be a teacher now' (Watson 2017:

26). Power relations, when researching *among* the children, seem to shift continuously. My standing with the children in the classroom remained fluid. They made their own constantly changing decisions about who I was and what that might mean for them.

Troubling the imperative to 'build rapport'

When researching *with* children, O'Kane (2008) suggests that establishing a degree of rapport with child participants, repositions them as participating subjects in the research process, rather than 'objects' of research. Sumsion (2003) argues for the need for humility and reciprocity when ethically researching with children. While these ideas are widely promoted and thought to endorse a mutual respect in all encounters, they do suggest a special positioning of children. Adults do not usually require rapport building foundations in adult-adult research. The question asked is, 'if children are competent social actors, why are special 'child-friendly' methods needed to communicate with them?' (Punch 2002: 321). Are children created as 'needy', or 'less' capable than adults, if we approach researching with them in a different or special way?

Creating a rapport and building relationships, centred on a particular research agenda, did not seem to be necessary for the children in this classroom study. In educational contexts, particularly in early childhood, children are very familiar with adults who ask questions, observe them, take photographs of them and make notes about them in the classroom. Children are skilled and conversant in their interactions with different adults; alternative or casual educators, parents, professionals and other visitors that regularly visit the setting. The idea of building rapport for a research agenda is somewhat troubled here. Research relationships based on an adult agenda, seemed to some degree, insincere and uncomfortable for me, and on further reflection, for the children. How does the adult researcher do this in an ethical way?

Some children were curious about my presence, as someone different and unfamiliar, but others showed little interest. Their interest in me changed all the time. As a researcher, would I only build rapport with those who seemed interested? Questioning the imperative of rapport building and its importance for children came about early in the research project when I met Matilda.

> As I sat in the sandpit several children approached me asking, 'Who are you?' I replied that my name was Karen and that I was a researcher. I asked them if they had seen a letter at home about a researcher visiting the classroom. Some of the children recalled the letter. Matilda joined the group on her arrival and announced that she had seen my photo on a letter that her dad had read to her. She said, 'Ok, I'm ready to get talking to you right now, what do you want to know?' (Watson 2017: 25)

Matilda positioned herself as a research participant on her arrival that day. She was informed. She had read (her father had read to her) the 'Participant Information Statement' provided for caregivers with the hope that they would explain my position to their children. I prepared in addition a picture version of the information statement to share with the children hoping to ensure their informed consent. Matilda reported her informed consent and positioned me as a researcher. It seemed there was no ambiguity for her about who I was or what she needed to do. The children were positioned throughout as the gatekeepers of their own participation and consent (Danby and Farrell 2005; Warming 2011). Consent remained open at all times for negotiation and renegotiation. Rapport or relationship building as a prerequisite to the research did not seem necessary for Matilda at that time. She positioned herself clearly as a participant ready to contribute.

Researching *among* children

While spending time *among* the children an 'informality' emerged and my 'less than a teacher' position evolved. The children became more 'cheeky' towards me, they buried me in the sandpit and they allowed me and encouraged me to hear them use 'naughty' words. They stopped asking for my support in upholding class rules. Initially they would wait to gauge my reaction, thinking that as a teacher/adult I might make a corrective comment about their words or actions, but when no comment was forthcoming, they started to regard me as different to a teacher.

Corsaro (1985) advocates that the researcher should let the children define and shape the ethnographer's role. How to go about this, involved a fluidity and it changed all the time for me. Often having no choice, the children continually 'played' with me and my ambiguous status:

> During morning indoor activity time Fleur and Frances asked me to record their song. They were playing with taping sticks and creating the song as they went along.
>
> FRANCES: (singing) 'Star tastic is some fun, makes me happy, makes me laugh.'
>
> FLEUR: 'And the sea and you swim in the sea with lights.'
>
> FRANCES: 'Makes me happy if I catch a fish.'
>
> FLEUR: (giggling) 'And her hair looks like wee.'
>
> ME: 'And the hair looks like wee, that sounds funny.'
>
> FLEUR: (more giggling) 'I want to do a funny bit.'
>
> FRANCES: 'Star tastic is a poo haircut.' (both giggling loudly now)
>
> FLEUR: 'And your eyeball looks like paint.' (looking at me)
>
> FRANCES: 'Your eyeballs fall out of the paint.'
>
> FLEUR: 'And your nostrils look like a pig.' (giggling but directing this at me)
>
> FRANCES: 'Star star tastic I do a wee.' (laughing loudly)
>
> FLEUR: 'Sea sea tastic if you poo in the sea.'
>
> FRANCES: 'Sea sea sea, if you do a poo in the sea.'
>
> FLEUR: (talking not singing) 'I always wee in the pool and I wee in swimming class.'
>
> FRANCES: (singing) 'If you swim in a class you do a poo in your pants and go to the toilet and ask your dad.'
>
> ME: 'This song is not getting any better.'
>
> FLEUR: 'Ok star star tastic if you vomit out your nose and poo comes out of your bottom.'
>
> ME: 'I think I'll turn off my recorder now, it's getting too rude.'
>
> FLEUR: 'No, no, we need it to be rude.' (Watson 2017: 27)

The children did not position me as a teacher, or as an authority, in this classroom. They created the song as they went along perhaps to test my position. I felt like they were trying to see if I would stop them or correct them, or ask them to sing another song. As I took a less authoritative position they positioned me as someone they could 'play around with'. I had been in the centre two days a week for about five weeks, so Fleur and Frances had become familiar with my presence, and had come to think of me as different to the teachers. Fleur sums it up at the end when she says 'we need it to be rude'. Their words exercised their power as these words might be considered, in this discursive context, 'forbidden' or at least not said in front of adults. I was positioned by them, as less than a teacher, and able to exercise less authority.

The children's positioning of me was always changing. The way I positioned them was also fluid and our interactions remained open-ended and always uncertain. The children were never obliged to participate and they moved in and out of conversations casually, at times refusing to engage at all, or changing their minds during conversations. I did not see myself as researching with children. I did not ask them to engage in any particular or prescribed activities. I watched and 'chatted' as events happened. I did not feel obliged to create a particular rapport with them, as most of them seemed relaxed with my presence in their space. I came and went in their lives, as they did in mine. Becoming a regular participant in the classroom offered me a view of everyday encounters and the words and actions used by the children, as they took up the dominant and normative discourses in their classroom and sanctioned ways of 'being' and 'not being'. 'Hanging out' in the children's space, observing their activities allowed for an examination of how they were being shaped by these discourses and how this shaping effected their inclusive and exclusive practices.

Children's understandings of difference and the 'normal'

Researching *among* children provides for opportunities to view young children's close encounters with difference. Robinson and Jones-Diaz (2006) concur that young children are aware of diversity and difference at a young age and are very capable of identifying what they understand as the 'normal' or the 'right way to be' in the classroom context. As they actively draw on the normalizing discourses in the early years classroom they make decisions about who might be the same or different to them. Children are not merely socialized by adults. They are not passive in their encounters with each other. Children readily exclude peers based on their difference in everyday interactions (Connolly, Smith and Kelly 2002). How do young children mediate inclusionary and exclusionary practices, as 'stakeholders' in the process, and members of the normal?

Drawing on a poststructural perspective, the observer's gaze settled on the un-interrogated 'normal' in the classroom and the children's understandings of it. 'Inclusive' early childhood education research most often employs a medical model perspective and tends to focus on the remediation and inclusion of the child with special or additional needs. In challenging this view, taken for granted understandings of the 'normal' in the early childhood classrooms, are argued to be governed by, and created within, medical and scientific knowledges. The knowledge within these disciplines has become so familiar, that there is no longer any reflection on it, or critique of it, with the 'normal' surfacing as a comfortable truth shared by all (Harwood and Rasmussen 2004). In the classroom, adults and teachers are engaged in a ceaseless inspection of those who may not fit the norm. Children are also attentive to the 'normal' and very capable of observing and scrutinizing each other according to it (Watson 2017). The children work to establish and maintain the 'normal' and any comparisons to it.

The 'normal' is established via multiple discourses and provides the 'expertise' and knowledge for understanding the individual, for diagnosing and categorizing them, while making available vocabularies to speak about the 'normal' or the 'not normal'. Rose (1999: 131), contends that 'normality is not an observation but a valuation'. The constructed 'normal' provides the guide and judgement about what is desirable, while also extrapolating that it is a goal that needs to be achieved or worked towards.

The following section deliberates the research 'tools' used to examine how these discursive understandings are constructed.

Research 'tools' for researching among children

Researching *among* children conjures up an image of the researcher being a part of the classroom action. Taking the time to note the numerous conversations and create the many observations of playground and playroom happenings, produces noteworthy meaning. Ethnography *among* children exposes the researcher to new understandings of everyday practices and flows of the classroom. As a research methodology, it involves the researcher spending months 'within the patterns of community life, moving in the spaces shaped by the community and taking part in its activities on its terms' (Traweek 1988: 10).

Whilst 'hanging out' *among* children in their community over time, their discursive understandings of themselves, as the 'normal' or Other, become more distinguished. These understandings are made obvious in the children's repeated 'subject' performances. How young children reiteratively take up certain available and sanctioned discourses that position them powerfully in their relations with others, is of interest and more assessable when the researcher becomes part of the study. Being a part of the research furthermore, involves a level of self-critique and reflexivity. Doing this necessitates not only an examination of the children's take up of discursive understandings of the 'normal' but as the researcher, a reflexive inquiry into one's own.

Using poststructural 'tools' to analyse the discursive 'normal' permits an interrogation of it, and its powerful effects on inclusionary and exclusionary practices among the children. Combining Foucault's conceptualizations of discourse, power and subjectivity, along with Harré and van Langenhove's (1999) analytical tool of positioning theory, and Davies' (1989) concept of category boundary work, opens up other ways of viewing the operations of power and inclusion in early years education (Watson 2017).

Discourses shape the way the children come to know themselves and others as discursive subjects, as they actively participate, negotiate and renegotiate within the multiple discourses in the classroom and the power relations that are produced. The concept of discourse is broader than just language (Foucault 1972) and is understood as social, material, historical and linguistic practices. As Foucault writes, discourses are 'practices that systematically form the objects of which they speak' (Foucault 1972: 49). Discourses produce ways of doing, being and thinking for subjects and also ways of not doing, not being and not thinking. One's discursive subjectivity becomes noticeable as it is performed within the situated discourses, produced and constrained by relations of power. Relations of power produce one's subjectivity, privileging some, while subjugating others.

As the children take up positions as classroom participants, they identify with others who are similarly positioned as the 'same', creating a category where membership is permitted to a particular kind of person, who knows how to belong and how to be correctly located as a member (Davies 1993). The category boundary is defined and defended. Positioning theory explores the interactions between people, from their own standpoint, and as representatives or exemplars of a particular group (Harre and van Langenhove 1999). Positions taken up by people are relational and having taken up one's position, one sees the world from that vantage point. Knowing how to belong and how to perform as a member, and how to maintain oneself that way, involves category boundary and maintenance work (Petersen 2004; Davies 1989). What work does the 'normal' do in the early years classroom?

Developmental discourses create membership positions

In the classroom multiple discourses shape the children's understanding of the diagnosed child. As the children negotiate difference they draw on the circulating discourses. Some of these discourses include child development, developmental psychology, special education, friendship and play discourses, regulatory discourses and competitive hegemonic discourses. As the children encounter the child with a diagnosis, they employ these discourses to understand themselves, while also using them to comprehend and speak about others. In the following scene, developmental discourses are taken up by the children as they come to understand the diagnosed child in their classroom.

In the early childhood classroom, the children use the terms 'big' and 'little' to describe and position themselves and others. These positions, made available in child development discourses, are taken up by the unmarked children to explain the Other. The discourses actively contribute to the production of the category of the 'normal'. The 'normal' come to position themselves as 'big'. To be 'big' is to be more adult-like, more developed and closer to a prescribed and created norm.

> As Hugo (a child with a diagnosis) arrives in the morning he moves down into the yard towards the cubby house. Hayley (a child without a diagnosis) follows him,

calling him. He appears to ignore her. She corners him at the garden seat and moves
her arms around him in a smothering way. The way she encircles her body around
his is as if he was a much smaller child and she the adult. He tries to move away
from her. Two teachers then arrive to 'rescue' Hugo from Hayley's attention. They
ask Hayley to give him some space. She moves away while they continue to talk to
Hugo saying to him how much Hayley likes him. He then moves away from the
teachers. I approach Hayley shortly after this and ask, 'Why did you cuddle Hugo?'
To which she replies, 'Cause he's my little best friend, because he's cute, and I'm five
and he's three.' (Watson 2017: 36).

Hayley moves in on Hugo as soon as he arrives. Hugo appears to ignore
her calling his name but she persists and then smothers him, corralling and
cuddling him. She positions herself performing an 'adult-like' role, possibly
mothering or trying to be the teacher, following him and attempting to
keep him close. Formative discourses circulate in the early childhood setting and it is through these discourses that young children are subjected as
they participate (Laws & Davies 2000: 207). They shape young children's
understanding of the right way to be, the right way to act, giving 'voice'
and privilege to those who are understood as 'correct'. Child development
and developmental psychology discourses produce positions via numerous
stated binaries which might include, but not limited to: big/little, helper/
helpless, to know/ to not know, already learnt/just learning, rational/irra-
tional, dependent/ independent, able/unable, rule follower/rule breaker,
play with others/play alone.

Hayley positions herself as the 'motherly carer' for Hugo on his arrival
and makes comments about Hugo being her best 'little' friend, referring to
him as 'cute'. She does not interact with the other unmarked children in this
way. She talks about being five and says that Hugo is three. Being five in the
early childhood classroom is significant. To be older in this development-
focused environment is produced as more powerful and more desirable.
Ageism is rampant, as age brings privilege and prestige. Age can function
as a resource to get what one wants and is used most often to mark out
power and social positioning (Löfdahl 2010). Children will sometimes
mention their age as soon as you meet them.

CHLOE: 'I'm five and I only have four and a half months till I finish preschool.'
HUNTER: 'I'm four, nearly five ... no not really five.' (Watson 2017: 37).

Age gives one credibility and legitimacy in the classroom.

DANIEL: 'I'm five and a half, five and a half is older than five.'
NOAH: 'I'm four and half, yeh, four and a half, that's older than four.' (Watson 2017: 37)

In another conversation the 'battle' to be the 'oldest' transpires amongst the unmarked children.

JENNA: 'I'm 12.'
ELLIOT: 'I'm 4.'
FAITH: 'I'm 48, 60.'
ME: 'You're what?'
FAITH: '48, 60.'
LUKE: 'I'm 15.'
JENNA: 'I'm 13.........no I'm 100.' (Watson 2017: 37)

Looking back to Hayley's comment about Hugo, she states that he is three. Hugo is not three, he is five. Hayley positions herself as older and more capable. The way she moves in to try and hold Hugo might indicate that she positions him as vulnerable and needy. Her body is much smaller than Hugo's but she positions herself as the bigger and older one. How is Hugo subjected in this classroom when his subjecthood is produced, but also limited by normative discourses? Hugo is discursively produced as 'younger', marked by the diagnosis bestowed on him by developmental and psychological knowledges and expertise.

Troubling the effects of developmental understandings

In early childhood education, for the most part, developmentalism circulates unquestioned (Walkerdine 1993; Cannella 1997; Soto & Swadener 2002). There has been a century-long domination of these perspectives in the field (Soto & Swadener 2002). Developmental and psychological discourses are deeply embedded and sanctioned, and are readily taken up by the children, marked and unmarked, and their teachers. More recently however there has been a growing recognition of alternative theoretical perspectives (Burman 2008; MacNaughton 2005; Bloch, Swadener and Cannella 2014). From this view, child development is acknowledged as a historical, social, political and cultural construction, produced in particular contexts, and used to legitimize the surveillance, measurement, control and categorizations of groups of people, children more specifically, as normal or deviant (Cannella 1997).

In child developmental discourse, performing being 'big', 'older', or more mature is considered adult-like, closer to the desirable norm. The adult position in the classroom, in relation to the child, is typically endowed with power. Cannella (1997) argues that child development 'is an imperialist notion that has fostered dominant power ideologies and produced justification for categorizing children' (158) rendering children in need of adult support, and among children, creating categories of those who need help and those who do not. Those who understand themselves as 'big' comprehend that they are different to those they position as being 'little'. Developmental and psychological discourses contribute to the regimes of truth (Foucault 1977) that govern the ways educators think about children and consequently deliver early childhood practice. These regimes of truth produce an authoritative consensus about what needs to be done and how it should be done (MacNaughton 2005) and what is of value and what is not of value.

Big and little, as developmental binaries, are discussed openly and 'naturally' by the unmarked children and their teachers and are instantly drawn upon to enhance their understandings and explanations of each other. The Other is younger, deficient and sometimes pathological. Binary thinking is expressed in the following statements made by the children: 'He's not a kid, he's a little boy', 'We're big kids, when the little kids scream and scream and scream they get a turn on the guitar to keep them down', 'What about the big kids in the little room and the little kids in the big room', 'No I'm a big girl and I stay inside', 'He can't talk and he's little' (Watson 2017: 39)

The above statements show how the 'normal' position themselves as the older. They refer to themselves in one example as 'kids' and not 'little'. They recognize themselves as more mature, as they do not show unbridled emotions, such as screaming in the classroom. They 'know' their place and what classroom they belong in. They position themselves as rational 'rule following', self-disciplined and autonomous subjects, who have developmentally appropriate skills. As 'big' kids, in these statements, they produce themselves as different from, and superior to, the 'little' kids.

As the authoritative discourse, developmental psychology delivers a way for adults to 'speak' about children. It also provides a potent way for children to 'speak' about themselves and about each other. The knowledge of the 'human' sciences and in particular 'the role of psychology, psychiatry and the other "psy" sciences' (Rose 1999: 7) re/produce this firmly entrenched discourse. The legitimate 'psy' science discourses provide the unmarked children with the approved language to talk about others who are different; the younger child or the child with a diagnosis.

Developmental psychology is a formative tool through which children are subjected (Burman 2008). As a science, psychology has produced taken-for-granted practices that have been considered as 'facts' (Walkerdine 1989) and these substantially contribute to the created conditions, limits and possibilities for becoming subjectivities, their relational power and agency. The measurement and categorizing achieved by the discipline of psychology inevitably constitutes 'subjects who can have no access to legitimate forms of power or agency' (Laws & Davies 2000: 207). What does this mean for Hugo who is created within this discourse? What does it mean for Hayley? How does Hugo's positioning as 'helpless' and exercising less power, shape his subjectivity and effect his participation? How does the developmental discourse shape Hayley's subjectivity as the helper, with access to legitimized power? What does it mean for inclusive practice?

Hayley performs her category membership of the 'normal' drawing on multiple discourses. As the more adult-like being, she positions herself as having a caring role, offering help to the 'younger' child. Her actions and member positioning mark Hugo as in need of 'help'. Hayley's category boundary work produces Hugo as a marginalized Other. 'Helping' the Other is a performance enacted by many of the children in this classroom, and is mostly supported by the teachers. While the 'act of helping' is of great public value in producing a caring society, it also has other effects. Problematizing the power of this practice and the way it constructs the marked child as Other is an effect that warrants further consideration.

The teachers' actions show some concern about Hayley's 'over-the-top' greeting and Hugo's rejection of her attention, as he tries to get away from her. The teachers watch Hayley and Hugo and then act on their understandings of Hugo's discursively constructed needs, rescuing Hugo from Hayley's 'over-caring'. In doing this however, they inadvertently reinforce Hugo's marking, as not capable of looking after himself, and in need of their help. Hugo appears to reject Hayley's 'helping' attention. He may not wish to be positioned as the 'little' one, in need of her help and 'mothering care'. As the teachers separate Hugo from Hayley they too engage in category boundary work reinforcing the binary of the 'normal' and the 'not normal'. Separation of the 'normal' and 'not normal' as an effect of the discourses in the classroom, persistently surfaced as significant in the larger study (Watson 2017).

As a former early childhood and early intervention teacher, turned researcher in this project, it became necessary for me to engage in my own struggle within the circulating discourses and to do this a degree of reflexivity was called for. To question the politics of my performance as a researcher in some way recognizes my part in it. As a participant in the research process I too was produced and constrained by discursive understandings of the classroom and its inhabitants.

Using reflexivity

> As I observed and noted the children's persistent statements about being 'big' and being 'little', I considered how I had positioned myself within this discourse, and how my previous ways of knowing had positioned children. I too would have rescued Hugo from Hayley's over helping. My knowledge and teaching practice was built on clinical and 'scientific' 'truth', and my understandings of the child were entrenched within 'the medical model of disability'. Developmental psychology positions the adult as privileged and adult ways of 'knowing' and 'doing' as superior and the child as the binary opposite, immature and deficient. Questioning developmental thinking illuminated for me the children's statements about themselves and others. What

once would have been very familiar and acceptable now seems uncomfortable and undesirable. As development was always presented to me, as a teacher, as a positive and something to be desired and worked towards, it was 'natural' that 'bigger' was better. Wasn't it? I lament the unquestioning and uncritical way I performed as a teacher and how I positioned myself. When I thought about the children that I had 'diagnosed' within these discourses as developing more slowly or differently, I always made the now dubious assumption that it was important for them to progress and catch up. I continue to grapple with these practices. How does one begin to interrupt these embedded ways of thinking? (Watson 2017).

Shifting the focus

The idea of examining inclusive and exclusive process in the classroom began with the ambition of finding better ways to include the diagnosed 'special' child. Researching *among* children provided for me, a way of viewing children's understanding of themselves and those they encounter. The children's observed authority in this context possibly challenges previous ideas around the vulnerability of children, as they participate in research. The direction of this study took a slight departure from researching with children, examining classroom discourses and their effects, as the research focus. Children are not positioned here as passive participants in their negotiations in the classroom. Investigating the way they take up or resist available discourses allows the researcher insight into their agency, their subjectivities and the power relations that position some children with privilege and others with subjugation.

This analysis offers no adjudication on the children or those who work diligently in classrooms everywhere. I am not proposing a critique of individual teachers or children as they work and play (Watson 2017). It is the uninterrupted and robust knowledges that I critique here and not the participants. Practices, words and actions taken up within the normative discourses are informed by embedded and pervasive knowledges that have effects. These knowledges surround us all shaping the possibilities of our becoming subjectivities and our agency in the context. Some knowledges are so well established in the early childhood classroom, that they have become a taken for granted and powerful 'truth' that we all feel we must abide by. However, as we abide by this 'truth' we inadvertently subjugate those we desire to support, those who we wish to include.

Spending time, inside the classroom among research participants, affords the opportunity to understand how classroom narratives shape what the children understand about difference. There is a chance to understand what participants find interesting and challenging, boring and funny, different and strange, 'right' and the 'wrong' ways of 'being' and 'doing', and how people and things fit together or don't fit together (Traweek 1988). Having these understandings of the 'inclusive' classroom assists in identifying exclusionary discursive practices. Thinking about how to do 'inclusion' better, is not the challenge, it is instead, learning 'how to detect, understand and dismantle exclusion as it presents itself in education' (Slee 2013: 905). This research *among* children has done this work, as it has detected how the 'normal' operates as a legitimate and oftentimes exclusionary authority. While the 'inclusive' classroom and its inhabitants continue to produce and reproduce meanings, which are firmly embedded in discourses that create difference as a problem, and difference as a deficit, inclusion will remain elusive. There might be promise of how we can shift the focus from objectifying participants in the classroom (Watson 2017) and begin to understand that we are all implicated in the making of ourselves as discursive subjects and in the making of each other.

References

Ailwood, J. (2010). It's about power: researching play, pedagogy and participation in the early years of school. In S. Rogers (ed.), *Rethinking Play and Pedagogy in Early Childhood Education*, pp. 19–31. New York: Routledge.

Alderson, P. (2008). Children as Researchers: Participation Rights and Research Methods. In P. Christensen and A. James (eds), *Research with Children: Perspectives and Practices,* pp. 276–290. New York: Routledge.

Bloch, M. N., Swadener, B. B., and Cannella, G. S. (eds) (2014). *Reconceptualising early childhood care and education: Critical questions, new imaginaries and social activism.* New York: Peter Lang.

Burman, E. (2008). *Deconstructing developmental psychology.* East Sussex: Routledge.

Butler, J. (1997). *Excitable Speech. A Politics of the Performative.* New York: Routledge.

Cannella, G. S. (1997). *Deconstructing Early Childhood Education: Social Justice and Revolution.* New York: Peter Lang.

Christensen, P. (2004). Children's participation in ethnographic research: Issues of power and representation. *Children and Society,* 18 (2), 165–176.

Christensen, P., and James, A. (eds) (2008). *Research with Children: Perspectives and Practices* (2nd ed.). London: Routledge.

Christensen, P., and Prout, A. (2002). Working with Ethical Symmetry in Social Research with Children. *Childhood,* 9 (4), 477–497.

Connolly, P., Smith, A., and Kelly, B. (2002). *Too Young to Notice? The Cultural and Political Awareness of 3–6 year olds in Northern Ireland.* Belfast: Community Relations Council.

Corsaro, W. A. (1985). *Friendship and Peer Culture in the Early Years.* Norwood, NJ: Ablex.

Danby, S., and Farrell, A. (2005). Opening the research conversation. In A. Farrell (ed.), *Ethical Research with Children,* pp. 49–67. London: Open University Press.

Davies, B. (1989). *Frogs and Snails and Feminist Tales: Preschool children and gender.* Sydney: Allen and Unwin.

Davies, B. (1993). *Shards of Glass: Children reading and writing beyond gendered identities.* Sydney: Allen and Unwin.

Foucault, M. (1972). *The archaeology of knowledge and the discourse on language.* New York: Pantheon.

Foucault, M. (1977). *Discipline and punish: the birth of the prison.* London: Penguin.

Foucault, M. (1982). The Subject and Power. *Critical Inquiry,* 8 (4), 777–795.

Gallacher, L., and Gallagher, M. (2008). Methodological Immaturity in Childhood Research? Thinking through participatory methods. *Childhood,* 15 (4), 499–516.

Harré, R., and van Langenhove, L. (eds) (1999). *Positioning Theory: Moral Contexts of Intentional Action.* Oxford: Blackwell Publishers.

Harwood, V., and Rasmussen, M. L. (2004). Studying schools with an ethic of discomfort. In B. Baker & K. Heyning (eds), *Dangerous Coagulations? The Uses of Foucault in the Study of Education,* pp. 305–321. New York: Peter Lang.

Laws, C., and Davies, B. (2000). Poststructuralist theory in practice: Working with 'behaviourally disturbed' children. *International Journal of Qualitative Studies in Education,* 13 (3), 205–221.

Löfdahl, A. (2010). Who gets to play? Peer groups, power and play in early childhood setting'. In L. Brooker and S. Edwards (eds), *Engaging Play*, pp. 122–135. Berkshire: Open University Press.

MacNaughton, G. (2005). *Doing Foucault in Early Childhood Studies: Applying poststructural ideas*. Abingdon, Oxon: Routledge.

Mayall, B. (2002). *Towards a Sociology for Childhood: Thinking from Children's Lives*. Buckingham: Open University Press.

Mayall, B. (2008). Conversations with Children: Working with Generational Issue. In P. Christensen and A. James (eds), *Research with Children: Perspectives and Practices*, pp. 109–123. New York: Routledge.

O'Kane, C. (2008). The Development of Participatory Techniques: Facilitating Children's Views about Decisions that Affect Them. In P. J. Christensen and A. James (eds), *Research with Children: Perspectives and Practices*, pp. 136–159. London: Falmer Press.

Petersen, E. B. (2004). *Academic Boundary Work: The discursive constitution of scientificity amongst researchers within the social sciences and humanities* (PhD). University of Copenhagen, Copenhagen.

Punch, S. (2002). Research with Children: The same or different from research with adults. *Childhood, 9* (3), 321–341.

Robinson, K. H., and Jones-Diaz, C. (2006). *Diversity and Difference in Early Childhood Education: Issues for theory and practice*. New York: Open University Press.

Rose, N. (1999). *Governing the Soul: The Shaping of the Private Self* (2nd edn). London: Free Association Books.

Slee, R. (2013). How do we make inclusive education happen when exclusion is a political predisposition?. *International Journal of Inclusive Education, 17* (8), 895–907.

Soto, L. D., and Swadener, B. B. (2002). Toward Liberatory Early Childhood Theory, Research and Praxis: decolonizing a field. *Contemporary Issues in Early Childhood, 3* (1), 38–66.

Sumsion, J. (2003). Researching with Children: Lessons in humility, reciprocity and community. *Australian Journal of Early Childhood, 28* (1), 18–23.

Traweek, S. (1988). *Beamtimes and Lifetimes – The World of High Energy Physicists*. London: Harvard University Press.

UNICEF. (1989). *Convention on the Rights of the Child*. New York: UNICEF.

Walkerdine, V. (1993). Beyond Developmentalism?. *Theory and Psychology, 3* (4), 451–469.

Walkerdine, V., and the Girls and Mathematics Unit, Institute of Education. (1989). *Counting girls out*. London: Virago Press.

Warming, H. (2005). Participant observation: a way to learn about children's perspectives. In A. Clark, A. Trine Kjørholt and P. Moss (eds), *Beyond listening: children's perspectives on early childhood services*, pp. 51–70. Bristol: Policy.

Warming, H. (2011). Getting under their skins? Accessing young children's perspectives through ethnographic fieldwork. *Childhood*, 18 (1), 39–53.

Watson, K. (2017). *Inside the 'Inclusive' Early Childhood Classroom: The Power of the 'Normal'*. New York: Peter Lang.

PART II

Innovative explorations of different forms of voice

MELANIE NIND

5   Multimodal listening and attending to children
    with complex disabilities in educational settings

This chapter addresses how we listen to the voices of children with complex disabilities in educational settings. It begins with arguments about why we need to attend to what these children might want to say, for the sake of their development and well-being, for our educational purposes, for research purposes, and related to these – because of their rights as children and disabled persons. A critical approach to the notion of voice is adopted alongside a multimodal approach to how we might approach voice. Practical examples from the author's research and other important studies are used to illustrate how children experiencing profound disability can contribute to research. This involves researchers and others attuning to children's modes of communication through sustained, attentive observation and by adopting an openness to dialogue and collaborative meaning making.

For the choice of disability terminology throughout the chapter, I mostly use the language of 'children with' as commonly used in educational settings in the UK; this is not to deny the position that these are 'disabled children' in the sense of being disabled by society (I would argue as well as – and in interaction with – their organic impairments). I use the term 'disabled learners' or 'disabled children' when I want to indicate a disabling process. I occasionally use the more internationally recognized terminology of 'intellectual impairments', but often want to emphasize the profundity, complexity or multiple nature of the impairment or disability. While 'profound and multiple learning *difficulties*' is the term used in the UK for children, I prefer the language of disabilities, which can be used for children or adults, is less euphemistic, and connects more with other disabilities.

The importance of listening and attending

This book takes an unashamedly rights-based approach to the subject matter of children's (here using the UK meaning of under-18s) participation, engagement and voice. I applaud this and yet, writing as an educationalist who spent the early part of her teaching career working on the realities of trying to open up communication with her students with profound intellectual impairments, I begin from a different place. In thinking about the importance of listening to such children and young people with complex and multiple disabilities in educational settings, I see first and foremost the importance of this for their development: If is it my job to teach you then I need to be able to reach you. Reaching across our differences as learners and teachers, disabled and not, is a reciprocal project which I argue begins with the teacher's attitude of listening and openness to dialogue.

In this chapter I discuss the educative priority first, moving on to the importance of listening for the well-being of learners, which I see as integrally linked to the educational endeavour, and then to the need to listen for research purposes, culminating in the rights of children and disabled persons to be involved in research as in all aspects of the social world. In the second part of the chapter I address the more practical questions of how we might follow through on the commitment. Throughout, I have in mind Tangen's (2008: 158) useful summary of the different concepts at work in relation to voice:

> The metaphorical term 'listening to children's voices' refers to different levels or aspects of meaning. First, when used in a context of educational research and practice, it refers to *research methodology and practitioners'* (and *policy-makers'*) *strategies and methods* for gathering and understanding children's experiences and views. Second, the term also refers to certain *phenomena* – i.e., children's or pupils' *experiences and future perspectives, and their views on daily routines and activities, or on particular issues.* Third, 'listening to children's voices' includes a reference to *the subjects* who are being listened to, as well as to the subject who is listening, and also to the relationship between the subjects.

The importance of listening and attending for learning

The importance of 'pupil voice' is well rehearsed in the literature. It is associated with a whole host of social and educational benefits as Cheminais (2008: 7) discusses: attending to pupil voice provides information for teachers, strengthens partnership between pupils and teachers, helps with setting priorities and understanding what matters from pupils' perspectives, creates a listening organization in which pupils feel valued and respected; it motivates, develops skills, and fosters a sense of belonging, creative thinking and so forth. Put like this it all seems so obvious. Listening to learners (I use learners to mean children and young people situated as pupils or students and not to imply that teachers are not learners too), and finding appropriate methods to do this, is in the interests of learners and teachers, just as it is in the interest of policy makers and researchers (Greene and Hill 2005). We might expect all schools to have action research projects to enhance their capacity to listen to pupils' voices.

Despite the obvious benefits of listening and attending to learners, there are as Fielding (2004) puts it, 'recalcitrant realities'. Schools have poor track records regarding listening and attending to pupils' voices, especially when it comes to learners with complex disabilities or challenging behaviour. I started teaching in special schools at a time when pupils with learning disabilities were subjected to intensive behavioural regimes in which they were to be moulded towards a more ideal type of pupil and a more normalized person. The idea of pupils having a voice, a view, or any real agency was an anomaly. Looking back at this (see 'for example Hewett and Nind, 1988), it is easy to see how much has changed with the promotion of the rights of children and disabled people through the United Nations Conventions, the advent of school councils, requirements here in the UK for pupil input into annual reviews of progress and so on. Applied Behaviour Analysis, though, is flourishing in the current decade. In special educational settings, where children undergo treatment-style interventions, there may be mixed messages surrounding the business of listening to children with complex disabilities. Similarly, the communication and attitudinal barriers to listening can be high; Watson, Abbott and Townsley (2007: 91) note that: 'Not only are children with complex healthcare needs rarely directly involved in research, but they are also not consistently being listened to by the professionals and services that support them'. Similarly, the views and experiences of young children are neglected (Clark, McQuail and Moss 2003). All this reinforces Corbett's (1998: 54) observation 'that some voices are difficult to hear because of a lack of conventional communication resources, a hesitant or inarticulate delivery and a marginalized social status'; to the list we might add assumptions about the child's value and the effort involved in listening.

Educational settings vary enormously in their inclusivity, their formality and their listening ethos. It is unsurprising perhaps that research has shown that young children communicate more freely at home than at school or pre-school (Tizard and Hughes 1985; Flewitt 2005; Nind, Flewitt and Payler 2011). While schools are concerned with the cognitive, communicative and social development of disabled children, families tend to be concerned with *attending* to children. As Flewitt (2005) explains, at home, children's knowledge is valued and worthy of good attention from the people around them. In contrast, they talk less in preschools where they are 'no longer supported by the shared understandings present in their homes' (p. 213). Moreover, often in early childhood education settings, the opportunities for communications and the pace and timing of exchanges are prescribed by established practices and routines rather than by the children. Ironically then, educationalist agendas can work against fostering communication, and educators and researchers would do well to take lessons from the nurturing of voice in children's homes.

As an educator of children with complex disabilities in the 1980s and 1990s, I was led to the arena of caregiver-infant interactions for a model of what proper attention to children's voices looks like in infancy. Multiple studies of these interactions have shown the qualities of the communicative spaces that are created when the focus is almost entirely on appreciating the infant. Here the pace is set by the child. The modes of communication are those that the child favours and uses freely. The routines are ones within which the child has the familiarity and feeling of safety from which to take risks with their voice. Communication here is for the sheer pleasure of it.

Rather than constitute the opposite of the communicative spaces in our school, our staff group saw that these could become the way of doing things for us as teachers and learners. Not least because the evidence was there that these spaces are optimal environments for learning (see Schaffer 1984 as a gateway to this literature). Intensive Interaction (Nind and Hewett 2005) was the result.

Colleagues and I developed Intensive Interaction as a teaching approach for learners experiencing disability such that they had not developed speech or other formal communication systems, had not learned how to be in the social world very effectively, and were largely cut off from positive learning interactions. The approach is based on five key principles for practice taken from the study of optimal caregiver-infant interaction:

- The creation of mutual pleasure and interactive games, being together with the purpose of enjoying each other;
- The teacher adjusting her/his interpersonal behaviours (gaze, voice, linguistic code, talk style, body posture, facial expression) in order to become engaging and meaningful;
- Interactions flowing in time with pauses, repetitions, blended rhythms; the teacher carefully scanning and making constant micro-adjustments, thus achieving optimum levels of attention and arousal;
- The use of intentionality, that is the willingness to credit the learner with thoughts, feelings and intentions, responding to behaviours as if they are initiations with communicative significance;
- The use of contingent responding, following the learner's lead and sharing control of the activity. (Nind 1996: 50)

This is, in many ways, was/is the epitome of listening and attending to learners with complex disabilities to support their learning. Prioritized in this way, this style of working, has been shown to benefit learners in their development of social and communication abilities (Nind 1996; Hutchinson and Bodicote 2015). I revisit this work in this chapter as it is the best argument I know for the importance of focusing on the stance of the teacher for releasing the communicative potential of the learner. It therefore offers aspects of a model for researchers wishing to involve people with complex disabilities.

The importance of listening and attending for well-being

The proliferation of the concern for the emotional well-being of learners came after our early work on Intensive Interaction (Nind 2011). Emotional well-being is succinctly defined as 'a holistic, subjective state which is present when a range of feelings, among them energy, confidence, openness, enjoyment, happiness, calm, and caring are combined and balanced' (Stewart-Brown 2000: 32). This is pertinent to the discussion of listening and attending to disabled children in that, as Katherine Weare a leading figure in the field explains, experiencing emotional well-being can come from feeling 'uniquely known, recognized, nurtured and valued' (Weare 2004: 25). This in turn can come from people listening and attending to you.

It is noteworthy that, whatever one's primary motivation for listening to disabled learners, the outcome may be a positive one for those learners' emotional well-being. There are plenty of accounts in the literature of the harm that education has done to 'special school survivors' and disabled learners whose experiences of mainstream education have not been consistent with authentic inclusive education (see e.g. Davis and Watson 2001). Yet an educational environment with a listening culture can have the opposite effect; it can be a healthy environment where communicating (about) emotions is normal and unthreatening (Weare 2004) and where staff are not over-whelmed by the feelings elicited in them by the behaviours of learners (Nind 2011). Properly attending to one another can foster mutual pleasure in interactions, supporting feelings of security needed for learning, and thereby sustaining a learning as well as healthy environment. It can be helpful to see emotion as embedded in the interactive space in that whether or not emotional well-being is an explicit goal of listening to learners, we would never intentionally want to do emotional harm.

The importance of listening and attending for research

At this point in the chapter it is timely to remind ourselves of some of the harm researchers have been known to do when they have not acted in ways promoted in this book. In some contexts this has been referred to as colonizing research; owing to the ways researchers have subjugated the knowledge of colonized peoples, making research become 'one of the dirtiest words in the indigenous world's vocabulary' (Smith 2012: xi). Feminist research arose in part in response to the ways in researchers both used women and failed to represent their diverse experiences (Bowles and Duelli Klein 1983). For many disabled people research has done similar harms, labelling and rejecting them (Townson et al. 2004), medicalizing and pathologizing them (Beresford and Wallcraft 1997). People with complex disabilities have largely been excluded from research because, as Booth and Booth (1996: 67) sum up, the exclusion of 'inarticulate subjects' is legitimized by the difficulties in interviewing them, seen 'in terms of their deficits rather than the limitations of our methods'.

Disabled children tend to be missing from research unless the research is specifically about them (Hill 2005) and even then it is rare to find educational research with children with complex disabilities. This neglectful treatment of disabled children is all about the power of the researcher over the research and the researched. There has, however, been a 'drive to redress wrongs, both past and present' (Nind 2014a: 17) by overturning invisibility and disrupting power relationships.

Researchers concerned to do better in terms of listening to the disabled people who have traditionally been the objects of their research have moved to talking about, and conducting, research in different ways as participatory, emancipatory, child-led and inclusive. Sometimes the discourse has been about sharing power, at others it has been about 'handing power over ... as if power were a commodity that can be passed around' (Nind 2014a: 21). At its most basic, the dynamic is about the drive encapsulated in qualitative research to explore how people understand, experience and voice their lived worlds (Hammersley 2013), but the drive towards democratization of ways of knowing extends further.

In participatory research the emphasis tends to be on finding methods that, 'rather than reinforce views of children's incompetence' facilitate exploration of their 'capacities, needs and interests from their own point of view' (Thomas and O'Kane 1998: 346). Also emphasized is the outlook of the researcher applying such methods, and the need to 'tune in' and 'adjust our listening' (Clark 2001: 333) such that even very young (or disabled) children contribute their knowledge to research directly, rather than through proxies. The aim is often to 'engage in meaningful partnerships with the researched', resulting in 'a de-privileging of "researcher-only" expertise' (Byrne et al. 2009: 68).

In emancipatory research, disabled people do much more than participate actively in the research, they control the entire process as 'a form of education and political action' working 'towards the achievement of their liberation' (French and Swain 1997: 28). Similarly, Kellett (2010: 42) has promulgated a form of child-led research in which 'every decision, every action, every word in every sentence' is 'sourced, discussed and approved by the young people to ensure their own voice [is] neither diluted nor distorted'. For children with complex disabilities the challenge in this may be too much. This is in part why the discourse of inclusive research has developed in which there is 'no one right way' to do things (Walmsley 2004: 69) as long as we are moving away from research that people experience as oppressive and towards researchers acting respectfully and listening to what people with learning disabilities want from research. In relation to children this means accepting 'children as persons' which means accepting their 'experiential life' as interesting (Greene and Hill (2005: 3) and accepting their rights to be represented in research.

The importance of listening and attending for children's rights

The human rights of disabled children constitute one of the key drivers in education settings for engaging learners' voices (Lundy 2007; Cheminais 2008); this sits alongside agendas of active citizenship, school improvement and personalization. Global moves to recognize the rights of children and young people are made explicit in the United Nations Convention of the Rights of the Child (1989). Articles 12 and 13 in particular have been taken on by national government policies and incorporated in Education guidance such as The Children Act (1989) in the UK and The National Children's Strategy (2000) in Ireland. Article 2 stresses that the rights apply to all children without discrimination. Hence hearing children's views and supporting their active participation in the activities of their communities is not just important from a rights-based perspective, but a legal necessity.

Enacting listening and attending: more and less than pupil voice

In this second half of the chapter I focus more on the question of how, rather than why, educationalists and researchers can listen and attend to children with complex disabilities. First though, I subject the notion of voice and pupil voice to some critique. This is crucial because, as Mazzei and Jackson (2009: 1) have persuasively argued, a whole discourse of 'giving voice', 'making voices heard' and so on has taken hold in qualitative research. This, they argue, reflects a kind of myth of 'voice as present, stable, authentic, and self-reflective ... "there" to search for, retrieve and liberate' (p.2). It is as if words from people's mouths are pure and it is the researcher's role to minimize any corruption of them. Turning to research with children, Todd (2012) notes the way that children's voices are often treated uncritically and the reductionist tendency to link children's voices with a single plane of experience – that of child. We need to remember the diversity among children, including disabled children, and the multiple voices that interact with and inform whatever they might express in research. While it is valuable to seek insider perspectives, rarely are insiders isolated from wider social cultures (Thompson and Gunter 2006; Thomson 2007). This reflects a key concept from Bakhtin's (1986) polyphony, that our speech is filled with the words of others.

Mazzei (2009) helpfully introduces questions of: when does voice happen, how does voice happen and where does voice happen? She encourages us to think about how we hear voices – not in the practical sense that I will move on to, but in the conceptual sense. 'We seek a voice that maps onto our ways of knowing, understanding, and interpreting' she argues (p.48). We are part of the meaning-making that transpires as we 'read' voices and silences, and this is inevitably limited in terms of knowing anything with certainty. I have found new researchers to be reluctant to read meaning into photographs and drawings, for fear of misinterpreting, yet unquestioning of their ability to read meaning from written transcripts. Being critical about voice means casting it all into uncertainty so that we are careful with our claims about voice – constructively mistrustful. In inclusive research there has sometimes been a rush to throw out, or at least quieten, the voices of academics in a privileging of the voices of disabled people, with the occasional critical stance that these need to be brought into dialogue (Nind and Vinha 2014).

Enacting listening and attending: a practical project

For me, dialogue is at the heart of doing research inclusively (Nind and Vinha 2014) and it is at the heart of inclusive and interactive pedagogy (Nind 2014b). Establishing dialogue is the core practical project for teachers and researchers. In the research context, if we are to build bridges between what we can know as academic researchers and what we can know at the grass roots then we need to foster dialogue (Nind and Vinha 2014). This does not just mean seeking marginalized voices, but really hearing them, and being willing to challenge them. Armstrong and Collis (2014) have talked about moving away from your space or my space into a new space. This is a space where we do not assume what the other knows or thinks, but where we genuinely want to know. This space may be physical or metaphorical but it is a space where dialogue happens. In an education context, if we are to build the kinds of relationships within which learning flourishes, teachers must be genuinely open to listening and entering into dialogue. Working with a school for girls who had been excluded from the mainstream we have observed this in action (Nind, Boorman and Clarke 2012) and the girls recognized it too, with Sam reflecting on the teachers, 'I don't think [they] really read my file. I think they got to know me for me' (p. 650).

The need for dialogue with children with complex disabilities raises multiple practical challenges: How do we get close enough to those children? How do we manage their lack of words and often their lack of interest in us? And how do we create new dialogic spaces? In the research literature, methods that might enable the inclusion of these children are limited to ethnographies and observational studies, mostly involving extended time with children, coming to understand them and their social worlds. Greene and Hill (2005: 8) suggest methods are needed that 'are suited to children's level of understanding, knowledge, interests, and particular location in the social world', that is, methods that are appropriate developmentally and to their stage in the life course. Finding guidance on doing research with children with profound or complex disabilities is especially challenging. For this we need to go to Simmons and Watson (2014) and to the work Ben Simmons did to find a research approach and set of methods that would allow him to understand the behaviours, communications and social experiences of Sam, a nine-year-old with profound and multiple disabilities, to hear his voice. This involved constructing meaning through a collaboration between Ben, Sam and significant people in Sam's life. It involved in part following the approach used by Morris (2003, cited by Simmons and Watson 2014: 140) of 'being with' Sam. This meant soaking up his social world, becoming sensitive to subtle changes in his interactions and unique behaviours and engaging with the multiple realities of the people who variously interpreted these. This latter part has echoes of Clark's (2001) Mosaic approach, which culminates in a similar kind of open, reciprocal exchange – a learning conversation or 'fusion of horizons' (Simmons and Watson 2014: 150).

The work of Ben Simmons with Sam, alongside the handful of other examples of work of this kind (Morris, 2003; Brewster, 2004; Goodley et al., 2004; Vorhaus, 2016), highlights the importance of observation, mostly sustained observation undertaken in an ethnographic tradition. In some ways, when children's disabilities are profound or complex, listening is observing, or as I prefer to put it, attending. It is by attending to someone that we get to know them intimately, and in this context, this is critical to getting to hear their voice. Participatory observation allows us to get to know a person. To this method, Ben Simmons added creating vignettes, which were detailed descriptions of small events including what Sam was doing and feeling and what was happening with his eyes, face, posture, movement and sound. These vignettes represented a dialogue between interaction and interpretation, which could be subjected to further reflection, dialogue and interpretation.

Intensive Interaction (Nind and Hewett 2005) is a helpful, holistic educational approach that similarly does this kind of dialogic space making work. There is a substantial body of work explaining the practicalities of this approach (see <www.IntensiveInteraction.co.uk>); here I just tease out the key parts of Intensive Interaction that provide practical guidance on listening and attending and thereby creating a sense of dialogue. This sits comfortably with a critical stance on voice as I am not arguing that this is a recipe for knowing unquestionably what a child with profound and multiple learning disabilities is feeling or wanting to say, but that it is a way of opening ourselves up, a way of attuning to what we might be able to read in them. In Intensive Interaction, practitioners do their listening through observing intently; we describe this as being 'tuned in' (Nind and Hewett 2005: 61) so that every change is scanned for, noticed and registered. This is supported by the use of video and reflection on that video and with colleagues. Tuning in means attending to actions, sounds, and body language, but also to tempo, mood and potential significance or meaning. Micro adjustments can be made then to the interaction or environment in a search for what is optimal for well-being and communication. In this way we are hearing the child's voice, that voice is having influence and that child is experiencing agency (see discussion in this volume of Lundy 2007). We communicate – by the quality of our focus on the child and what is happening for them – how much that child matters to us. This is the educational, well-being work in dialogue with the research work.

Enacting listening and attending: multimodality

In this final section of the chapter, I build connections between the approaches I have described, which can seem like a very specialist departure in education and research to a more mainstream movement towards a concern with multimodality. The concept of multimodality highlights our multiple means (modes) of making meaning/ communicating/ interacting and the synergies between them, as the modes appear and work together. The emphasis in the study of multimodality is on the 'integrated, multimodal whole' (Jewitt, Bezemer and O'Halloran 2016: 2). Multimodality differs from the work on multi-sensory approaches more familiar in special education, because of the attention multimodal researchers pay to the cultural and social resources for meaning making. Rooted in social semiotics (as well as conversation analysis), multimodal researchers focus on the active process of sign-making which is bounded by the social context (Dicks et al. 2011), but in which people as social actors have agency, as well as the different modes available in that context having different affordances (Jewitt et al. 2016: 9).

Educational/early childhood researcher, Rosie Flewitt has led the way in recent work researching the meaning making interactions of young disabled children, where 'adopting multimodal concepts', as Jewitt et al. (2016: 5) put it, has proven useful. Flewitt (2005) explains that young children supplement their linguistic resources with non-verbal signs; different modes are used to negotiate ideas, get responses, establish turn-taking and so on. As 'language is almost always part of a bigger whole' (Jewitt et al. 2016: 24), limited or no language is not a problem in multimodal research. Just as children's silences have come to be understood as communicative (Lewis 2010), so too has stillness in the world of communication going on in children's hands (Nyland, Ferris and Dunn 2008). The central premise in this kind of research is that 'all modes of expression carry meaning and that different modes can contribute to meaning making in specific ways' (Flewitt 2005: 209).

Flewitt (2005) concludes from her ethnographic case studies of young children that lack of talk does not mean lack of meaning-making. A multimodal lens, she argues, avoids pathologizing lack of talk, with multimodal analyses illustrating co-constructed meanings through gaze, facial expression and body movement' (p.220). In our work together (e.g. Flewitt, Nind and Payler 2009) multimodal analysis has informed the holistic way in which we have approached making field notes and analysing video. It has kept our attention on children's agency as they experience and interact with the world, and it has been helpful in illustrating the different modes and the ascription of intent and meaning to them in the different social contexts of home, inclusive and special early childhood education settings (Nind, Flewitt and Payler 2011). It has ensured that we attune to all that is going on communicatively, and this is a way of listening and attending to children with complex disabilities in research that I am happy to advocate.

Multimodality and attending go hand in hand. Vorhaus (2016: 2016) advocates a 'preparedness' to look for signs of responsiveness in someone with profound and multiple learning disabilities and 'to go on (and on) looking'. Goode (1994) advocates vigilance in listening and observing to conversations between bodies when someone has multiple impairments. Clark recognized this with young children too, arguing in relation to the Mosaic approach that researching the perspectives of young children 'requires a readiness to tune into different modes of communication' (Clark 2011: 311). She reminds us that choosing modes, like choosing research methods, supports agency in 'the co-construction rather than extraction of meaning' (p.313). For children with complex disabilities, this need for practitioners and researchers to 'tune in' is intensified, not just for research but for all communication. Listening to children does not necessitate that the researcher interviews children, it requires that the researcher approaches, questions and attunes to their meaning making. A great example of this is Clark's research question in her Living Spaces study – 'what does it mean to be me in this place?' There is a lot that researchers can do to enter into dialogue with children with complex disabilities to understand their experiences of their social worlds.

Conclusion: attending is everything

This book is about researching children's participation, engagement and voice and this chapter has turned the focus to what this means for research with children with complex disabilities. I have argued that we need to listen and attend to children, however profound their impairments, for the purposes of education, well-being and research. I have discussed some of the ways in which we can make this a reality. In conclusion, I want to stress the importance of the recurrent theme throughout of attending to children. I thank my doctoral student, Bernard Andrews for placing this at the forefront of my mind as I write. Focusing on how to know what is right when teaching children with social, emotional and mental health difficulties, he reflects:

> When we pay attention to our students, it is necessarily painful if they are in pain. This is more than empathy, because to look at someone empathetically is to see their lives in terms of our own. To pay attention is to remove ourselves from our thought entirely. (Andrews 2018:161)

I like the selflessness in this concept, which is emphasized in the same thesis when the following from a letter from Simone Weil to a friend is cited (Andrews 2018: 69): 'Attention is the rarest and purest form of generosity' (Weil and Bousquet 1982: 18). While I stress entering into dialogue with children's multimodal voices, I think we need to do so in this generous spirit.

References

Andrews, B. (2018). *How Can a Teacher of Students with SEMHD Unhide Moral Values?* PhD thesis, University of Southampton.

Armstrong, A., and Collis, A. (2014). Lessons for (new) inclusive researchers and discussion, Presentation at the National Centre for Research Methods 2014 Research Methods Festival. Retrieved from: <http://eprints.ncrm.ac.uk/3540/>.

Bakhtin, M. (1986). *The Dialectical Imagination: Four Essays*. Austin, TX: University of Texas Press.

Beresford, P., and Wallcraft, J. (1997). Psychiatric system survivors and emancipatory research: Issues, overlaps and differences. In C. Barnes and G. Mercer (eds), *Doing Disability Research*, pp. 66–87. Leeds: Disability Press.

Booth, T., and Booth, W. (1996). Sounds of Silence: Narrative Research with Inarticulate Subjects. *Disability and Society*, 11, 55–69.

Bowles, G., and Duelli Klein, R. (eds) (1988). *Theories of Women's Studies*. London: Routledge and Kegan Paul.

Brewster, S. J. (2004). Putting Words into their Mouths? Interviewing People with Learning Disabilities and Little/No Speech. *British Journal of Learning Disabilities*, 39, 166–169.

Byrne, A., Canavan, J., and Millar, M. (2009). Participatory Research and the Voice-centred Relational Method of Data Analysis: Is it worth it? *International Journal of Social Research Methodology*, 12 (1), 67–77.

Cheminais, R. (2008). *Engaging Pupil Voice to Ensure that Every Child Matters: A Practical Guide*. Abingdon: Routledge.

Clark, A. (2001). How to Listen to Very Young Children: The Mosaic Approach. *Child Care in Practice*, 7 (4), 333–341.

Clark, A. (2011). Multimodal Map Making with Young Children: Exploring Ethnographic and Participatory Methods. *Qualitative Research*, 11 (3), 311–330.

Clark, A., McQuail, S., and Moss, P. (2003). *Exploring the Field of Listening To and Consulting With Young Children*. London: Thomas Coram Research Unit/ University of London Institute of Education/Department for Education and Skills.

Corbett, J. (1998). Voice' in emancipatory research: imaginative listening. In P. Clough and L. Barton (eds), *Articulating with Difficulty: Research Voices in Inclusive Education*, pp. 54–63. London: Paul Chapman.

Davis, J. M., and Watson, N. (2001). Where are the Children's Experiences? Analysing Social and Cultural Exclusion in 'Special' and 'Mainstream' Schools. *Disability and Society*, 16 (5), 671–687.

Dicks, B., Flewitt, R., Lancaster, L., and Pahl, K. (2011). Multimodality and ethnography: working at the intersection. *Qualitative Research*, 11(3), 227–237.

Fielding, M. (2004). Transformative Approaches to Student Voice: Theoretical Underpinnings, Recalcitrant Realities. *British Educational Research Journal*, 30 (2), 295–311.

Flewitt, R. (2005). Is Every Child's Voice Heard? Researching the Different Ways 3-year-old Children Communicate and Make Meaning at Home and in a Preschool Playgroup. *Early Years*, 25 (3), 207–222.

Flewitt, R. S., Nind, M., and Payler, J. (2009). 'If She's Left with Books She'll Just Eat Them': Considering Inclusive Multimodal Literacy Practices. *Journal of Early Childhood Literacy*, 9, 211–233.

French, S., and Swain, J. (1997). Changing Disability Research: Participating and Emancipatory Research with Disabled People. *Physiotherapy*, 83 (1), 26–32.

Goode, D. (1994). *A World Without Words: The Social Construction of Children Born Deaf and Blind*. Philadelphia, PA: Temple University Press.

Goodley, D., Lawthom, R., Clough, P., and Moore, M. (2004). *Researching Life Stories: Method, Theory and Analyses in a Biographical Age*. London: RoutledgeFalmer.

Greene, S., and A. Hill. (2005). Researching children's experience: Methods and methodological issues. In S. Greene, S. and D. Hogan (eds), *Researching Children's Experience: Methods and Approaches,* pp. 1–21. London: Sage.

Hammersley, M. (2013). *What is Qualitative Research?* London: Bloomsbury Academic.

Hutchinson, N., and Bodicote, A. (2015). The effectiveness of Intensive Interaction, a systematic literature review. *Journal of Applied Research in Intellectual Disabilities,* 28(6), 437–454.

Jewitt, C., Bezemer, J., and O'Halloran, K. (2016). *Introducing Multimodality.* Abingdon: Routledge.

Kellett, M., with original research contributions by young people with a learning disability: Allan Aoslin, Ross Baines, Alice Clancy, Lizzie Jewiss-Hayden, Ryan Singh and Josh Strudgwick (2010). WeCan2: Exploring the Implications of Young People with Learning Disabilities Engaging in their Own Research. *European Journal of Special Needs Education,* 25 (1), 31–44.

Lewis, A. (2010). Silence in the Context of Child 'Voice'. *Children and Society,* 24, 14–23.

Lundy, L. (2007). 'Voice' is Not Enough: Conceptualising Article 12 of the United Nations Convention on the Rights of the Child. *British Educational Research Journal,* 33 (6), 927–942.

Mazzei, L., A. (2009). An impossibly full voice. In A. Y. Jackson and L. A. Mazzei (eds), *Voice in Qualitative Inquiry,* pp.45–62. London: Routledge.

Mazzei, L. A., and Jackson, A. Y. (2009). Introduction: The limit of voice. In A. Y. Jackson and L. A. Mazzei (eds), *Voice in Qualitative Inquiry,* pp. 1–13. London: Routledge.

Morris, J. (2003). Including all Children: Finding Out about the Experiences of Children with Communication and/or Cognitive Impairments. *Children and Society,* 17, 337–348.

Nind, M. (2011). Intensive Interaction, emotional development and emotional well-being. In D. Hewett (ed.), *Intensive Interaction: Theoretical Perspectives,* pp.22–38. London: Sage.

Nind, M. (2014a). *What is Inclusive Research?* London: Bloomsbury Academic.

Nind, M. (2014b). Inclusive Research and Inclusive Education: Why Connecting Them Makes Sense for Teachers' and Learners' Democratic Development of Education. *Cambridge Journal of Education,* 44 (4), 525–540.

Nind, M., Boorman, G., and Clarke, G. (2012). Creating Spaces to Belong: Listening to the Voice of Girls with Behavioural, Emotional and Social Difficulties through Digital Visual and Narrative Methods. *International Journal of Inclusive Education,* 16 (7), 643–656.

Nind, M., Flewitt, R. S., and Payler, J. (2011). Social Constructions of Young Children in 'Special', 'Inclusive' and Home Environments. *Children and Society,* 25 (5), 359–370.

Nind, M., and Hewett, D. (1988). Interaction as Curriculum. *British Journal of Special Education*, 15 (2), 55–57.

Nind, M., and Hewett, D. (2005). *Access to Communication: Developing the Basics of Communication with People with Severe Learning Difficulties through Intensive Interaction* (2nd ed.). London: David Fulton.

Nind, M., and Vinha, M. (2014). Doing Research Inclusively: Bridges to Multiple Possibilities in Inclusive Research. *British Journal of Learning Disabilities*, 42 (2), 102–109.

Nyland, B., Ferris, J., and Dunn, L. (2008). Mindful Hands, Gestures as Language: Listening to Children. *Early Years*, 28 (1), 73–80.

Schaffer, H. R. (1984). *The Child's Entry into a Social World*. New York: Academic Press.

Simmons, B., and Watson, D. (2014). *The PMLD Ambiguity: Articulating the Life-Worlds of Children with Profound and Multiple Learning Disabilities*. London: Karnac.

Tuhiwai Smith, L. (2012). *Decolonizing Methodologies: Research and Indigenous Peoples* (2nd edn). London: Zed Books.

Stewart-Brown, S. (2000). 'Parenting, wellbeing, health and disease'. In A. Buchanan and B. Hudson (eds), *Promoting Children's Emotional Well-being*, pp. 28–47. Oxford: Oxford University Press.

Tangen, R. (2008). Listening to Children's Voices in Educational Research: Some Theoretical and Methodological Problems. *European Journal of Special Needs Education*, 23 (2), 157–166.

Thomas, N., and O'Kane, C. (1998). The Ethics of Participatory Research with Children. *Children and Society*, 12, 336–348.

Thomson, F. (2007). Are Methodologies for Children Keeping Them in Their Place?. *Children's Geographies*, 5 (3), 207–218.

Thomson, P., and Gunter, H. (2006). From 'Consulting Pupils' to 'Pupils as Researchers': A Situated Case Narrative. *British Educational Research Journal*, 32 (6), 839–856.

Tizard, B., and Hughes, M. (1984). *Young Children Learning: Talking and Thinking at Home and at School*. London: Fontana.

Todd, L. (2012). Critical Dialogue, Critical Methodology: Bridging the Research Gap to Young People's Participation in Evaluating Children's Services. *Children's Geographies*, 10 (2), 87–200.

Townson, L., Macauley, S., Harkness, E., Chapman, R., Docherty, A., Dias, J., et al. (2004). We are All in the Same Boat: Doing 'People-led Research'. *British Journal of Learning Disabilities*, 32, 72–76.

Walmsley, J. (2004). Inclusive Learning Disability Research: The (Nondisabled) Researcher's Role. *British Journal of Learning Disabilities*, 32, 65–71.

Vorhaus, J. (2016). *Giving Voice to Profound Disability*. Abingdon: Routledge.

Watson, D., Abbott, D., and Townsley, R. (2007). Listen to Me, Too! Lessons from Involving Children with Complex Healthcare Needs in Research about Multi-agency Services. *Child: Care, Health and Development*, 33 (1), 90–95.

Weare, K. (2004). *Developing the Emotionally Literate School*. London: Paul Chapman.

Weil, S., and Bousquet, J. (1982). *Correspondence*. Lausanne: Editions l'Age d'Homme.

6 The phenomenology of intersubjectivity and research with profoundly disabled children: Developing an experiential framework for analysing lived social experiences

Introduction

Whilst there is some terminological variation when referring to people with profound intellectual impairment, this chapter uses the term 'profound and multiple learning disabilities' (PMLD) because it is the preferred term within the geographical and professional context of the study being reported (i.e. schools in England). Furthermore, this chapter specifically discusses '*children* with PMLD' to signal that all participants were under the age of 16 and thus not legally recognized as adults in England.

It is estimated that between 9,000 (Salt 2010) and 14,700 (Emerson 2009) school-aged children have PMLD in England. Historically, the concept of PMLD is rooted in developmental psychology and refers to students said to experience global developmental delay stemming from neurological impairments (Scope 2013). A review of the literature in this field has demonstrated that the cognitive abilities of children with PMLD are often compared to those of the neonate or infant insofar as children with PMLD are described as operating at the preverbal stages of development (Simmons and Watson 2014). For example, children with PMLD are understood as being pre-volitional (they lack free will or agency and cannot move with intent) (Farrell 2004); pre-contingency aware (they do not show awareness of cause-effect relationships) (Ware 2003); pre-intersubjective (they do not represent other people as subjects 'like me', and cannot differentiate between

subject and object); pre-symbolic or pre-intentional (they do not intentionally communicate meaning to others) (Coupe O'Kane and Goldbart
1998); and stereotypic in behaviour (they display reflexive, non-volitional
behaviour) (Tang et al. 2003). In addition to profoundly delayed cognitive
development, children with PMLD are also said to experience a range of
additional impairments, including physical impairments (Neilson et al.
2000) and sensory impairments (Vlaskamp and Cuppen-Fonteine 2007).

Research in the PMLD field has traditionally drawn conceptual
resources from behaviourist and cognitivist psychology to develop assessment tools and intervention strategies. Whilst behaviourist research has
aimed to support the functional or adaptive skills of children with PMLD,
cognitivist research has aimed to support children's emerging object cognition and social awareness (Simmons and Watson 2014). Methodologically,
researchers have drawn from post-positivist forms of philosophy to develop
experiments anchored in behavioural observation methods (e.g. applied
behaviour analysis). Criticism has been levelled at interventionist research
which treats children as objects of research rather than subjects to be consulted. Proponents of the latter view have drawn from constructivist philosophy to develop assessment tools such as 'talking mats' that are said to
reveal the preferences (likes and dislikes) of children with PMLD (Simmons
and Watson 2017).

The current author has developed an alternative research approach to
exploring the lived experiences of children with PMLD. This richly interpretivist methodology is rooted in longitudinal, participatory observation
methods, working collaboratively with children with PMLD and teaching
staff in context, and writing storied fieldnotes or 'vignettes' about the daily
lives of children with PMLD (Simmons and Watson 2014, 2017). The aim
of this chapter is to build on this approach by developing an experiential
framework for analysing vignette data pertaining to lived intersubjective
experiences. Put differently, the aim is to develop and apply a phenomenological description of what it is like to experience the other as a social
being, to engage with the other as a social being, and to be experienced
as a social being by the other. In doing so, it is hoped that we can develop
our methodological toolkit for exploring the lived social experiences of
children with PMLD.

Project

Vignette data discussed in this chapter comes from a three-year research project[1] funded through a British Academy Postdoctoral Fellowship (2014–2017) which investigated the social inclusion of children with PMLD who experienced both special and mainstream educational opportunities. The research aimed to (1) investigate how different educational settings (mainstream and special) afforded different opportunities for social interaction, (2) examine how children with PMLD respond to different opportunities, and (3) explore how different opportunities impact on the growth of social awareness and communication skills of children with PMLD. The aim here is not to present the findings of the research, but to present data excerpts in order to illustrate how a phenomenological framework can make the data intelligible.

The methodology was designed to in order to develop understanding of the meaning of children's actions. Seven children participated in the research (aged 5–13). Each child was observed one day a week in a mainstream school and one day a week in a special school over a ten-week period. Given the individualized behavioural repertoires of children with PMLD who participated in the study, the research required acts of interpretation and coming to know children through processes of familiarization and engagement with the children over extended periods of time. It also required open and reciprocal dialogue with significant others (parents, teaching staff etc.) who knew the children intimately and could share their understandings of children's actions. The following sections describe the project, which made use of participatory and non-participatory observations, pre-observation focus groups and on-going dialogue with staff and parents. This approach has been described in more detail elsewhere (see Simmons and Watson 2014, 2017).

---

1   The project received ethical approval from the University of Bristol's Research Governance Office, and the National Social Care Research Ethics Committee / Health Research Authority (REC Reference 15/IEC08/0006).

Pre-observation focus groups and semi-structured interviews

Prior to undertaking fieldwork, the researcher facilitated a pre-observation focus group involving key members of school staff for each child (e.g. teachers, teaching assistants, speech and language therapists, etc.). The researcher also conducted a semi-structured interview with the parents of each child. The aim of the focus groups and interviews was to explore each child's interests, abilities and methods of communication by consulting those who knew the children intimately. This allowed for the development of an initial lens through which to interpret and understand actions of the child when observed. For example, staff and parents for one child ('Billy') described the subtle difference between rocking in distress and rocking in excitement. When rocking in distress, Billy's actions were intensive and accompanied by angry vocalizations, stiff limbs and his bottom being raised off the wheelchair seat. By contrast, when rocking in excitement Billy would be slouched and look directly at the exciting event or person. Both of these rocking behaviours were differentiated from Billy's generalized convulsive (tonic-clonic) seizures, which were described by his parents as 'uncontrollable frantic wobbles' involving the whole body, with his lips sometimes turning blue. Concrete descriptions of children's behaviours by significant others helped guide the researcher's observations and make the children's individualized behavioural repertoires more intelligible in the early days.

Participatory observation

Observation in the PMLD field typically involves a distant-observer stance where the researcher employs a structured observation schedule. By contrast, the project being described in this chapter employed participatory observation methods. Participatory observation involves the researcher acting or participating in the lives of those he or she is trying to understand. By immersing himself or herself in the daily routines and activities of the children's lives, the researcher can become intuitively familiar with the routines and children's responses and experiences of them.

During the project, the researcher engaged in on-going participatory observation by acting as a teaching assistant for the children one day a week in a mainstream school and one day a week in a special school. The purpose of this participation was to allow for alternative ways of 'getting to know' the children involved in the study by 'being with' them (Morris 2003). Interacting with the children and supporting their learning in context alongside other teaching staff was one way of becoming familiar with the children's day (e.g. routines, interventions, behaviours etc.). This kind of observation also helped to develop trust and rapport between members of staff (Cohen, Manion and Morrison 2011) and provided opportunities for informal discussion with staff in real time. These informal conversations were central in developing interpretation insofar as the researcher was able to share and discuss his interpretations with staff members, ask questions and seek out staff members' expertise and wisdom (e.g. to resolve confusion about the meaning of newly observed or unexpected behaviours).

Non-participatory observation and vignette-writing

Fieldwork data was composed of 'vignettes' written during periods of non-participatory observation. Vignettes are rich and prosaic renderings of fieldnotes about social interactions. They have a story-like structure and adhere to chronological flow. Vignettes are restricted to a particular place, time and agent (or group of agents), and can vary from a few lines of descriptions to the length of a chapter (Miles et al. 2014). Erickson (1986) defined the vignette as:

> ... a vivid portrayal of the conduct of an event of everyday life, in which the sights and sounds of what was being said and done are described in the natural sequence of their occurrence in real time. This moment-to-moment style of description in a narrative vignette gives the reader a sense of being there in the scene. (149–150)

When opportunities for children with PMLD to engage in social interaction were observed the researcher would write detailed, descriptive accounts of the observation as the interaction unfolded, paying attention to who initiated the interaction and how, the actions of the interactive participants over time and contextual variables such as place and time of interaction, the items involved in the interactions. Vignettes included micro-descriptions of children's changing facial expressions and body movements, which were crucial in the early research stages as they helped the researcher develop a basic awareness of how a child expressed his or her emotions. This involved writing about where the child was looking, whether his or her eyebrows were raised, the shape of his/her mouth, how his/her head was tilted, what his/her arms and legs were doing, the noises he/she was making, etc.

Vignette-writing as research method is borne from an ethnographic tradition that avoids universal, objective truth and realism and is closer to the postmodern view of research which embraces a view of reality as participative and collectively constructed through shared engagement. To these ends, the vignettes were written to offer a rich, thick, descriptive piece of writing co-constructed out of the interplay between children's interactions with the world (which included the researcher) and both the researcher's and staff member's interpretation of that interaction. For methodological and ethical reasons it was important to locate subjective understandings in the written text as this was discussed with significant others in order to avoid potentially misrepresenting the children. The vignettes were read by others who knew the children or who observed the event, and the readers offered their own interpretation through informal conversations (e.g. between lessons or in the playground) which were essential to help deepen understanding of the observations.

Hundreds of vignettes were written and, through this on-going member-checking process, the researcher learned to 'see' the children from the perspectives of others who worked with them. However, this process of interpretation operated bi-directionally insofar as the researcher's interpretations presented to staff challenged their preconceptions which led them to reconsider and reconstruct their own understandings. This led to on-going, reflective dialogue during the course of the research and negotiations of interpretations.

Two examples of vignettes are given below. The first person narration is kept in order to keep a sense of authenticity. The aim of the presentation of vignettes is not to present conclusions about the findings of the research, but to provide a space in which to 'test' an emerging phenomenological framework developing later in the paper.

Vignettes

The two vignettes below are excerpts of field notes written during 2015–2016. They involve 'Amy' who was five years old, and 'Finn' who was eight. Both attended a PMLD unit in a special school, and went to age-appropriate mainstream classes one day a week for the purpose of the research project. In each of the vignettes I felt that I was engaged in an interaction that revealed the social awareness of the children.

VIGNETTE I: AMY

Lovely interaction with Amy this morning! I entered the classroom and began walking to the cloakroom. I noticed Amy out the corner of my eye (to the right of me) – head up, back straight, big wide eyes as if she was saying 'Hello! Look at me!' I sensed that she was trying to pull me into her world before I could [verbally] acknowledge her presence (well done, Amy!) I turn, but before I say 'hello' she gives me a big beautiful smile which makes me smile back. My words come out jumbled (I was about to say 'Good morning, Amy' but for some reason changed part way through in order to comment on Amy's smile, and it came out 'Good-smile-gailly'. I laugh at myself (felt a little embarrassed) and Amy laughs out loud, which makes me laugh even more. We chuckle together. TAs [Teaching Assistants] turn around and comment on what a lovely mood Amy is in today. She stares at me with bright, sparkly eyes, as if anticipating that I will do something amusing. I dump my coat and bag beside her and start chatting. She maintains eye contact and groans excitedly. I waffle a bit then see the blue spikey rubber ball on the floor (same as Caleb's), give it a shake and show Amy. The ball flashes and she turns her head to face away and remains still so I thought that I'd lost her attention. She then starts snorting as if trying to hold in a laugh. I move and sit beside her so I can see her face – her face is red, saliva bubbles froth out of her mouth and she howls with laughter! (Ha!) I ask if she's teasing me but she refuses to make eye contact. Happy moans. She then appears to phase out and rubs her nose. It's time for register so she is wheeled to the table. [Have I been teased like this before?]

VIGNETTE 2: FINN

Finn's TA asked me to help Finn with his lip balm. Staff have been keen to develop Finn's sense of agency (as a learning objective) and have been encouraging him to apply his own lip balm. This involves rubbing the balm on Finn's finger and encouraging him to raise it to his lips and apply it independently. The TA places a small pot of strawberry balm near Finn's nose and encourages him to smell it. 'Oh strawberry, Finn! Your favourite!' No sign of nostrils moving, but he arches his back, takes his feet off the footplates and straightens his legs (was this in response to the sweet strawberry smell?). TA saw him licking his lips (I missed this). TA tells Finn that I will be helping him today: 'Show Ben how good you are, Finn!'. I chat to him too – tell that I'm excited to see him. Happy groan from Finn. Following TA's instructions, I rub Finn's finger in the lip balm (his arm was resting on the tray attached to his wheelchair). I hold Finn's forearm and slowly guide it to his mouth. What was interesting is that I *felt* him accept me and our bodies appeared to negotiate bodily space. When I first moved Finn's arm he recoiled a bit (moved his arm towards his chest briefly – startle response?) I spoke to him and he almost instantly relaxed and let me *help him* guide his arm. He was moving roughly in the right direction (from chest to mouth) and I could feel him trying to move, but he also relaxed and let me guide him at times in a sort of 'toing and froing' motion, like we were both trying to traverse some sort of motor space between his chest and his mouth, or like he was trying to incorporate my movements into his. It was like he couldn't connect the two spaces independently but was happy to be steered back on track. When the finger touched his lips he licked the balm rather than rub his lips with his finger. We repeated the exercise several times. Teacher comes over to watch and explains that he is happy to open his mouth but doesn't seem to know what to do with the balm when it gets to his lips.

In the following sections a phenomenological framework will be developed. The framework will then be applied to the above vignette later in order to examine the extent to which it illuminates the structure of intersubjectivity contained in the vignettes.

Developing a phenomenological framework for understanding intersubjectivity

A phenomenological description of intersubjective awareness may appear paradoxical: it involves articulating something which, in essence, is pre-personal and operates *beneath* reflective consciousness in order to give rise to meaningful experience (which can be the object of reflection after the fact). In other words, the phenomenology of intersubjectivity is one that attempts to describe that which is tacitly presupposed, that which gives origin, structure and meaning to experience, and that which is not in itself directly experienced but rather *discovered* upon reflection. It is important to note here that the aim of this chapter is not to discover structures of experience, but to develop a framework based on contemporary literature in the phenomenology of sociality (e.g. Szanto and Moran 2016). This in turn can inform reflection insofar as it allows the current author to trace the emergence of experiential moments where it is simply 'known' that the other (in this case, the child with PMLD) is intersubjectively aware of the current author in the context of the author's research project. It is suggested that if this tracing can be possible, the phenomenological framework can help validate or authenticate how and why the author feels that something is the case, rather than simply ascertain that something is the case because the author experienced or felt it to be so. To put it differently, the aim is to explore how the structure of the researcher's intersubjective awareness during engagement with children with PMLD can provide an experiential form of evidence that children with PMLD are intersubjectively aware.

In the following discussion a thematic review of the literature regarding the phenomenology of intersubjectivity will take place in order to develop an experiential framework to analyse the vignettes above.

Non-inferential awareness

A key theme in the phenomenology of intersubjectivity is that experience of the other's social being is a *non-inferential form of awareness*, meaning that we do not typically cognize or calculate the existence of self-awareness in others. Rather, we automatically recognize it through perception of the other's actions, what Schutz (1972) refers to as 'signitive apprehension' (100). When observing another person '[m]y intentional gaze is directed right through my perceptions of his bodily movements to his lived experiences lying behind them and signified by them' (ibid.).

Being-in-the-world

Furthermore, we do not simply perceive individuals in abstraction from their environments, but instead perceive people directly as a power to perform in a given situation. The basic unit of social experience is the other person as a *being-in-the-world*. Being-in-the-world is a concept that relates an embodied subject to his or her tasks. The world is made meaningful to the subject in terms of how it affords particular kinds of actions, and my perception of the other is one that is *situated*, as Romdehn-Romluc (2011) states: '[...] I am aware of the other's body and environment as complementary parts of one whole' (139).

Part of the reason why we perceive the behaviour of the other as meaningful is because we immediately experience that action as an intelligent way of engaging with the world. As Merleau-Ponty (2002) notes, the self perceives the other through the body, and in doing so discovers that the other's body is 'a miraculous prolongation of my own intentions, and a familiar way of dealing with the world' (412). Observing the behaviour of the other can transform the observer's experience of the world:

> No sooner has my gaze fallen upon a living body in processes of acting than the objects surrounding it immediately take on a fresh layer of significance: they are no longer simply what I myself could make of them, they are what this other pattern of behaviour is about to make of them. (Merleau-Ponty 2002: 411–422)

We experience the other's agency as a kind of pull or drag – the body of the other presents as a 'vortex' (ibid.: 412) which my own world is sucked into, and in doing so the world emerges as something that is shared. The behaviour of the other is thus not simply a 'mere fragment of the world' (ibid.) but a way of elaborating the world, or a certain viewpoint. In other words, social experience can be mutually elaborating – the experience of the other can change my experience of my world and vice versa.

So far discussion has explored non-inferential dimensions of intersubjectivity. This has focused on what may be dubbed a passive dimension of experiencing other people. However, there is a dimension that is very much active, and through which originality and creativity flourish leading to a new sense of a self and other. We do not simply watch others and non-inferentially grasp their meanings – we engage and communicate with others.

Unpredictability and shared control

When we engage in a conversation with another person, we do not know exactly how the conversation will unfold and the direction it will take (unless we are reading from a script). In fact, a key theme in the phenomenological literature concerns both joint affect and *limited or shared control* I experience during social interactions. For example, in the experience of dialogue, 'there is constituted between the other person and myself a common ground; my thought and his are inter-woven into a single fabric' (Merleau-Ponty 2002: 413). This intertwining of subjectivities into a third space, or common ground 'of which neither of us is the creator' (ibid.), hints not just at the co-constitution of a space, but the way in which such a space influences our thoughts and actions. What is important here is the idea that the shape and meaning of interaction is co-constituted in the moment, that our words and thoughts are drawn from us during the dialogue and that the process and content of the dialogue are shared. 'We have here a dual being, where the other is for me no longer a mere bit of behaviour in my transcendental field, nor I in his; we are collaborators for each other in consummate reciprocity' (ibid.). We can observe the other interacting with the world, and even focus on bits of behaviour (which, in essence, is at the heart of scientific methodology in the PMLD field e.g. applied behaviour analysis), but by *interacting* with the other person a shared space emerges and even a shared being emerges. As Merleau-Ponty

(2002) puts it: 'Our perspectives merge into each other, and we co-exist through a common world (ibid.)'. He also states: '[w]hat we do in effect is to iron out the I and the Thou in an experience shared by a plurality, thus introducing the impersonal into the heart of subjectivity and eliminating the individuality of perspectives' (144). Such interactions can lead to new experiences and draw 'thoughts which I had no idea I possessed' (ibid.). It is only after the interaction, upon reflection, that I integrate the experience into the singular and recognize the thoughts as 'mine' as opposed to 'ours'.

Mutual incorporation

Fuchs and De Jaegher (2009) explain the above in terms of social interaction having two centres of gravity. Centres of gravity oscillate between dominance and submission during the interaction. When two people interact, it is possible that the co-ordination of movements, gestures, gazes, etc. overrides individual intent resulting in a shared sense-making act. This may be experienced as the interactive process gaining its own centre of gravity: 'Each of them behaves and experiences differently from how they would do outside of the process, and meaning is co-created in a way not necessarily attributable to either of them' (476). Fuchs and De Jaegher (2009) refer to this process in terms of *mutual incorporation*, defined as 'a reciprocal interaction of two agents in which each lived body reaches out to embody the other' (474). For example, mutual incorporation can be used to described eye contact which takes the form of a 'fight of gazes': I may feel the other's gaze as a pull, a suction, or also as an arrow that hits me and causes a bodily tension; I may feel his gaze right on my face (e.g. when blushing with shame); I may be fascinated by the gaze or withstand it, 'cast it back' etc. How I react (e.g. blushing) to the gaze of the other begins to shape his next action. This non-inferential process is immediate; it does not rely on internal representations and mental simulation of the other's anger. Rather, we immediately feel tense, angry or threatened by the impact of the gaze.

Gesture and symbolic communication

For Merleau-Ponty, a gesture tacitly becomes symbolic when it affects the behaviour of the other in such a way that the other's behaviour becomes an extension of the behaviour of the self who is gesturing:

> The sense of the gestures is not given, but understood, that is, recaptured by an act on the spectator's part. The whole difficulty is to conceive this act clearly without confusing it with a cognitive operation. The communication or comprehension of gestures comes about through the reciprocity of my intentions and the gestures of others, of my gestures and intentions discernible in the conduct of other people. It is as if the other person's intention inhabited my body and mine his. (Merleau-Ponty 2002: 215)

Marratto (2012) explains that what enables a gesture to become a sign is that it comes to function as a reliable indicator of another's subsequent movement. This requires that the person making the gesture is able to recognize another person's movement as a sequel to the previous gesture. This happens because the previous gesture motives the gesturer's own continuation of action.

A/symmetry and the power to reckon with the possible

Finally, symmetry and asymmetry are core themes in Merleau-Ponty's (2002) phenomenology of intersubjectivity. The experience of intersubjectivity is the experience of being one of many selves who share a world. 'Our perspectives merge into each other, and we co-exist through a common world (413)'. Romdehn-Romluc (2011) argues that, to experience the other as a subject (rather than an object) I must experience the other like I experience myself: 'Merleau-Ponty seems to understand symmetry to require that I experience myself and others as being the same sort of beings, and that my experience does not present either of us as privileged' (137).

While symmetry plays an important part in the experience of the other, there are also times of asymmetry, or the 'power to reckon with the possible' (Romdehn-Romluc 2011: 93). The physical world becomes an environment (*Umwelt*) when we make sense of it and ourselves through action, for example in terms of how the environment affords us opportunities to interact. However, we can choose to act or not act, we have agency and a degree of freedom. We are always already in communication with the social world, but we can also choose to shy away from it, ignore it and disengage. Because we are part of the social world we can turn away from it, and self-consciousness is this expression (Romden-Romluc 2011). Furthermore, whilst experiential symmetry is a core feature in interaction contexts, breakdowns in symmetry can occur when unforeseen events cause us to reflect about the interaction event (Fuchs and De Jaegher 2009). In other words, during the interactional flow symmetry can break and we are reminded of our own individual subjectivities – we may be conversing, but the other's opinions starkly contrast with our own and force us to reflect.

Application of phenomenological framework

In the previous section a thematic review of the phenomenology of intersubjectivity was performed in order to develop a framework for analysing lived intersubjective experience. This framework will now be applied to the two vignettes presented earlier in the chapter to assess the efficacy of this framework.

Vignette 1 begins with a sense of the researcher being sucked into an interaction with the participant called Amy. The researcher noticed Amy in his peripheral vision and immediately changed his originally intended direction and purpose – from heading to the cloakroom to turning towards Amy in order to greet her. ('I noticed Amy out of the corner of my eye [...] head up, back straight, big wide eyes as if she was saying 'Hello! Look at me!' I sensed that she was trying to pull me into her world before I could [verbally] acknowledge her presence'). Amy's gesture (her smile) automatically elicits a smile from the researcher. The researcher is surprised by Amy's alertness and it is as if she draws from the researcher a different verbal greeting from the one that he attempted to deliver: instead of saying

'Good morning', the researcher attempted to compliment Amy's smile part way through the sentence. The researcher uttered 'Good-smile-gailly' and felt embarrassed after. All of this happens in a matter of seconds. The researcher and Amy enter into a phase of shared emotions – they both laugh and each person's enjoyment enriches the other ('I laugh at myself [...] and Amy laughs out loud, which makes me laugh even more'). Arguably, what emerges here is a sense of symmetry. Following Zahavi and Salice (2016), it appears that the researcher and Amy were both laughing at the researcher's vocalization – there was interdependence, joint affect, and the emotion was experienced as being shared (the researcher and child were laughing together). There is a limited sense of control during the interaction, at least on the researcher's behalf, hence his fumbling phraseology and surprise at being teased. This is perhaps the first time that Amy has teased the researcher ('Have I been teased like this before?'). During the interaction the researcher felt that Amy was staring at him 'as if anticipating that I will do something amusing [...]'. The researcher shows Amy a spikey blue ball and Amy looks away ('She stares at me with bright, sparkly eyes' [then] 'turns her head to face away and remains still'). The researcher feels that Amy has lost interest in him and/or the ball, but she then 'starts snorting as if trying to hold in a laugh' until she eventually erupts with laughter. 'I ask if she's teasing me but she refuses to make eye contact' and emits 'happy moans'. For Fuchs and De Jaegher (2009), the meaning that emerges from social interaction is original in the sense that no single individual can lay claim to it. Rather, it is created through the interaction process itself. This is what Fuchs and De Jaegher (2009) consider to be authentic joint or participatory sense-making and give humour as an example. Humour, they say, can arise from a 'counter-intentional event in the interaction, for example a mishap or mismatch. Think of a child handing over an object to her father and, because of his hesitation, quickly taking it back. In this way, a game of teasing may emerge' (477). In Vignette 1 It is unclear if the researcher is the catalyst for the teasing sequence or whether Amy is practising a behavioural sequence learned elsewhere. However, the researcher felt that she was teasing, though she may have been simply declining the object then laughed at the researcher's presence once more.

Compared to Amy's interaction in Vignette 1, Finn's interaction with the researcher in Vignette 2 is qualitatively different in nature. It involves the researcher helping Finn by dabbing lip balm onto Finn's finger, and guiding his finger to his lips. The interaction is not built around a teasing game, but is of an intercorporeal nature and involves a sharing physical space. The researcher is left with a distinct impression of sharing or negotiating movement. For Merleau-Ponty (2002), in the same way that the parts of my body together make a complete system – the 'corporeal schema' (164) -, my body and the body of the other also make a complete system – what may be dubbed the 'intercorporeal schema'. The researcher observing Finn had previously seen TAs (Teaching Assistants) guide Finn's finger to his lips and perform this daily routine. As a distant rather than a participatory observer the researcher assumed that Finn was largely *passive* during the routine. However, on becoming a participant the researcher's understanding of Finn was enriched through his embodiment. Using concepts derived from the phenomenological framework developed above, we see several key features at work. At first Finn is largely passive – he lets the researcher rub the balm on Finn's finger, but when the researcher begins to raise Finn's arm and Finn recoils it is unclear whether this is a 'startle response', a volitional movement, or an intentional/symbolic signal meaning 'no'. However, upon hearing the researcher's voice Finn 'almost immediately relaxes' and lets the researcher guide his arm. Soon enough a sense of mutual incorporation emerges (a sense of two lived bodies reaching out to embody the other). When Finn moves his fingers towards his mouth the researcher stops guiding Finn, but when Finn begins to move off-track, the researcher gently guides Finn and Finn lets the researcher take over the movement before picking it up again. ('I felt him accept me, and our bodies appeared to negotiate bodily space […] in a sort of to-ing and fro-ing motion, like we were both trying to traverse some sort of motor space between his chest and his mouth'). This sense of intertwined volitions is strong and surprises the researcher – Finn is incorporating the trajectory of the researcher's movement into his own and vice-versa. Through this a sense of a third space emerges which emanates from Finn and the researcher and yet neither of the interactive partners are in complete control. There is a sense of the researcher's gesture becoming symbolic insofar as the researcher can read his gesture in Finn's bodily movements and sees Finn's movement as a continuation of the researcher's movement. (This begins when Finn relaxes after hearing the researcher's words and continues in the way Finn takes up the researcher's suggested direction of movements). Similarly, it may be argued that Finn's willingness to move independently and the researcher's willingness to stop steering Finn is confirmation that Finn's gestures (i.e. his volitional powers) are recognized as symbolic by the researcher's body. Whilst the feeling or awareness of the agency of Finn is non-inferential and accompanies an emerging sense of 'we', the vignette also demonstrates that the researcher is partly forced back into himself as a reflective subject when the researcher questioned the meaning of Finn's behaviours (and the efficacy of the researcher's own attempts to guide Finn). This was discussed above in terms of experiential symmetry and asymmetry. It may be argued that Finn's initial recoil demonstrates his powers to reckon with the possible.

Concluding discussion

This chapter has attempted to develop and examine a phenomenological framework that can guide reflection about lived intersubjective experience. It is the first attempt at developing such a framework in the PMLD field and is motivated by a desire to challenge deficit-based accounts of children with PMLD whilst legitimizing the researcher's intuitive experiences of children with PMLD as socially aware. The strength of the chapter lies in the extent to which it articulates a novel framework for guiding reflection about the structure of social experience in order to explain how and why we immediately experience children with PMLD as social. In doing so, it is hoped that we can build an experiential evidence base regarding the social awareness of children with PMLD.

Whilst the idea of a framework is novel (at least in the PMLD field), the framework itself has not been significantly developed. In addition to the need for further synthesis of phenomenological literature on the topic (to draw out more themes), there is a need to apply the framework to more data excerpts in order to test the framework's explanatory power. Furthermore, the framework is being applied at the end of the data collection phase of a research project which, methodologically, has involved intensive and richly interpretivist forms of working with people with PMLD in context over 10-week blocks (Simmons and Watson 2014, 2017). Given this, there is a need to theorize how the process of familiarization and working with children and teaching staff in context shapes our experiences, and how this directly influences the experience of sociality of children with PMLD. Phenomenologically, this has been described by Taipale (2016) as a shift from typification to individuation, meaning that whilst we rely on stereotypical identities to inform our empathic relation with strangers on a daily basis, we learn to see through typified identities and develop intimate, personal knowledge through regular engagement with others. This intimate knowledge becomes sedimented in our experience and leads to an enriched and personalized empathic stance with those that we know well. How this relates to the framework has yet to be theorized and will be one area to be developed in the future.

References

Bates, E., Camaioni, L., and Volterra, V. (1975). The acquisition of performatives prior to speech. *Merrill-Palmer Quarterly of Behavior and Development*, 21, 205–226.

Cohen, L., Manion, L., and Morrison, K. (2011). *Research Methods in Education* (7th edn). London: Routledge.

Coupe O'Kane, J., and Goldbart, J. (1998). *Communication Before Speech: Development and Assessment* (2nd edn). London: David Fulton.

Emerson, E. (2005). Underweight, obesity and exercise among adults with intellectual disabilities in supported accommodation in northern England. *Journal of Intellectual Disability Research*, 49, 134–143.

Erickson, F. (1986). Qualitative methods in research on teaching, in Wittrock M., C. (ed.) *Handbook of research on teaching* (3rd ed.). New York: Macmillan.

Farrell, M. (2004). *Inclusion at the Crossroads*. London: David Fulton.

Fuchs, T., and De Jaegher, H. (2009). Enactive intersubjectivity: Participatory sense-making and mutual incorporation. *Phenomenology and the Cognitive Sciences*, 8, 465–486

Gibson, J. (1979). *The ecological approach to visual perception*. Boston: Houghton Mifflin Co.

Koo, J. (2016). Concrete interpersonal encounters or sharing a common world: which is more fundamental in phenomenological approaches to sociality?. In T. Szanto, and D. Moran (eds), *Phenomenology of Sociality: Discovering the 'we'*. London: Routledge.

Marratto, S. (2012). *The Intercorporeal Self: Merleau-Ponty on Subjectivity*. New York: SUNY Press.

Merleau-Ponty, M. (2002). *Phenomenology of Perception*. London: Routledge.

Miles, M. B., Huberman, A. M., and Saldaña, J. (2014). *Qualitative Data Analysis – A Methods Sourcebook*. London: Sage Publications.

Morris, J. (2003). Including all children: finding out about the experiences of children with communication and/or cognitive impairments. *Children and Society*, 17, 337–348.

Neilson, A., Hogg, J., Malek, M., and Rowley, D. (2000). Impact of surgical and orthotic intervention on the quality of life of people with profound intellectual and multiple disabilities and their carers. *Journal of Applied Research in Intellectual Disabilities*, 13, 216–238.

Romdenh-Romluc, K. (2011). *Merleau-Ponty and Phenomenology of Perception*. London: Routledge.

Salt, T. (2010). *Salt review: independent review of teacher supply for pupils with Severe, Profound and Multiple Learning Difficulties (SLD and PMLD)*. Nottingham: Crown Copyright.

Schutz, A. (1972). *The Phenomenology of the Social World*. Evanston, IL: Northwestern University Press.

Scope (2013). Profound and Multiple Learning Disabilities/Difficulties (PMLD). Retrieved from: <www.scope.org.uk/services/education-and-learning/schools/meldreth-manor/pmld>.

Simmons, B., and Watson, D. (2014). *The PMLD ambiguity: articulating the lifeworlds of children with profound and multiple learning disabilities*. London: Karnac.

Simmons, B., and Watson, D. (2017). From Individualism to Co-construction and Back Again: Rethinking Research Methodology for Children with Profound and Multiple Learning Disabilities. In B. Kelly and B. Byrne (eds), *Valuing Disabled Children and Young People: Research, Policy and Practice*. London: Routledge.

Szanto, T., and Moran, D. (eds). (2016). *Phenomenology of Sociality: Discovering the 'We'*. London, Routledge.

Taipale, J. (2016). From Types to Tokens: Empathy and Typification. In Szanto, T. and Moran, D. (eds), *Phenomenology of Sociality: Discovering the 'We'*. London: Routledge.

Tang, J. C., Patterson, T. G., and Kennedy, C. H. (2003). Identifying specific sensory modalities maintaining the stereotypy of students with profound multiple disabilities. *Research in Developmental Disabilities*, 24, 433–451.

Vlaskamp, C., and Cuppen-Fonteine, H. (2007). Reliability of assessing the sensory perception of children with profound intellectual and multiple disabilities: a case study. *Child: Care, Health and Development*, 33, 547–551.

Ware, J. (2003). *Creating a Responsive Environment for People with Profound and Multiple Learning Difficulties* (2nd edn). London: David Fulton.

MIRIAM TWOMEY

7 Embodying voice: Children speak through their bodies

> Movement forms the I that moves before the I that moves forms movement.
>
> — MAXINE SHEETS JOHNSTON (2011)

Could there be a connection between how children with autism experience the world and how they move? What if the voice of the child is illustrated in some part through movement? Can we think differently about disabled children's bodies and minds and view movement as a means of expression, or as embodied voice? Placing the child with autism in a research context frequently represents them as objects, and describes them in terms of cognitive, social, or communicative deficits, or in terms of assessment, diagnosis or intervention. It is acknowledged in the literature that children with autism fail to express embodied, social actions and communicative behaviours similar to their peers and are challenged in developing social relationships. This may be further exacerbated by the emergence of asymmetrical relationships in the context of increasingly nuanced forms of language associated with later childhood. This chapter will explore the need to consider voice differently. For children with Autism Spectrum Disorders (ASD) who communicate differently and who may not voice their needs and desires audibly, this chapter will propose that the emphasis should be on affective engagement, as well as the role of the body and embodied experience. It will describe a research project conducted in the Republic of Ireland that discovered that children's participation and engagement can be facilitated through the use of the Creative Arts. It will describe how children with and without the label of autism were consulted. This chapter presents obstacles children with autism experience in terms of sensory motor disruption, its potential impact on social relatedness, and the need to focus on embodied experiences. It will explore the contribution of interactive exchanges and expression through movement and imitation facilitated by the Creative Arts.

Policies of childhood and voice

Article 12 of the United Nations Convention on the Rights of the Child (UNCRC 1989) recognizes children as active participants in society with the right to say what they think about decisions that affect their lives and have those views heard and respected. This raises many challenges for researchers, professionals and parents, if we are to acknowledge that not all children with autism who communicate nonverbally have a voice. It demands that we change our understanding of what voice is, and how it can be expressed (Gallagher and Gallagher 2008).

Conceptualizing voice differently requires that we also prioritize Article 13 of the UNCRC: The right for children to express themselves in different ways (talking, drawing, writing, photography) but also that we move beyond these methods by acknowledging embodied voice and recognizing new frameworks for understanding the role of embodied social interactions. A paradigm shift acknowledging the child as autonomous and agentic calls for a participatory framework, where constructivist efforts at researching with children, not on children, requires collaboration and consultation with children. In the absence of audible voice, we need to look at ways of seeing and hearing the child who doesn't communicate verbally (Smith 2016: 182). This chapter suggests that whatever form children's needs and intents are expressed should be regarded as realization of voice.

Philosophies of childhood

Ireland is emerging from a period of harsh austerity and lacks a well-established Early Years philosophy. The recent Early Years initiative Brighter Outcomes Better Futures (Department of Children and Youth Affairs

[DCYA] 2014) is the first overarching national policy framework for children and young people (aged zero to twenty-four years), where Early Intervention is regarded as a key transformational goal (DCYA 2014). Support at preschool level is now implemented through the Access and Inclusion Model (AIM) which is implemented where needed in an inclusive way (DCYA 2016). In the absence of an early years philosophy, this chapter draws on a new philosophy of Early Childhood established by Nordic theorists including Lenz-Taguchi (2009), Borgnon (2007) and Olsson (2009), from the field of Early Childhood Studies. These authors counter traditional views of childhood understood in linear terms where progress is indicated by movement towards developmental milestones and predetermined outcomes. This new theorizing shifts from a narrow perspective on what the child could become, towards a more holistic perspective of how the child can be. It also provides a transformational lens with which to view Early Intervention, education and inclusion, where difference can be interpreted through understandings of children and their subjectivities as learners and where children who do not fit into pre-established schemes of development and learning are included.

Olsson (2009) draws upon a Deleuzo-Guatarrian (1987, 2004) perspective and illustrates how the philosophers of difference' concepts of 'flows', 'energies', 'fluidity' and 'movement' provide us with fresh thinking in what were previously staid early childhood pedagogies and practices. Of particular interest are the elements that challenge fixed or predetermined outcomes. This philosophy is particularly useful in avoiding and displacing dualist or binary notions of disability and normality. Operationalizing this philosophy, Olsson (2009) suggests that children and adults meet around a problem, negotiating 'lines of flight'. 'Lines of flight' according to Deleuze and Guattari, lead a person's life in a new direction; the trajectory or course more important than the destination. This can be applied to the education for children with Special Educational Needs (SEN) where we draw attention to the 'process' rather than the 'position', as positioning may hamper movement (Olsson 2009). This suggests that pedagogical inventiveness and creativity should remain open ended and in movement. Borgnon (2007) describes the construct of the 'becoming child' by superimposing the image of Stella Nona her infant niece, who is learning to walk, over that of a surfer catching a wave. Using a metaphor of movement, and that of an apprentice surfer, Stella Nona disrupts the adult/child binary with rhizomatic thinking associated with Deleuze and Guatarri displacing typical perceptions of childhood comprising ages and stages.

Movement and being moved

The development of self and self other relatedness appear to have their onset in early interaction patterns in the parent child dyad. Zahavi (2012) notes that exploration of the self in Autism Spectrum Disorders has not received enough attention. Phenomenologists consider the embodied experience as central to self other relating (Samaritter and Payne 2013). Movement is a central feature of relationships and is acknowledged in early infancy research as a core element of intersubjectivity (Trevarthen 1979; Stern 2010). Spontaneous movement of a child is described by Sheets-Johnstone (2011) as constitutive of agency and selfhood. Our very beginnings are movement orientated or movement derived. The infant moves in order to survive, and early consciousness is formed through tactile-kinaesthetic interactions with the world (Sheets-Johnstone 2011). The role of the body and embodied experience is crucial to an understanding of affective engagement that begins in early childhood. Schore (2011), Trevarthen (1979) and Stern (1985, 2010) describe movement that is intrinsic to development in the context of relationships between the child, the caregiver and the environment. Mother–infant communication studies by Trevarthen (1990) proposed that the original human experience of dialogue emerges in the first few weeks of life, as parent and child engage in a dance of 'emotional attunement' by means of facial gestures, voices, hand gestures in the present moment. Stern (1985 and 2010) refers to the emergence of self through 'vitality affects', which prioritize movement and comprise elements of time, force, space and directionality. Vitality forms and vitality affects characterize personal feelings as well as dynamics of movements.

Trevarthen and Dellafield-Butt (2013) in their review of ASD and sensory motor challenges describe how for children with autism, thwarted sensorimotor control affecting movement acts as a barrier to social engagement, learning socioemotional understanding and regulation. The authors speculate that if it is an intrinsic disruption to timing that affects the perception of others' forms of vitality, then this ought to be able to be learned, or remediated, once a relational connection is established between the child with ASD and a communicative partner. The authors recommend Intensive Interaction, Music Therapy, and imitation therapies to establish this affective connection. These form an intersubjective resonance by adjusting movement timing, where social understanding and learning can grow.

Being moved by others, according to Reddy in *Moving Others Matters* (2012), is fundamental to human life. Drawing on two seminal papers '*On Being Moved*' by Bråten (2007) and Hobson's (2007) chapter *On Being Moved in Thought and Feeling*, Reddy recalls Adam Smith's famous example of spectators' unconscious imitation of the movements of the tightrope artist as they watched from below. This form of inner imitation was referred to by Lipps in 1903 as '*Einfuhling*' which means 'feeling into' describing the process of inner knowledge of another's feelings.

This raises the essential conundrum relating to what happens when we are not moved [physically and emotionally] by others. Being moved by others is an innate human capacity (Reddy 2012). From the field of social psychology, Bråten (2007) refers to the ability to be centred in another's body as 'alter-centric' and regards it as fundamental for experiencing people as people, with their subjective orientations of the world. Hobson (2007) refers to how we identify with the other. His thesis is that being moved by others in a subjective orientation is a central feature to understanding the thoughts, feelings and attitudes of others.

Sensory motor disruption and social relatedness

Sensory problems are included as core features in the Diagnostic and Statistical Manual of Mental Disorders (DSM V AMA 2013). Prior to that empirical findings by Baranek, David, Poe, Stone and Watson (2006) found that pre-schoolers with autism had high rates of sensory difficulties (60 to

100 percent). More recently research reviews by Marco, Hinkely, Hill and Nagarajan (2011) and Baum, Stephensen and Wallace (2015) account for the differences in underlying neural processing of sensory and social communication. Sensory difficulties therefore, may cause young children with autism to experience the world in a dysregulated way and consequently they may have disruptions in intersubjective connectedness. Importantly the work of DeGangi, Breinbauer, Roosevelt, Porges, and Greenspan (2000) highlights the connection between regulatory and developmental problems presenting in infancy with later impoverished development of social interactions, highlighting the need for early intervention in these areas. Children with autism progress from sensori-motor and pre-symbolic movements (spinning, rocking, overstimulation), where according to Prizant, Weatherby and Rudell (2000), they are striving for emotional regulation to a space where they can connect in one to one interactions in significant relationships.

Movement and bodily expressed experiences

The role of movement has been particularly important in phenomenology. In a well-known work of the 'Primacy of Movement' Sheets-Johnstone (2011) argues rather for a holistic, qualitative concept of motion: '... a temporal-spatial-energetic dynamic, a kinetic aliveness that is in play throughout the course of our everyday lives' (ibid.: 29). Torres et al. (2013) explore the relevance of micro-movement in ASD and highlight a spectrum of adaptive volitional control and intentionality. The authors explain that in the typically developing young child, movements can be performed under voluntary control or occur spontaneously. Spontaneous movements are embedded in natural movement and entrained socially through adult speech and interaction (Torres et al. 2013). Torres et al. describe the adaptation of typical neonates where young children adapt and navigate flexibly through spontaneous and intentional acts of behaviour. Children with autism experience difficulties with volitional control of their movements and frequently there is a disconnect between their intentions and actions (Robledo et al. 2012).

Trevarthen and Dellafield-Butt (2013) suggest that early prenatal failure of systems that control movement, timing, and coordination that regulate affective evaluations of experiences are evident in motor sequencing, attention, affective expression and intersubjective engagement when the child with autism gets older. According to the authors this supports the need for the use of non-verbal, non-cognitive activities which sensitively encourage engagement through relational or creative therapy. Similar to early attachment experiences or the unfolding of intersubjectivity emerges through the caregiver infant relationship.

A phenomenological perspective on autism

The research described in this chapter considers challenges relating to movement and sensory motor development, as it opens up thinking to include a mind body association and include perspectives from contemporary phenomenology as that advocated by Fuchs and de Jaegher (2009) and de Jaegher (2013).

A phenomenological approach considers autism as a disorder of primary or embodied intersubjectivity (Fuchs 2015). It prioritizes the notion of a 'mindbody' connection suggesting a non-representational, enactive and embodied concept of intersubjectivity where a mental representation (Fuchs and De Jaegher 2009: 466) or cognitive theory of sociality may not be applicable. It accounts for difficulties in the bodily expressed world of children. As a psychological and phenomenological theorist, De Jaegher (2013) promotes an enactive account of autism and suggests that people perceive their environment and events within it, in terms of their ability to act on it.

Developing this view, De Jaegher explores how embodiment and sense-making connect, that is, autistic distinctiveness of movement, perception, and emotion relate to how people with autism make sense of their world. Therefore a child's unique sensory, motor and nonverbal communication repertoire may influence how he/she understands or responds to the world around them. However, De Jaegher (2013) suggests that a greater attention

to detail, preference for repetition and sameness may have significant meaning for people with autism and should not be considered as inappropriate
behaviours. Social interaction processes are considered high end cognitive
processes which may prohibit children's engagement. This suggests that
we need to be open to expressions at a bodily level and less focused on
advancing children's higher level repertoires. Other researchers suggest
that the child with autism has a lesser tendency to perceive, respond to
and engage with the bodily expressed attitudes of another (Garcia-Perez,
Lee and Hobson 2007). Hobson (1993, 2002), Hobson and Lee (1999),
and Hobson and Meyer (2005) note that children with ASD cannot identify with the actions of others. They can't register or assimilate the bodily
anchored psychological stance of another person.

   According to Marsh et al. (2013) individuals with ASDs have significant
visuomotor processing difficulties. Even if perception and visual timing is
intact, there can be problems with motor responses and understandings – a
feeling of not being grounded in the world and not properly partaking in
the rhythms of the world by moving their own bodies to pace themselves to
it. The authors describe it as similar to catching a merry-go-round when we
cannot run fast enough to jump on (Marsh et al. 2013). Regarding children
with ASD the authors suggest that action and movement 'are necessary in
order to learn about the world, the flow of the world and our relationship
with it' (ibid.: 2). The authors suggest that viewing autism from a Gibsonian
(1979) ecological theory of perception and a dynamical systems approach
to action (Warren 2006), we learn of the significance of action in learning.
They promote a simple analogy to describe interactions; that we are pulled
into the natural orbit of another's movement rhythms, that we match these
movements and are responsive to them (Marsh et al. 2013). The authors also
suggest that the severity of autism may impact on matching speech as well as
the rhythm of movement. It is possible therefore that motoric differences,
including fine and gross motor, postural control, balance differences, difficulties synchronizing one's gestures with another, may underlie social or
affective engagement. Many social tasks require a high degree of coordination of movement – eye gaze, gesture, attention, gestural positioning, key
to any success is that the child is interested (Torres and Donnellan 2015).

   So what are the implications of this knowledge? The child with autism
engages with the world and other people differently; their differences in

sensing, movement, perception and nonverbal communication indicate that their embodiment and sense making may be at a bodily level.

Exploring creative methodologies

Can children tell us how they feel nonverbally? Is there a voice that is seen and not heard? It was with these questions in mind, that the present study was designed to explore children's thinking around inclusion, play and belonging. It sought to explore if creative methods could encourage the affective engagement and participation of children with autism through imitation and movement. This research also sought to enquire how a child with autism navigates through and subjectively experiences inclusion in the day-to-day world of the classroom. It supported the concept of listening to children in making decisions with them not for them (Dahlberg and Moss 2005). Using qualitative, longitudinal case studies, non-verbal and movement-based experiences, the research sought to explore if creative methodologies could facilitate or elicit embodied voice? This research was mindful of Komulainen's (2007) claim that voice may embrace forms of communication that are challenging for disabled children.

Acknowledging the challenges involved in facilitating intersubjectivity and engagement, this research utilized creative approaches which were sensitively developed to facilitate non-verbal children with autism. A portfolio of methods was developed during the research that was subtly and interchangeably discerning to the receptive and expressive language difficulties associated with ASD, but also considerate of the ages of the children and their ability to communicate (Lewis, Robertson and Parsons 2005).

The central theme guiding these research methods was of finding ways to engage children with autism rather than focusing on their developmental deficits. Kellet and Nind (2003) refer to engagement as the most crucial code defining social communicative development in children with ASD. Reducing verbal input and increasing visual supports was crucial to the methods adopted in this research. This research noted the particular difficulties disabled children experience in articulating voice (Lewis and Porter

2007). Innovative work by Jones and Gillies (2010) and Long, McPhillips, Shevlin and Smith (2012) was particularly relevant to this research in its approach to the encouragement of creative technologies to sensitive investigation in the context of inclusive groups of children. Recognizing the importance of Article 13 of the Convention, a combination of talk and impromptu drawing was used. During the early stages of the research attention was also given to listening carefully to children by using sensitive cues as well as using multi-method tools to encourage non-verbal children to express themselves. Shaughnessy (2012) developed drama for children with autism and refers to the need for engaged and participatory practices to engage mind with body. Tortora (2005) claims, that we can uncover information about children's social, emotional, physical, communicative and cognitive development by observing their non-verbal expressions.

Imitation

The research methods used in this project were based on long standing work on imitation and its effects on children with autism. Nadel and Peze (1993) observed that imitation was crucial in the child's social cognitive development and that it established a sense of shared experience. Research by Field, Field, Sanders and Nadel (2001) showed that imitation by an adult had an enhancing effect on the social behaviour of children with autism. Nadel and colleagues (2000) previously adapted the still face paradigm to demonstrate that children with autism developed expectant behaviours such as looking and touching an adult following imitation. The authors' work on imitation changed nonverbal engagement in children with autism. Escalona, Field, Nadel and Lundy (2002) showed that after imitation children with autism had improved distal and proximal social behaviours. The current research was particularly interested in the distal communicative attempts of looking and vocalizing and proximal effects of moving close to and touching that emerged in research by Field, Nadel and Ezell (2011). Nadel (2015) however draws the distinction between imitation which requires matching one's motor patterns to that of another. This is possible when these actions are possible in terms of the child's motor abilities. If the child can match and develop a synchrony with the movements of others then this may move beyond imitative learning and communication and develop some level of intentionality or agency.

Puppetry

Puppetry has been used previously with children with autism. Rapport and engagement were greatly enhanced by puppets in studies by Schrandt, Buffington-Townsend and Poulson (2009), Dwight-Salmon (2005) and Epstein, Stevens, McKeever, Baruchel and Jones (2008). This research adopted a 'least adult role' (Warming 2012) where puppets conducted role plays and later focus group interviews. This research invited children to contribute as researchers (Jones and Gillies 2010). Trimingham (2010) adopted a phenomenological and embodied approach to puppetry to theorize on the puppet's role as a surrogate communicator and facilitator with children who lack communication skill, but also to address how neurological patterns are developed through physical interaction and how puppets, as innocuous but controllable physical objects, may have a therapeutic role in re-establishing disrupted patterns. She explores the use of puppets as Winnicott's (1971) 'transitional objects' operating in a 'transitional space'. Using Winnicott's notion of a bridge between the inner world that we control, and the external world, which we do not, these activities are linked to a creative 'space' of mind. Puppets operate in this space. Neilson, Slaughtor and Dissanayake (2012) suggest that children with autism may imitate object directed actions that have tangible, functional outcomes with less emphasis on social motivations.

Concerns about the representation of children's voice for children with severe disabilities are of the utmost importance. Who decides what voice is and how it is represented needs to be addressed. This is significant when we attempt to represent the views and wishes of children with severe communication difficulties where adults act as intermediaries. For the purposes of this study, due to the children's young age and communicative impairment, parents were approached regarding consent. Confidentiality and anonymity were explained to all participants. Participants were advised in written form and were verbally reassured that their names would be anonymized and any distinguishing features relating to children, school setting or locality would be dealt with confidentially. Anonymization in the form of removing names and any other form of identification was explained.

Regarding ethical procedures relating to children's participation, confidentiality was also described and dealt with in a way that children could understand. While children's participation is increasingly ambiguous and contested (Graham and Fitzgerald 2010), this research was fully supported by visual aids [Objects of Reference] and pictorial representations in consultation with the Speech and Language therapist, including Picture Exchange Communications System (PECS) and the Irish signing system LAMH. Similar to Smith, Taylor and Gollop (2000) listening to children's voices and encouraging them to actively participate was integral to the research design. The researcher held the belief that children can communicate their views and intentions if adult partners are sensitive to their perspectives. This research invited children to participate but also developed child centred research methods where children themselves were actively designing their own topics, giving them more agency in the approach to ethical dilemmas (Holland, Renold, Ross and Hillman 2008). An ethics-in-practice approach was constantly observed. Even when the child was unable to give informed consent, there were opportunities for assent and dissent to ensure that their inclusion in the study was voluntary and that they were not being coerced (Lewis and Porter 2007). Children with autism were provided with communication tools as opportunities to participate or withdraw from the research. Like Tozer (2003) children with autism had a stop card and a change card symbol to signal their ability to allow them to discontinue.

AARON

Aaron was a four-year-old boy with autism, sensory defensiveness, severe communication difficulties and emotional regulation challenges. Like many children Aaron relied on his senses to perceive and understand everyday experiences, however sensory disruption meant that Aaron had difficulty processing everyday information such as sounds, sights and smells. He was challenged by the disintegrated semantics of these senses, failing to absorb information in a coherent, systematic way. As a form of expression, Aaron sometimes repeated single words using echolalia. His movements were similar to echolalic speech. Not so much a disturbance of movement but a truncation of movement, moving differently. Mismatch of gaze, gesture, and interrupted timing meant that Aaron moved in rigid and repetitive ways; evidential of the unrelenting sameness he craved; repeating the same expressive form, over and over again.

Research project

At the beginning of each session, I encouraged Aaron's teacher to incorporate strategies recommended by the Occupational Therapist implementing Di Gangi et al.'s (2000) emphasis on physiological regulation preceding emotional regulation. During the early stages of the research I used sign Aaron was familiar with [Irish Sign Language] and visual supports as well as nonverbal gesturing, to facilitate communication and guide Aaron's understanding and actions. I reduced my language and demonstrated responsiveness through matching Aaron's movements (Caldwell 2006) in initiating a co-regulated state between adult and child.

This research invited children to contribute as researchers (Jones and Gillies 2010). Rapport was greatly enhanced with Aaron's peers by the introduction of two puppets. The children named the puppets 'Pretty Girl' and Pretty Boy' (Shown in Picture 1). The puppets engaged the class group in role play (Schrandt, Buffington-Townsend and Poulson 2009; Dwight-Salmon 2005; Epstein, Steven, McKeever, Baruchel and Jones 2008). The puppets (as co-researchers) conducted focus groups; following with role-play about thematic topics such as 'play', 'friendship', 'feeling included' 'joining in', and 'feeling left out'. The format of the class was initially in theatre style. It allowed children to extend other children's answers; their responses prompting each other, reaching deeper into peer and school culture (Lewis 2002). An analysis of the videos involved member checks with the classroom staff and opinion from an interobserver who was expert in the field of movement and autism.

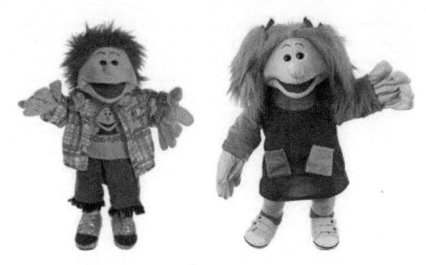

Figure 7.1

The research comprised of four phases over a 15-month period. Children in the classroom were included in all four phases (See Table 7.1). This chapter will describe the experiences of one child Aaron.

Table 7.1. Phases of Research

Aaron [Pseudonym]	Setting	Intervention	Analysis
Phase 1	Resource Room with small group of children including buddies	'Talk and draw' PECS. Supported by Julie	Observation, video-analysis [inter-observer]
Phase 2	Large multi-grade mainstream, classroom – seated next to buddy	PECS/Puppet role play Supported by Julie	Observation, video-analysis [inter-observer]
Phase 3	Large multi-grade mainstream, classroom – seated next to buddy	PECS/Puppet role play/ Puppet intervention Supported by Julie	Observation, video-analysis [inter-observer]
Phase 4	Large multi-grade mainstream, classroom – seated next to buddy	PECS/Puppet role play/ Puppet intervention Supported by Julie	Observation, video-analysis [inter-observer]

Ethical considerations

During each visit to the school adjacent to the Early Intervention Unit, I accompanied Aaron and Julie (Aaron's Special Needs Assistant) to his new classroom. As part of the school's First Steps integration programme, Aaron attended a new mainstream classroom adjacent to his Early Intervention unit. A primary objective was to engage Aaron in the research with the other children in the classroom. While puppetry was introduced to the class through focus groups and role play, one of the puppets 'Pretty Girl' approached Arron and imitated him. As stage two of the research progressed, Aaron found the puppets' presence increasingly tolerable. This research was mindful of Gernsbacher et al.'s (2003) findings of sensory over-reactivity to social visual stimuli. The puppet's face was less threatening resulting in Aaron's willingness to engage in social activities. Adapting Gernsbacher et al.'s (2003) observations on eye gaze, the puppets' gaze circumvented the room full of children and was not singularly directed towards Aaron. The puppet also served Aaron's preference for a preferred non-transient, visual, environmental stimulus (Quill 1997), providing a visual-constant modality over time that did not change dynamically.

The puppet initially followed Aaron's lead, imitating him, but alternating this with the stop/freeze methods pioneered by Nadel et al. (2000) and Escalona et al.'s (2000) spontaneous interaction by the adult. As the project extended during phase 3, Aaron's distal behaviours [attention and imitation] improved and the proximal effects [touching] also progressed. It was easy to keep the puppet's body and face still; allowing for Aaron's adaptation of Caldwell's (2006) use of dyadic interaction and playful imitation where 'tuning in', and 'repeating' the child's activities was used.

Aaron's story (based on researcher's field notes):

> In the initial stage of the research project Aaron did not seek out others, and though he watched peers, he rarely sought their attention and did not initiate interaction. He did not understand their bodily communication, gestures or invitations to play. Failing to respond, he appeared distant and aloof. His blue eyes gazed fixedly at objects. He loved counting and early maths was his passion. Aaron was not interested in the talk and draw phase of the research. He continued writing his favourite letters of the

alphabet and numbers 1–10 on the work sheet. He chose not to become involved,
though Amy his buddy persisted in her efforts to include him; reassuring him that she
would remain beside him ... At the start of the second phase of the research, Aaron
briefly glanced at the puppets; quickly averting his gaze to a number chart fixed on
the opposing wall. Aaron mostly ignored the puppets during the initial role play. Amy
chatted to Aaron, continually checking to see if he needed his fidget toy. As the focus
groups started, Aaron remained ambivalent. His body remained still and fixed when
the puppet moved towards him. While 'Pretty Boy' addressed the group, 'Pretty Girl'
approached Aaron appearing to observe his movements. Aaron moved suddenly, dis-
concerted by the untoward advances of the puppet. While Aaron moved, the puppet
remained still. Immediately afterwards the puppet imitated Aaron's actions. Aaron
glanced upwards observing the puppet's movements, feeling less threatened when the
puppet once again became still and looked away focusing on the other children ...
During phase 3, Aaron began to respond to the puppet's movements. A circular relationship developed incorporating reciprocal chains of movement. When the puppet
imitated his movements, Aaron began to imitate the puppet's movements. Puppet
interventions were maintained over a number of sessions. When the researcher was
not present, the class teacher implemented puppetry. These class sessions lasted 20–30
minutes and included an entire class group over a period of 3 months. Aaron's reactions
were demure but became visually and gesturally more enthusiastic. Amy sat beside
Aaron encouraging his interactions with the puppet. Despite his fascination with
objects, Aaron had warmed to 'Pretty Girl' ... During phase 4 of the research a real
functioning microphone was introduced. The puppet chatted to the class as usual but
now encouraged them to respond through the microphone. The children ran towards
the puppet reaching to take hold of the microphone, begging to go first. A flicker of
animation was observed in Aaron's eyes during the class focus group. Increasingly
Aaron vocalized with more clarity and intention. He gestured enthusiastically – his
gaze becoming steady and consistent, looking expectantly at the puppets and reaching
towards the microphone purposefully. The puppet gave the microphone to Aaron,
Aaron vocalized ... the children responded enthusiastically.

Discussion of findings

This final section of this chapter seeks to interpret findings in terms of
the central tenets of this book where themes of participation and engagement were facilitated through the use of the Creative Arts. Imitation was a

valuable support for Aaron who was not connected to others, who had little continuity of interaction or experience and who feared change and uncertainty. Due to strong sensory proclivities, Aaron avoided touch and often did not seek out support and regulation from others. In fact, he actively resisted the attempts of others to regulate him. Aaron was vulnerable in a world of social interaction and relationships. In the overwhelming and unpredictable world of the classroom, DiGanghi et al.'s (2000) sensory integration strategies was utilized prior to the intervention. While Aaron showed reluctance he was dependent on caregivers to regulate his physiological and emotional needs. Aaron gradually became more content in the mainstream classroom.

During the puppet interviews, Aaron frequently became dysregulated when faced with conflicting social and sensory stimuli. Imitating his movements enhanced co regulation (Caldwell 2006; 2010). As the interviews progressed with the class group, implementation of the school's Buddy system successfully encouraged Aaron to participate. Aaron's engagement increased following imitation by the puppet. While 'Pretty Girl' moved, she appeared to subjectively move Aaron. Aaron moved in response to the puppet's movement. Aaron not only moved physically towards the puppets, he appeared to be moved in terms of orientation and intent. The puppet's intervention validated the work of Nadel et al. (2000) and Escalona et al. on imitation, but also affirmed principles of Intensive Interaction and Caldwell's imitation strategies. Imitating Aaron's actions, the puppet embodied a voice that said 'I can see what you are doing. I can do the same thing ...', in essence attaching value to that movement.

These movement and imitation patterns eventually developed a synchrony, demonstrating evidence of a 'moving self' and 'moving others' (Foolen 2012). What became obvious was a mutuality between Aaron's movements and increased engagement. There appeared to be a connection between motion and emotion (Foolen 2012; Hobson 2007; Trevarthen 1979). A phenomenological view would suggest that the ability to move is a precondition for the ability to perceive the world (Overgaard 2012).

When recognizing that the puppet imitated his actions, Aaron experienced a sense of validation and connectedness. Aaron moved beyond mirroring and imitation to engaging in reciprocation and mutual recognition during interactions. The puppet's imitation was regarded as successful in engaging Aaron over a period of time. However the introduction of a microphone was the most engaging element for Aaron and the rest of the class group. This contests the relationship between imitation and agency.

In agreement with the literature, Aaron experienced difficulty with social relating (Hobson 1993; Hobson et al. 2007), understanding the intentions and feelings of others (Baron-Cohen 1989; Baron-Cohen, Leslie and Frith 1985) and making sense of the world. He did not engage with the typical language and communication repertoires representing sociality in the mainstream classroom. Aaron's efforts were to the untrained eye stilted, lacking in intentionality, comprising social, communicative and motor difficulties. What must be realized is that the obstruction may be ours, in terms of how we understand and perceive Aaron's expressiveness. Using de Jaegher's enactive approach we may interpret his increased meaning making during encounters with the puppet and the microphone.

While Aaron was described as autistic, what was of particular note was the intensity of challenges with which he perceived the world and how difficult it was to overcome them. However, this research illuminates the increasing intensity of Aaron's engagement when he was interested and involved. As the research progressed Aaron moved from a dysregulated state with severe disruption in intersubjective connectedness to a smoother synchrony, where he co-constructed meaning. Through movement and imitation, communicative attempts by the child with autism showed evidence of a shift from isolation to connectedness. The puppet adjusted to Aaron's engagement level; in effect becoming an intermediary of engagement; revealing evidence of a competent and agentic child.

Children's insights and understandings

This research identified with newer philosophies of childhood particularly that from Nordic research (Borgnon 2007; Olsson 2009; Lenz Taguchi 2008). Findings in this research affirmed the need for a rethinking of childhood where identity does not have fixed ends in sight (Olsson, 2009) but comprise possibilities (Deleuze and Guatarri 1987 and 2004). What was of particular interest in this research was the process of engagement and the role of bodily centred movement, expressions and interactions, which are not typically associated with voice.

Reconfiguring voice

Aaron presented with imbalances of communication and behavioural repertoires; confounding his role as agentic or meaningful. This begs the question if bodily expression counts as legitimate? When Aaron's distress was noteworthy or when competing stimuli in the form of students' and teachers' voices were apparent, his autism became more visible. Conceivably there were other incoming stimuli dominating his classroom experience. A question arising from this research is if these stimuli precluded Aaron's attempts to interact socially? Was Aaron unable to move and be moved by others (Hobson 2007) or were many experiences available to him but a successful response to one stimulus resulted in failure to respond to others? Aaron's efforts at achieving a more regulated state may have prohibited him from engaging in social interaction. The concern is: did his poorly articulated social language entrench a medical view?

What it means to be included

Lessons learned from children's experiences include the importance of engagement and the significant role of imitation and movement when working with young children with autism. In this research children's views on being included, belonging and playing were sought by puppets. While the class group responded to puppet interventions, for one child, the use of imitation by the puppet was more significant. The use of creative methods including drama may inform practitioners, parents and researchers about the importance of engagement.

For children with disabilities a deeper concern lies in the absence of audible voice; how do children make their needs known? This research affirms the role of new thinking in the field of enactive phenomenology (De Jaegher 2015), mind science including cognitive linguistics (Foolen 2012; Reddy 2012), and intersubjectivity (Fuchs and De Jaegher 2009) in relation to nuanced presentations of voice. It also serves to elucidate that the language we have for our bodies can adequately explain or give voice to thoughts, feelings and intentions. It is important that parents, caregivers and teachers understand that language and communication systems that are represented by the body may be misconstrued if children remain dysregulated, cannot participate and are not engaged. The challenge is to facilitate regulation prior to participation and engagement and recognize the presence of children's pre-verbal 'intentional' behaviour.

Returning to Hobson's (2007) question, 'what happens in the absence of being moved by others?' Reddy's (2012) construct is compelling, 'If I can move, I can move others'. This reaffirms the interpersonal nature of mind and language. In the absence of voice, more specific research needs to investigate phenomenological relationships between movement and engagement in the context of intersubjectivity and nuanced presentations of voice. If the movement of a child with autism embodies emotions, needs and desires, parents, teachers and caregivers need to know it.

References

American Psychiatric Association (2013). Diagnostic and Statistical Manual of Mental Disorders (DSM-5) (5th edn). Washington, DC: American Psychiatric Association Publishing.

Baranek, G. T., David, F. J., Poe, M. D., Stone, W. L., and Watson, L. R. (2006). Sensory Experiences Questionnaire: discriminating sensory features in young children with autism, developmental delays, and typical development. *Journal of Child Psychology and Psychiatry*, 47 (6), 591–601.

Baron-Cohen, S. (1989). The autistic child's theory of mind: a case of specific developmental delay. *Journal of Child Psychology and Psychiatry*, 30 (2), 285–297.

Baron-Cohen, S., Leslie, A. M., and Frith, U. (1985). Does the autistic child have a 'theory of mind'?. *Cognition*, 21, 37–46.

Baum, S. H., Stevenson, R. A., and Wallace, M. T. (2015). Behavioral, perceptual, and neural alterations in sensory and multisensory function in autism spectrum disorder. *Progress in Neurobiology*, 134, 140–160.

Borgnon, L. (2007). Conceptions of the Self in Early Childhood: Territorializing identities. *Educational Philosophy and Theory*, 39 (3), 264–274.

Bråten, S. (2007). *On Being Moved: From Mirror Neurons to Empathy*. Amsterdam: John Benjamins Publishing Company.

Caldwell, P. (2006). *Finding You, Finding Me: Using Intensive Interaction to Get in Touch with People Whose Severe Learning Disabilities are Combined with Autistic Spectrum Disorders*. London: Jessica Kingsley.

Dahlberg, G., and Moss, P. (2005). *Ethics and politics in early childhood education*. London: RoutledgeFalmer.

Dahlberg, G., Moss, P., and Pence, A. R. (2007). *Beyond quality in early childhood education and care: languages of evaluation* (2nd edn). London: Routledge.

De Jaegher, H. (2013). Embodiment and sense-making in autism. *Frontiers in Integrative Neuroscience*, 7, 15.

DeGangi, G. A., Breinbauer, C., Roosevelt, J. D., Porges, S., and Greenspan, S. (2000). Prediction of childhood problems at three years in children experiencing disorders of regulation during infancy. *Infant Mental Health Journal*, 21 (3), 156–175.

Deleuze, G., and Guattari, F. (1987). *A thousand plateaus: capitalism and schizophrenia*. London: Athlone Press.

Deleuze, G., and Guattari, F. (2004). *EPZ Thousand Plateaus*. London: Bloomsbury.

Donnellan, A. M., Hill, D. A., and Leary, M. R. (2012). Rethinking autism: implications of sensory and movement differences for understanding and support. *Frontiers in Integrative Neuroscience*, 6, 124.

Dwight Salmon, M. (2005). *Script Training with Storybooks and Puppets: A Social Skills Intervention Package across Settings for Young Children with Autism and Their Typically Developing Peers*. Columbus, OH: Ohio State University.

Epstein, I., Stevens, B., McKeever, P., Baruchel, S., and Jones, H. (2008). Using puppetry to elicit children's talk for research. *Nursing Inquiry*, 15 (1), 49–56.

Escalona, A., Field, T., Nadel, J., and Lundy, B. (2002). Imitation effects on children with autism. *Journal of Autism and Developmental Disorders*, 32, 141–144.

Field, T., Field, T., Sanders, C. & Nadel, J. (2001). Children with autism display more social behaviors after repeated imitation sessions. *Child Development*, 5, 317–323.

Field, T., Nadel, J., Ezell, S. (2011). Imitation therapy for children with autism. In Williams, T. (ed.), *Autism spectrum disorders from genes to environment*, pp. 287–299. Retrieved from: https://www.intechopen.com/books/autism-spectrum-disorders-from-genes-to-environment

Foolen, A. (2012). *Moving Ourselves, Moving Others: Motion and Emotion in Intersubjectivity, Consciousness and Language.* Amsterdam: John Benjamins Publishing Company.

Fuchs, T. (2015). Pathologies of Intersubjectivity in Autism and Schizophrenia. *Journal of Consciousness Studies*, 22, 1–2, 191–214.

Fuchs, T., and de Jaegher, H. (2009). Enactive intersubjectivity: Participatory sense-making and mutual incorporation. *Phenomenology and the Cognitive Sciences*, 8 (4), 465–486.

Gallagher, L. A., and Gallagher, M. (2008). Methodological immaturity in childhood research? Thinking through participatory methods. *Childhood*, 15 (4), 499–516.

Garcia Perez, R. M., Lee, A., and Hobson, R. P. (2007). On Intersubjective Engagement in Autism: A Controlled Study of Nonverbal Aspects of Conversation. *Journal of Autism and Developmental Disorders*, 37, 1310–1322.

Gernsbacher, M. A., Davidson, R. J., Dalton, K., and Alexander, A. (2003). *Why do persons with autism avoid eye contact?* Paper presented at the Annual Conference of the Psychonomic Society, Vancouver, BC.

Gibson J. J. (1979). *The Ecological Approach to Perception.* Boston, MA: Houghton Mifflin.

Graham, A., and Fitzgerald, R. M. (2010). Progressing children's participation: exploring the potential of a dialogical turn. *Childhood*, 17 (3), 343–359.

Government of Ireland (2014). Better Outcomes Brighter Future: The National Policy Framework for Children and Young People 2014–2020. Dublin: Stationary Office. Retrieved from: <http://www.dcya.gov.ie/documents/cypp_framework/BetterOutcomesBetterFutureReport.pdf>.

Department of Children and Youth Affairs (2016). *Access and Inclusion Model: A New Model for Supporting Access to Early Childhood Care and Education (ECCE).* Dublin: Stationery Office.

Hobson, R. (1993). *Autism and the Development of Mind.* Hove: Lawrence Erlbaum.

Hobson, R. P. (2007). On Being Moved in Thought and Feeling: An Approach to Autism. In P. M. G. J. Martos Pérez, M. Llorente Comí and, C. Nieto (eds), *New Developments in Autism: The Future Is Today.* London: Jessica Kingsley.

Hobson, R. P., Lee, A., and Hobson, J. A. (2007). Only connect? Communication, identification, and autism. *Social Neuroscience*, 2 (3–4), 320–335.

Hobson, R. P., and Meyer, J. A. (2005). Foundations for self and other: a study in autism. *Developmental Science*, 8 (6), 481–491.

Jones, P., and Gillies, A. (2010). Engaging young children in research about an inclusion project. In R. Rose (ed.), *Confronting obstacles for inclusion – international responses to developing education*, pp. 123–136. London: Routledge.

Kellett, M., and Nind, M. (2003). *Implementing Intensive Interaction in Schools*. London: David Fulton.

Komulainen, S. (2007). The ambiguity of the child's 'voice' in social research. *Childhood*, 14(1), 11–28.

Lenz Taguchi, H. (2008). An 'Ethics of resistance' challenges taken-for-granted ideas in Swedish early childhood education. *International Journal of Educational Research*, 47 (5), 270–282.

Lewis, A. (2002). Accessing through research interviews the views of children. *Support for Learning*, 17 (3), 110–116.

Lewis, A. (2010). Silence in the Context of 'Child Voice'. *Children and Society*, 24 (1), 14–23.

Lewis, A., Newton, H., and Vials, S. (2008). Realizing child voice: the development of Cue Cards. *Support for Learning*, 23 (1), 26–31.

Lewis, A., and Porter, J. (2007). Research and Pupil Voice. In L. Florian (ed.), The SAGE Handbook of Special Education. London: SAGE Publications Ltd.

Lewis, A., Robertson, C., and Parsons, S. (2005). *DRC Research Report – Experiences of disabled students and their families: Phase 1*. University of Birmingham: Disability Rights Commission.

Long, L., McPhillips, T., Shevlin, M., and Smith, R. (2012). Utilising creative methodologies to elicit the views of young learners with additional needs in literacy. *Support for Learning*, 27 (1), 20–28.

Marco, E. J., Hinkley, L. B. N., Hill, S. S., & Nagarajan, S. S. (2011). Sensory Processing in Autism: A Review of Neurophysiologic Findings. *Pediatric Research*, 69 (5 Pt 2), 48–54.

Marsh, K. L., Isenhower, R. W., Richardson, M. J., Helt, M., Verbalis, A. D., Schmidt, R. C., and Fein, D. (2013). Autism and social disconnection in interpersonal rocking. *Frontiers in Integrative Neuroscience*, 7, 4.

Nadel, J. (2006). Does imitation matter to children with autism? In S. J. Rogers and J. H. G. Williams (eds), Imitation and the Social Mind: Autism and typical development, pp. 118–137. New York: Guilford Press.

Nadel, J. (2014). *How imitation boosts development in infancy and autism spectrum disorder*. Oxford: Oxford University Press.

Nadel, J., and Peze, A. (1993). What makes immediate imitation communicative in toddlers and autistic children? In J. Nadel and L. Camaioni (eds), *New perspectives in early communicative development*, pp. 139–156. London, New York: Routledge.

Nadel, J., Croue, S., Kervella, C., Mattlinger, M., Canet, P., Hudelot, C., et al. (2000). Do children with autism have expectations about the social behavior of unfamiliar people? *Autism*, 4, 133–145.

Nadel, J., Revel, A., Andry, P., and Gaussier, P. (2004). Toward communication: First imitations in infants, low-functioning children with autism and robots. *Interaction Studies*, 5, 45–74.

Nadel J., Aouka, N., Coulon, N., Gras-Vincendon, A., Canet, P., Fagard, J., and Bursztein, C. (2011). Yes they can! An approach to observational learning in low functioning children with autism. *Autism*, 15, 421–435.

Neilson, M., Slaughter, V., and Dissanayake, C. (2012). Object-Directed Imitation in Children With High-Functioning Autism' Autism Research, 6 (1), 23–32.

Olsson, L. M. (2009). Movement and experimentation in young children's learning: Deleuze and Guattari in early childhood education. New York: Routledge.

Prizant, B., Wetherby, A., and Rydell, P. (2000). Communication intervention issues for children with autism spectrum disorders. In A. Wetherby and B. Prizant (eds), *Autism spectrum disorders: A transactional developmental perspective (volume 9)*. Baltimore, MD: Brookes.

Quill, K. A. (1997). Instructional considerations for young children with autism: The rationale for visually cued instruction. *Journal of Autism and Developmental Disorders*, 27, 697–714.

Reddy, V. (2012). Moving others matters. In A. Foolen, U. M. Lüdtke, T. P. Racine and J. Zlatev (eds), Moving Ourselves, Moving Others, pp. 139–164. Amsterdam: John Benjamins Publishing Company,

Renold, E., Holland, S., Ross, N. J., and Hillman, A. (2008). Becoming Participant: Problematizing 'Informed Consent' in Participatory Research with Young People in Care. *Qualitative Social Work*, 7 (4), 427–447.

Robledo, J., Donnellan, A. M., and Strandt-Conroy, K. (2013.) An exploration of sensory and movement differences from the perspective of individuals with autism. *Frontiers in Integrative Neuroscience*, 16 (6) 107.

Samaritter, R., and Payne, H. (2013). Kinaesthetic Intersubjectivity: A dance informed contribution to self-other relatedness and shared experience in non-verbal psychotherapy with and example from Autism. *Arts in Psychotherapy*, 40 (1), 163–170.

Schore, A. N. (2001). Effects of a secure attachment relationship on right brain development, affect regulation, and infant mental health. *Infant Mental Health Journal*, 22, 7–66.

Schrandt, J. A., Townsend, D. B., and Poulson, C. L. (2009. Teaching empathy skills to children with autism. *Journal of Applied Behavior Analysis*, 42 (1), 17–32

Shaughnessy, N. (2012). *Applying Performance: Live Art, Socially Engaged Theatre and Affective Practice*. Basingstoke: Palgrave Macmillan.

Sheets Johnstone, M. (2011). *The Primacy of Movement*. Netherlands. John Benjamin's Publishing Company.

Smith, J. C. (2016). The embodied becoming of autism and childhood: a storytelling methodology. *Disability and Society*, 31 (2), 180–191, DOI: 10.1080/09687599.2015.1130609.

Smith, A. B., Taylor, N. J., and Gollop, M. M. (2000a). *Children's Voices: Research, Policy and Practice*. New Zealand: Pearson Education.

Stern, D. N. (1985). *The interpersonal world of the infant: a view from psychoanalysis and developmental psychology*. New York: Basic Books.

Tisdall, E. K. M. (2012). The Challenge and Challenging of Childhood Studies. *Children and Society*, 26, 181–191.

Tortora, S. (2005). *The Dancing Dialogue: Using The Communicative Power Of Movement With Young Children*. New York: Paul H. Brookes Publishers

Torres, E. B. (2015). Commentary on: An exploration of sensory and movement differences from the perspective of individuals with autism. *Frontiers in Integrative Neuroscience*, 9, 20.

Torres, E. B., Brincker, M., Isenhower, R. W., Yanovich, P., Stigler, K. A., Nurnberger, J. I. and José, J. V. (2013). Autism: the micro-movement perspective. *Frontiers in Integrative Neuroscience*, 7, 32.

Torres, E. B., and Donnellan, A. M. (2015). Editorial for research topic Autism: the movement perspective. *Frontiers in Integrative Neuroscience*, 9, 1.

Tozer, R. (2003). *Involving children with ASD in research about their lives: Methodological issues in interviewing children and young people with learning difficulties*. University of Birmingham: ESRC 2001–2003.

Trevarthen, C. (1979). 'Communication and cooperation in early infancy: A description of primary intersubjectivity. In: M. Bullowa (ed.), *Before speech*, pp. 321–348. Cambridge: Cambridge University Press.

Trevarthen, C. (1990). Signs before speech. In T. A. Sebeok and J. Umiker-Sebeok (eds), *The semiotic web*, pp. 689–755. Berlin: Mouton de Gruyter.

Trevarthen, C., and Delafield-Butt, J. (2013). Autism as a developmental disorder in intentional movement and affective engagement. *Frontiers in Integrative Neuroscience*, 7, 49.

Trimingham, M. (2010). Objects in transition: The puppet and the autistic child. *Journal of Applied Arts and Health*, 11 (3), 251–265

Tronick, E., Als, H., Adamson, L., Wise, S., and Brazelton, T. (1978). The infant's response to entrapment between contradictory messages in face-to-face interaction. *Journal of American Academy of Child Psychiatry*, 17, 1–13.

United Nations (1989). UN Convention on the Rights of the Child (UNCRC). Geneva: United Nations.

Warming, H. (2012). Theorizing (Adults' facilitation of) Children's Participation and Citizenship. In C. I. Baraldi, V. (ed.), *Participation, Facilitation, and Mediation: Children and Young People in Their Social Contexts*. New York: Taylor and Francis.

Warren W. H. (2006). The dynamics of perception and action. *Psychological Review*, 113, 358–389.

Winnicott, D. W. (1971). Playing and reality. New York: Basic Books.

Zahavi, D. (2012). Complexities of Self. *Autism*, 4 (5), 547–551.

MARTINE M. SMITH

8   Accessing the voices of children who use augmentative and alternative communication: Merits and perils of co-construction

Introduction

One of the most remarkable of children's achievements is mastery of the spoken language of their community. This mastery involves the insight that it is possible to influence the thoughts of others through uttering sounds. It involves working out how a continuous sound stream can be segmented to abstract individual units of meaning and storing those units in a way that the sound form can be easily retrieved and reproduced, while also storing information about how that specific sound form or word works within a phrase. While linguists (e.g., Chomsky 1986; Jackendoff 2002; Pinker 1994; Tomasello 2003) strive for theories to explain the structure of language and how it is acquired, children as young as three seem able to abstract and implement the rules of the language(s) of their environment without any formal instruction. Externalising those linguistic rules in order to communicate using speech involves transforming underlying ideas and concepts into rule-based language forms, mapping those units onto speech forms that ultimately must be translated into motor impulses, so that individual muscles move the speech articulators in one of the most rapid motor activities available to humans. For the majority of children, this mastery proceeds with such rapidity that it appears unremarkable.

Despite the ease with which most children accomplish this feat, some children encounter difficulties and a proportion of these children do not develop speech that can be easily understood by others, even by their parents. For many of these children and young people, speech production is not the only aspect of communication that is affected. Their ability to use gesture, manual signs, to effectively control facial expression and even eye gaze may all be compromized. For this group, providing a way to communicate usually involves recruiting other modalities and introducing new ways of communicating. Augmentative and alternative communication (AAC) refers to the use of modalities other than speech to augment or enhance speech that is difficult to understand or to replace speech as a mode of communication, both for expressive purposes and/or to support comprehension or understanding. AAC modes of communication are categorized as either aided or unaided. Unaided modes involve the use of a person's own body, with no external supports; gestures, facial expression, manual signs are all examples of unaided modes. Aided communication modes draw on external physical resources, including pictures, graphic symbols mounted in communication books or displayed on communication boards, as well as computer-based systems and tablet technologies that may incorporate voice output, as well as text and/or symbols.

Using alternative modes of communication introduces new challenges for all participants in interactions. Communicating using aided means is effortful, involving cognitive, linguistic and often also motor demands. Unlike in spoken language interactions, children who use aided communication must focus not only on their intended communication message and their interaction partner, but they must also attend to the external communication aid and to the process of message formulation. For example, if asked about their favourite film or book, children who use aided communication (like their peers without disabilities) must first decide on the film or book and retrieve the appropriate name from memory. However, they must then consider whether or not their external communication aid has the relevant vocabulary to name the film or book and if so, work out how to select that vocabulary. This process often involves navigating through several pages of a device in order to locate the relevant folder and vocabulary item, all the while retaining in memory the target lexical item and its relevance to the question. Even simple messages may take several minutes of navigation and searching, with all the implicit working memory and attention demands this search entails. If the specific vocabulary item is not available (often a problem in instances of highly specific vocabulary such as names of things, places and even people) children have to work out how to give clues that are sufficiently specific for their interaction partner to be able to hazard a reasonable guess. Throughout this process, they must monitor their interaction partner's attention and understanding of their attempts at communication, provide feedback to guide partner attempts at interpretation and persist in the face of incorrect guesses.

Even for adults without disabilities, these demands can disrupt interaction, as the following extract from Smith, McCague, O'Gara and Sammon (Smith et al. 2016: 280) illustrates. In this interaction, two university students are interacting with a peer (PA2) who is using a communication board that contains a combination of words, letters of the alphabet and graphic (i.e., picture-based) symbols. The students are discussing post-Christmas food traditions in their respective families. PA3 and PA4 are using natural speech. PA2 (in italics below) is using aided communication, pointing to spell words or select words on her communication board. The notation '< >' indicates overlap of speaker turns within the discourse.

Extract 6.1

6.1	PA4	The sandwich, this is a tradition in my family
6.2	PA3	God
6.3	*PA2*	*4*[1]
6.4	PA4	Four?
6.5	*PA2*	*5*
6.6	PA4	Five?
6.7	*PA2*	*d-a-y-s*[2]
6.8	PA3	four or five \<days\>
6.9	PA4	\<days\>
6.10	*PA2*	*DOG DOG DOG DOG DOG*[3] (pointing with emphasis)
6.11	PA4	you're getting a dog?

1   Numbers selected by pointing on the communication board.
2   Lower case letters separated by hyphens indicate spelling (see von Tetzchner and Basil, 2011).
3   Upper case italicized forms indicate selection of a whole word or graphic symbol.

6.12	*PA2*	*NO* (shakes head vigorously)
		a-f-<t>
6.13	PA4	<u>do you have</u> a dog?
6.14	*PA2*	*e-r*
6.15	PA4	After
6.16	*PA2*	*4(...)5*
6.17	PA3	Forty-five?
6.18		(all laugh)
6.19	PA4	after forty-five, four forty-five
6.21	*PA2*	(vocalizes, waves hand)
		a-f
6.22	PA4	af?
6.23	*PA2*	*t*
6.24	PA4	ter?
6.25	*PA2*	*4*
6.26	PA4	<u>four</u>
6.27	PA3	<u>four</u>
6.28	*PA2*	*o-<r ʃ>*
6.29	PA3	<u>or five</u>
6.30	*PA2*	*d-a-<y-s>*
6.31	PA4	<u>days</u>
6.32	*PA2*	*DOG DOG DOG DOG* (pointing with emphasis)
6.33	PA4	Dog
6.35	*PA2*	*DINNER DINNER DINNER* (pointing with emphasis)
6.36	PA3	Oh: it's for you to use the food for the dog's dinner! Yea, we give it to the cat

This extract illustrates the challenges of all participants in navigating this conversation successfully, as PA2 strives to time her aided communication contributions to fit with the conversation flow and PA 3 and PA4 work to make sense of those contributions, offering what seem like reasonable interpretations (e.g., 'you're getting a dog') and seeking constant confirmation about the accuracy of their suggested interpretations. It is not difficult to imagine how much challenging similar situations are for young children, who are in the process of learning the language of their community as well as how to use their aided communication system and who may have significant motor difficulties, as well as limited literacy skills to draw on to disambiguate and repair conversational breakdown.

Two issues are explored in this chapter. The first focuses on the inclusion of children's voices in decisions related to their own multimodal communication systems – what their 'voice' should look and sound like; the second relates to the opportunities and risks in interpreting co-constructed meanings in interactions using these voices. Although in this chapter, the focus is on children (that is, primarily those in the pre-adolescent stage of development), the issues raised are equally relevant to adolescents and young adults and are not age-limited.

Including children's voices in decisions about communication systems

Communication styles are unique to individuals, from the pitch of a speaker's voice to the use of gesture, to the specific phrases and mannerisms that identify each speaker as an individual. These identifying traits may be more easily apparent to others than to the speaker; they may emerge with little conscious attention or may be cultivated with care to project a particular persona. Children with significant speech impairments who use aided communication face many significant barriers in projecting their unique identity through their communication. Although children without disabilities may from time to time be required to communicate in a particular way, to adopt a particular tone of voice or to use (or not use) specific vocabulary, the extent to which 'others' control the concrete realization of the voice of children who use aided communication, is without parallel. Children are usually provided with communication aids that have been designed for them by others, incorporating vocabulary selected by others; that vocabulary may be displayed using symbols and organizational structures over which they have little control or choice. The voice that speaks their vocabulary may bear little resemblance to their own perceptions of their desired voice and may be unlike the voices of other children of the same age, gender or cultural background; other children who use aided communication may use exactly the same voice. One partial solution is to record the voice of an age-matched peer, at least for some messages, but the intelligibility of recorded digitized speech of young children can be problematic in terms of intelligibility (Drager and Finke 2012) while choosing a specific peer to act as a voice may be problematic in itself.

Attempts to date at accessing children's views to inform decisions about communication aid design and communication system configuration fall into two main categories: research that explores how children without disabilities can guide design decisions related to communication aids and research that explores the perspectives of children who use aided communication about their own communication systems.

Including children's voices in designing communication systems

One line of research aimed at ensuring that aided communication systems are tailored to the unique needs of children and optimized in terms of functionality has involved recruiting children without disabilities to explore some of the operational demands implicit in aided communication. Such research has focused for example on what types of symbols children find easiest to learn and retain (e.g., Dada et al. 2013; Drager and Light 2010; Mizuko 1987, Yovetich and Young 1988); how best to organize symbols on a display to minimize processing and working memory demands (Drager et al. 2004; McCarthy et al. 2006); exploration of developmental changes in children's ability to cope with aided communication configurations (Drager et al., 2003, Light et al., 2004a); the potential value of applying colour coding to symbols to facilitate location and access (e.g., Thistle and Wilkinson 2009; Thistle and Wilkinson 2017).

Another, more limited line of research has explored the views of children without disabilities on how aided communication systems should be designed to make them child-friendly and motivating (Light et al. 2004b; Light et al. 2007). This latter line of research highlights some of the features that children view as important that may not be as obvious to adults (Light and Drager 2007). For example, in the study by Light et al. (2007), six children without disabilities, aged between seven and ten years, drew or constructed inventions to support the communication of a fictional young child with severe speech and motor impairments and were then interviewed about the design decisions they made. In their discussions, children projected an image of a communication aid as a friend or companion, and created innovative names such as *Mind O'Matic 2000*, in order to make the invention appealing to young children. They incorporated multiple bright colours and lights into their inventions and used a range of materials including soft, squeezable options so that inventions could be hugged or so that children could 'take out their anger' on the device (Light et al. 2007: 280). Their designs involved devices that were either light and portable or large, but the latter were designed to move independently to follow the user around ensuring access at all times. What is striking about these features is that few if any are incorporated into the design of communication devices – even those that have no cost or design implications, such as assigning creative child-friendly names.

Children in Light et al.'s (2007) study also emphasized the importance of ensuring that a communication device was *cool* and supported self-esteem and social image. They stressed the function of their invented communication devices as tools to support interactive play activities, rather than simply to deliver messages. As noted by Light and colleagues, their inventions 'provided the user with *something to do* with others as well *as something to say* to others' (p. 283). This emphasis on the social interaction context and the prioritization of aesthetic appeal are features that even now are only marginally incorporated into device design. Communication aids are often designed from the perspective of adults without disabilities and construed as what Higginbotham and colleagues (Higginbotham et al. 2016, p. 204) term a 'sender-based vocabulary delivery system' rather than an interaction tool. Although the advent of tablet technologies has created new opportunities and drawn communication aid technology into the mainstream, the underlying framing of a communication device as a 'vocabulary delivery system' may create additional barriers to device use for young children, especially when that use entails significant cognitive and motor effort. Research of this kind highlights the importance of asking children for their views on the communication systems may be expected to use.

Incorporating children's perspectives on use of aided communication

Despite their many shortcomings, communication aids represent one way for children with very limited communication options to have a voice, to express themselves and to be heard. The question arises as to whether the effort required to become competent at using aided communication is worth the investment. The limited research available to date highlights a relatively high level of device abandonment or under-utilization, with up to one third of devices not being used with any regularity. Discussions with adults who use aided communication have highlighted that frequency of use is not always a good proxy measure for perceived importance (McCall et al. 1997). Some of the adults interviewed by Smith and Connolly (2008) ranked their aided communication system as critical even though they used it only infrequently, because the situations in which they used aided communication were high-stake situations, where autonomy in communication was critical. There have been few similar attempts to explore the views of young children towards their communication systems, with most research focused on family (Bailey et al. 2006; Crisp et al. 2014; Jonsson et al., 2011; Cress 2004), teacher (Soto et al. 2001; Kent-Walsh et al. 2008) or therapist (Johnson et al. 2006) views about aided communication.

In one of the few studies that directly sought the views of young children about their communication systems, Clarke and colleagues (Clarke et al. 2001) interviewed children (median age twelve years) and young adults about their communication systems and experiences. Of the seventeen children who were interviewed who used aided communication, many expressed views similar to those of the children without disabilities who participated in the study by Light et al. (2007). They articulated a desire to be able to design and tailor a system for themselves. Many valued the control that aided communication afforded ('lets me say anything', 'makes people listen') (p. 111). Their concerns centred on issues such as operational challenges (devices being too heavy, difficult, unreliable); on issues of self-image and identity ('[it is] embarrassing', '[using a symbol book means someone else speaks the words, it is] not my voice' (p. 111); or on problems in interaction, particularly the slow pace of aided communication and the impact of that pace on interaction. Similarly, the adolescents who participated in an anthropological study by Wickenden (2011) talked about adverse reactions from other people, lack of awareness in the wider community of alternative ways of communicating and negative attention related to use of assistive technology that was critical to their independence and autonomy. In contrast to the aspirations of the children who participated in the study by Light et al. (2007), the children interviewed by Clarke et al. (2001) who relied on aided communication, described their communication systems as *uncool, boring.* While tablet technologies may bring greater cachet to the communication situation, and get around some of the *uncool and boring* barriers, such technologies are not suitable for all children who need aided communication. Even with tablet technology, the physical effort involved in communicating is significant, rate of communication is slow and reliability is a concern.

Just as a speaking voice represents only one dimension of the communication identity of children and adults without disabilities, aided communication is only one component in a multimodal communication system for most children with severe communication impairments. There is a significant body of research that indicates that, even for very competent users of communication devices, aided communication is neither the most frequently used mode, nor the preferred mode of communication (Allaire et al. 1991; Andzik et al. 2016; Bailey et al. 2006; Cockerill et al. 2013; Crisp et al. 2014; Smith and Connolly 2008). However, becoming competent at using aided communication takes time and practice. Young children may find that communication partners prescribe use of certain communication modes (that is, certain types of voice), specifying 'say it on your board' or 'use your device', even when a message has been communicated, and has clearly been understood (Smith 2003). Conversely, communication partners can constrain the communication options available to a child who uses multimodal communication, simply by removing a communication book, by switching a device off, or by failing to switch it on.

Choices about where aided communication might be used or how systems are configured are largely outside the control of the children whose voices they are intended to represent. Many children who use aided communication are not physically able to set up their devices and rely on others to position a device or communication boards, to attach switches, turn on a device and ensure set-up meets the child's needs. Once a device or communication board is positioned out of reach, it is no longer an accessible communication option. Use of aided communication may be confined to specific contexts, most often school (Allaire et al. 1991) or therapy environments (Raghavendra et al. 2012). Even within school environments, there may be few opportunities for a child to actively communicate using aided communication (Andzik et al. 2016) and those opportunities are largely dictated by those around them, rather than by the individual child who uses AAC.

Together, these three themes highlight the fact that the voices of children who use aided communication can be muted and distorted in real and concrete ways. They have little choice over the design and configuration of the elements of their voice and often little control over where and with whom they can use that voice. Nonetheless, many children develop remarkably creative ways of navigating conversations in order to develop and assert their identities, to tell and share their stories and to build relationships. Within these interactions, the process of co-construction is a key pillar.

Co-construction in interactions involving aided communication: Hearing and honouring children's voices

Children who use aided communication must make many decisions about what they chose to communicate using symbols or words and what is more efficiently and effectively communicated using eye gaze, vocalization or body movements. These decisions must be nuanced with reference to the specific communication partner. Body movements that are readily interpretable by a very familiar adult may look more like involuntary motor reflexes to an unfamiliar partner, who may therefore not even attempt to ascribe meaning to the very same behaviour. Thus, children who have significant communication impairments must tailor their voice to the competencies of their communication partner, if communication is to be successful.

Although meaning within all interactions is co-constructed, in interactions involving aided communication the extent and nature of this co-construction differs qualitatively and quantitatively. Take the following example taken from Brekke and von Tetzchner (2003: 184) from an interaction between Sander (S), aged 5;10 years, and his teacher (T) using a book containing just under 300 graphic symbols:

Extract 6.2

S   *TALK*[4]
T   *What do you want to talk about?*
S   *UNIT*
T   *Do you want to talk about what happened in the unit?*
S   'Yes' (mouth movements)
T   *Tell me*
S   *LOTTO*
T   *Did you play lotto?*
S   'Yes' (mouth movements)
T   *Who did you play with?*
S   *KITCHEN*
T   *Did you play in the kitchen?*
S   'No' (mouth movements)
T   *Can you indicate the name ... Do you have the name on your board? Can you see the person you played with?*
S   (looks at the kitchen door)
T   *Did you play with Mari who works in the kitchen?*
S   'Yes' (mouth movements)

---

4   *UPPER CASE ITALIC FONT* is the convention used to signal use of a graphic symbol (von Tetzchner and Basil, 2011).

This extract illustrates a number of features of co-construction. The interaction is led by Sander, and his output is constructed over several turns, in what Scollon (1976) classically characterized as a vertical construction. Interspersed between Sander's contributions, his teacher recasts and extends his one-symbol contribution, putting flesh on the bones of the contribution to clarify exactly what meaning is intended, co-constructing the story of what occurred that day. Second, the teacher's familiarity is pivotal in two particular ways. One is her sensitivity and familiarity with Sander's nonverbal communication, his mouth movements that she apparently can reliably distinguish to interpret yes and no responses. The second relates to Sander's gaze towards the kitchen door, which she not only noticed, but could process to interpret a reference to a specific individual, an interpretation critically reliant on familiarity not just with Sander's ways of communicating but also with his world and the people within that world. It is not difficult to imagine a less familiar partner being able to recognize the same communication signals, but being unable to offer an interpretation to match Sander's communicative intent.

This structure of discourse is very common in interactions involving aided communication, where selection of a specific symbol or word is often only a starting point for negotiating intended meanings. Sometimes this kind of explicit negotiation is needed because the vocabulary available in a device or on a communication board does not match the intended message. On another occasion, Sander was discussing a boat trip with his teacher and selected three symbols *GUN, AFRAID* and *ILL*. In the open boat trip, he had felt unwell, was afraid of the swell and experienced the situation as dangerous. Lacking a symbol for 'dangerous', he selected *GUN* as the closest and most relevant symbol (Brekke and von Tetzchner 2003: 183). Successful flexible use of symbols relies not only on the creativity of the individual child, but also on the openness of communication partners to explore how a symbol might be relevant (Sperber and Wilson 1996) and on partners' willingness to engage in guessing and to persist with the negotiation, without imposing their own interpretation.

Dyads can be remarkably successful in co-constructing an agreed interpretation of meanings in these interactions. For example, in the following extract taken from Smith (2015: 216), a young student, J, is interacting with his teaching assistant (P), describing a video clip he just watched while she was out of the room. In this extract, J is using a voice output device and selecting each word individually.

Extract 6.3
J *'bad'*
P *oh, bad*
J *'boy' 'yellow' 'down'*
P *oh, oooh no, J. When you say yellow, is it something that's yellow?*
J *'yes'* (signals yes)
P *ahh, does the bad boy make somebody fall down?*
J *'yes'* (signals yes)
P *on a banana?*

From minimal output, the communication partner in this instance managed to co-construct a remarkably complete narrative, so that the sequence *bad boy yellow down* was interpreted as a narrative about a boy making someone fall on a banana. While such examples point to the extraordinary creativity of all those involved, the process of constructing elaborated interpretations from sparse communication offerings also poses risks. One is the risk of failure – an inability to resolve how a particular symbol is to be interpreted or glossed to represent the target meaning. For example, Jagoe and Smith (2016: 236) describe an extensive interaction lasting almost seven minutes between a young boy, Noel, and his teaching assistant, as Noel attempted to describe a picture that was not visible to the teaching assistant. The symbols he selected shared visual similarities with the picture to be described, but his partner focused on the written label of the symbols and so was unable to interpret how the symbols could be relevant to the conversation. For anyone who could see the picture, Noel's attempts made perfect sense; for his partner who did not have access to that background information, the symbols he selected were impossible to connect to a plausible scenario. While communication is often grounded in familiar territory, non-routine events, unexpected experiences or novel occurrences are also important communication triggers. In fact, it may be that unexpected personal experiences are critically important for children to be able to communicate to a trusted partner, precisely because that partner was not present at the time of the experience.

A second risk of relying heavily on partner familiarity to gloss interpretations of messages is that this strategy limits the range of communication partners likely to be able to successfully engage in interactions. Glossing the units of meaning offered often relies on having extensive shared background knowledge in order to make sense of the communication. For example, Smith et al. (2018: 50) describe an interaction between a mother and a young girl using a voice output communication device, as she relays to her mother the contents of a video clip she has just viewed of a mother jumping into a pool, while her children stood on the edge of the pool and laughed. To open the conversation, the young girl selected a pre-stored sentence in her device *I've made my first communion*, to which her mother responded *when we went swimming? Is it something about swimming?* This example illustrates not only the creativity of the young girl in finding a way to set the topic of the conversation through re-using an existing message, but also the ability of her mother to recognize that the message was relevant and should be interpreted as such, prompting her to think beyond a literal meaning to what the utterance could mean beyond the meaning of the words. However, other communication partners, no matter how skilful, might fail in this interaction, due to their lack of shared experiences. Linguistic communication offers a crucial bridge between environments and experiences. If children using aided communication rely on communication partners' knowledge of their experiences, they become vulnerable to self-limited social networks (e.g., Raghavendra et al. 2012), creating future risks of isolation (e.g., Oscar described in Smith, 2014) and potential silencing.

A third risk of rich co-construction in interactions involving aided communication relates to ownership of what is communicated. For children whose voices are reliant on the glossing and articulation of others, co-construction that applies layers of meaning and of grammar can transform messages in ways that may enhance the message but that may move some distance from the original intended communication. If a child accepts a gloss as an acceptable interpretation of their intended meaning, it is reasonable to infer that the glossed words are an accurate representation of what they would have said themselves? If a child agrees that is what they *meant*, does that mean that is what they *said*? There may be many reasons why a child might accept a glossed interpretation of their message even if the match with their intended communication is less than perfect. One reason might be that agreement is simply the easier option. Unless the communication involves high-stake outcomes, it may not be worth the effort of trying again to arrive at a closer match to the intended message. Alternatively, the proposed interpretation may be a much more interesting one and accepting that interpretation may extend an interaction that is pleasurable and rewarding. A third reason may be an over-developed tendency to comply with adult suggestions. This feature is cited as a risk factor for children with intellectual disability (Wissink et al. 2015) linked to their extended dependency on adults and it seems likely that the even greater dependence needs of children who use aided communication might lead to similar patterns of compliance. The vulnerability of young people who rely on aided communication and partner co-construction is exemplified in controversies such as those surrounding Facilitated Communication (Biklen 1992; Crossley, 1994; Schlosser et al. 2014), more recently referred to as Supported Typing or the Rapid Prompting Method (e.g., Tostanoski et al. 2014). At the core of the controversies surrounding these interventions is the question of ownership and authorship of communication messages (Mirenda 2017, Schlosser et al. 2014). The importance of being able to rigorously identify authorship is particularly critical where communication relates to personal safety and protection from harm (Travers et al. 2014).

Conclusion

The skills of communication partners in interpreting and co-constructing messages in interactions involving aided communication represent both opportunities and risks for children who use aided communication. Silencing the voices of aided communicators is remarkably easy. In fact, ensuring that their voices are authentically heard is far more difficult.

Balancing the demands of creating and supporting successful communication interactions, while promoting autonomy and independence in what
might be an effortful communicative process requires constant attention
and vigilance. There are rich opportunities to draw children's voices into
the discussions about how communication systems should be designed
and configured and there are indications that their insights are important
and unique. Their input into their own communication systems, their
own voices may be key to supporting them to invest the required effort to
master the operational and linguistic demands of aided communication.
Ultimately, questions about the ownership, authorship and autonomy of
their communication will be best addressed through enabling them to
become independent communicators, for whom co-construction operates
as it does interactions for most speakers: a useful oil for conversational flow,
but owned equally by all participants in the interaction.

References

Allaire, J., Gressard, R., Blackman, J., and Hostler, S. (1991). Children with severe
    speech impairments: caregiver survey of AAC use. *Augmentative and Alterna-
    tive Communication,* 7(4), 248–255.
Andzik, N., Chung, Y.-C. and Kranak, M. (2016). Communication opportunities for
    elementary school students who use augmentative and alternative communica-
    tion. *Augmentative and Alternative Communication,* 32 (3), 272–281.
Bailey, R., Parette, H., Stone, J., Angell, M., and Carroll, K. (2006). Family members'
    perceptions of augmentative and alternative communication device use. *Language
    Speech and Hearing Services in Schools,* 37 (1), 50–60.
Biklen, D. (1992). Typing to talk: Facilitated communication. *American Journal of
    Speech-Language Pathology,* 1 (1), 15–17.
Brekke, K. M., and von Tetchner, S. (2003). Co-construction in graphic language
    development. In S. von Tetzchner, S. and N. Grove (eds), *Augmentative
    and Alternative Communication: Developmental Issues,* pp. 176–210. London:
    Whurr.
Chomsky, N. (1986). *Knowledge of language: Its nature, origins and use.* London:
    Praeger Press.

Clarke, M., McConachie, H., Price, K., and Wood, P. (2001). Views of young people using augmentative and alternative communication systems. *International Journal of Language and Communication Disorders,* 36 (1), 107–115.

Cockerill, H., Elbourne, D., Allen, E., Scrutten, D., Will, E., McNee, A., Fairhurst, C., and Baird, G. (2013). Speech, communication and use of augmentative communication in young people with cerebral palsy: The SHandPE population study. *Child: Care, health and development,* 40 (2), 149–157.

Cress, C. (2004). Augmentative and alternative communication and language: Understanding and resopnding to parents' perspectives. *Topics in Language Disorders,* 24 (1), 51–61.

Crisp, C., Draucker, C., and Ellett, M. (2014). Barriers and facilitators to children's use of speech-generating devices: a qualitative study of mothers' perspectives. *Journal for Specialists in Pediatric Nursing,* 19 (3), 229–237.

Crossley, R. (1994). *Facilitated communication training.* New York: NY Teacher's College, Columbia University.

Dada, S., Huguet, A., and Bornman, J. (2013). The iconicity of Picture Communication Symbols for children with English as an additional language and mild intellectual disability. *Augmentative and Alternative Communication,* 29 (4), 360–373.

Drager, K., and Finke, E. (2012). Intelligibility of children's speech in digitised speech. *Augmentative and Alternative Communication,* 28 (2), 181–189.

Drager, K. D. and Light, J. (2010). A comparison of the performance of 5-year-old children with typical development using iconic encoding in AAC systems with and without icon prediction on a fixed display. *Augmentative and Alternative Communication,* 26 (1), 12–20.

Drager, K. D., Light, J. C., Carlson, R., D'Silva, K., Larsson, B., Pitkin, L., and Stopper, G. (2004). Learning of dynamic display AAC technologies by typically developing 3-year-olds: effect of different layouts and menu approaches. *Journal of Speech Language and Hearing Research,* 47 (5), 1133–1148.

Drager, K. D., Light, J. C., Speltz, J. C., Fallon, K. A., and Jeffries, L. Z. (2003). The performance of typically developing 2 1/2-year-olds on dynamic display AAC technologies with different system layouts and language organizations. *Journal of Speech Language and Hearing Research,* 46 (2), 298–312.

Higginbotham, D. J., Fulcher, K., and Seale, J. (2016). Time and timing in interactions involving individuals with ALS, their unimpaired partners and their speech generating devices. In M. Smith, and J. Murray (eds), *The Silent Partner? Language, interaction and aided communication,* pp. 199–229. London: JandR Press.

Jackendoff, R. (2002). *Foundations of Language: Brain, meaning, grammar, evolution.* Oxford: Oxford University Press.

Jagoe, C., and Smith, M. (2016). Relevance, multimodality and aided communication. In M. Smith, and J. Murray (eds), *The Silent Partner? Language, interaction and aided communication*, pp. 229–246. London: JandR Press.

Johnson, J. M., Inglebret, E., Jones, C., and Ray, J. (2006). Perspectives of speech language pathologists regarding success versus abandonment of AAC. *Augmentative and Alternative Communication*, 22 (2), 85–99.

Jonsson, A., Kristofferson, L., Ferm, U., and Thunberg, G. (2011). The ComAlong communication boards: Parents' use and experiences of aided language stimulation. *Augmentative and Alternative Communication*, 27 (2), 103–116.

Kent-Walsh, J., Stark, C., and Binger, C. (2008). Tales from school trenches: AAC service delivery and professional expertise. *Seminars in Speech and Language*, 29 (2), 146–154.

Light, J., and Drager, K. (2007). AAC technologies for young children with complex communication needs: State of the science and future research directions. *Augmentative and Alternative Communication*, 23 (2), 204–216.

Light, J., Drager, K. D., McCarthy, J., Mellott, S., Millar, D., Parrish, C., Parsons, A., Rhoads, S., Ward, M., and Welliver, M. (2004a). Performance of typically developing four and five year old children with AAC systems using different language organisation techniques. *Augmentative and Alternative Communication*, 20 (1), 63–88.

Light, J., Drager, K. D., and Nemser, J. (2004b). Enhancing the appeal of AAC technologies for young children: Lessons from the toy manufacturers. *Augmentative and Alternative Communication*, 20 (2), 137–149.

Light, J., Page, R., Curran, J., and Pitkin, L. (2007). Children's ideas for the design of AAC technologies for young children with complex communication needs. *Augmentative and Alternative Communication*, 23 (3), 274–287.

McCall, F., Marková, I., Murphy, J., Moodie, E., and Collins, S. (1997). Perspectives on AAC systems by the users and by their communication partners. *European Journal of Disorders of Communication*, 32 (3), 235–256.

McCarthy, J., Light, J., Drager, K., McNaughton, D., Grodzicki, L., Jones, J., Panek, E., and Parkin, E. (2006). Re-designing scanning to reduce learning demands: The performance of typically developing 2-year-olds. *Augmentative and Alternative Communication*, 22 (4), 269–283.

Mirenda, P. (2017). Values, practice, science and AAC. *Research and Practice for Persons with Severe Disabilities*, 42 (1), 33–41.

Mizuko, M. I. (1987). Transparency and ease of learning symbols represented by Blissymbols, PCS, and Picsyms. *Augmentative and Alternative Communication*, 3 (2), 129–136.

Pinker, S. (1994). *The language instinct. The new science of language and mind*. London: Allan Lane, The Penguin Press.

Raghavendra, P., Olsson, C., Sampson, J., McInerny, R., and Connell, T. (2012). School participation and social networks of children with complex communication needs, physical disabilities and typically developing peers. *Augmentative and Alternative Communication, 28* (1), 33–43.

Schlosser, R., Balandin, S., Hemsley, B., Iacono, T., Probst, P., and von Tetzchner, S. (2014). Facilitated Communication and authorship: A systematic review. *Augmentative and Alternative Communication, 30* (4), 359–368.

Scollon, R. (1976). *Conversations with a one year old.* Honolulu: University Press of Hawaii.

Smith, M. (2003). Environmental influences on aided language development: the role of partner adaptation. In S. von Tetzchner, and N. Grove (eds), *Augmentative and Alternative Communication: Developmental Issues,* pp. 155–175. London: Whurr.

Smith, M. (2014). Adolescence and AAC: Intervention challenges and possible solutions. *Communication Disorders Quarterly, 36* (1), 112–118.

Smith, M., and Connolly, I. (2008). Roles of aided communication: perspectives of adults who use AAC. *Disability and Rehabilitation: Assistive Technology, 3* (5), 260–73.

Smith, M., McCague, E., O'Gara, J., and Sammon, S. (2016). '... this is not going to be like, you know, standard communication?': Naturally speaking adults using aided communication'. In M. Smith, and J. Murray (eds), *The Silent Partner? Language, interaction and aided communication,* pp. 269–288. London: J and R Press.

Smith, M., Batorowicz, B., Dahlgren Sandberg, A., Murray, J., Stadskleiv, K., van Balkom, H., Neuvonen, K., and von Tetzchner, S. (2018). Constructing narratives to describe video events using aided communication. *Augmentative and Alternative Communication, 34,* 40–53. DOI: 10.1080/07434618.2017.1422018

Soto, G., Muller, E., Hunt, P., and Goetz, L. (2001). Critical issues in the inclusion of students who use augmentative and alternative communication: An educational team perspective. *Augmentative and Alternative Communication, 17* (1), 62–72.

Sperber, D., and Wilson, D. (1996). Précis of Relevance: Communication and Cognition. In H. Geirsson, and M. Losonsky (eds) *Readings in Language and Mind,* pp. 460–486. London: Blackwell.

Thistle, J., and Wilkinson, K. (2009). The effects of color cues on typically developing preschoolers' speed of locating a target line drawing: Implications for augmentative and alternative communication display design. *American Journal of Speech-Language Pathology, 18,* 231–240.

Thistle, J., and Wilkinson, K. (2017). Effects of background color and symbol arrangement cues on constrution of multi-symbol messages by young children without disabilities: implications for aided AAC design. *Augmentative and Alternative Communication, 33* (3), 160–169.

Tomasello, M. (2003). *Constructing a language: A usage-based theory of language acquisition*. London: Harvard University Press.

Tostansoki, A., Lang, R., Raulston, T., Carnett, A., and Davis, T. (2014). Voices from the past: Comparing the rapid prompting method and facilitated communication. *Developmental Neurorehabilitation*, 17 (4), 219–223.

Travers, J., Tincani, M., and Lang, R. (2014). Facilitated communication denies people with disabilities their voice. *Research and Practice for Persons with Severe Disabilities*, 39 (2), 195–202.

von Tetzchner, S., and Basil, C. (2011). Terminology and notation in written representations of conversations with Augmentative and Alternative Communication. *Augmentative and Alternative Communication*, 27 (2), 141–149.

Wickenden, M. (2011). Talking to teenagers: Using anthropological methods to explore identity and the lifeworlds of young people who use AAC. *Communication Disorders Quarterly*, 32 (2), 151–163.

Wissink, I., van Vugt, E., Moonen, X., Stams, G.-J., and Hendriks, J. (2015). Sexual abuse involving children with an intellectual disability (ID): A narrative review. *Research in Developmental Disabilities*, 36 (1), 20–35.

Yovetich, W., and Young, T. (1988). The effects of representativeness and concreteness on the "guessability" of Blissymbols', *Augmentative and Alternative Communication*, 4 (1), 35–39.

CLARE CARROLL

9   Let me tell you about my rabbit! Listening to the needs and preferences of the child in early intervention

We all go about our day to day lives interacting within our different contexts, for example, home and work. We can freely share with others what is important to us and we make choices and decisions about who we interact with and what activities we want to do. A child goes about his/her day to day routines within his/her familiar contexts (home/childcare/school) interacting with the people, objects, animals and places that are important to them. He/she too makes choices and decisions. A child lives in the context of a family system and the child's parents and siblings also go about their day to day routines interacting in their different contexts. The transactional model of development stresses that the child and their contexts shape each other and that this complex interaction impacts on development (Sameroff 2009). We are learning more about how the contexts of a child's world are extremely important and about how the day to day lives of the child and family are interdependent. We recognize that knowing more about the contexts in which a child interacts, in particular the distal influences, such as family, childcare and education is needed. Being mindful of the transactional model, let us think about a child with a neurodevelopmental disorder who needs the support of a team of early intervention practitioners to reach his/her potential. This child has significant developmental challenges that impact on their personal, social, educational or occupational functioning, for example, global developmental delay, intellectual disability, autism spectrum disorder. The early intervention practitioners cannot support the child and family without knowing their contexts, interests and needs. Therefore, the child and family and professionals become a unit/team and each team member needs a space to be heard and included.

Article 3 of the United Nations Convention on the Rights of the Child (UNCRC) established the principle that all children should enjoy the 'freedom to seek, receive and impart information and ideas of all kinds' (Office of the United Nations High Commissioner for Human Rights 1989). Hearing the voices of children who use early intervention services will not only facilitate everyone who supports the children in understanding their experiences but will also help embed the child's voice in collaborative practice.

Considering the child's ecological system (Bronfenbrenner 1979) we must understand the macrosystem of where their early intervention service is situated. Within the macrosystem, legislation and policies guide each country on the delivery of services and demonstrate a country's commitment to listening to children and families. In Ireland, at the start of the new millennium, the National Children's Strategy emphasized that a child's voice will be heard and that they will receive quality supports and services to reach their potential (Department of Health and Children 2000). This Strategy reinforced the UNCRC, specifically Articles 23 and 24, which focus on the right of children with disabilities to care, education and training and on the right to the access to services respectively (Office of the United Nations High Commisioner for Human Rights 1989). Currently, the National Policy Framework for Children and Young People 2014–2020 in Ireland, 'Better Outcomes Brighter Future' (Government of Ireland 2014) sets out six transformational goals which include supporting parents, listening to children, strengthening efforts to support children in expressing their views. All children and young people's services are informed by the principles of rights, family-oriented, equality, evidence informed and outcomes focused (Government of Ireland 2014). In Ireland, the commitment to focus on respecting and listening to children is signified further with the publication of Ireland's first 'National Strategy on Children and Young People's Participation in Decision-making' to ensure that children have a say in decisions that affect their lives (Department of Children and Youth Affairs 2015). This strategy aims to ensure that children will have a voice in decision-making was launched progressing the values and principles of participation and inclusion further (Daly et al. 2015).

Within the child's exosystem in Ireland, there is a wide variation in how services to young children with neurodevelopmental disorders are delivered (Carroll et al. 2013). A national programme called 'Progressing Disability Services for Children and Young People' is guiding the delivery of services for children with neurodevelopmental disorders whereby Children's Disability Network Teams support children with complex needs. For these services to work well for children and families they must be informed by the perspectives of all who use them. Yung (2010) recognizes that interventions must work well for both the child and their family for the child to reach their potential. Collaboration and relationships underpin Early Intervention (EI) services (Matthews and Rix 2013; Carroll and Sixsmith 2016a).

We recognize that there is a pressing need to include children with neurodevelopmental disorders as participants in research and practice in order to understand their micro and mesosytems. Because voices of children with disabilities have been overlooked in research (Kelly 2007; 2017) their voices have been excluded. We need to respond to our ethical responsibility and explore ways to make their participation a reality (Merrick 2011) in order to understand their experiences and to maximize their participation and that of their families (Department of Health and Children 2000). If we are to understand true family-centred services we need to hear the child and family perspectives. Parents' views are extremely important and they are fundamental to facilitate their child in reaching their full potential (Bailey et al. 2006; Bruder 2010). However with research advancing and the recognition of children as competent social actors it is not enough to rely on adult proxies (Beresford 1997; Markham and Dean 2006; Markham, van Laar, Gibbard, and Dean 2009). Nevertheless, it is important to recognize the role that parents play in supporting the interpretations of their child's communicative signals (Press et al. 2011; Carroll and Sixsmith 2016a). The following section will present some data from a pilot study on which a larger study was developed. The pilot study aimed to ascertain if young children with neurodevelopmental disorders could partake in the research process, namely data collection, and if so how could their views be included in a bigger study (please see end of chapter for Carroll and Sixmith (2016a)). The bigger qualitative study aimed to understand what supports and hinders early intervention services in Ireland from the perspectives of children, parents and professionals (Carroll and Sixmith 2016b; O'Shaughnessy Carroll 2016). Drawing on the pilot study with three children with neurodevelopmental disorders carried out by the author it was evident that although we want to hear the voices of young children with neurodevelopmental disorders in research accessing these children can be challenging.

Accessing young children with developmental disabilities: An example

The author wanted to explore how young children aged between three and five years with neurodevelopmental disorders could participate in the research process. For the pilot, the author wanted a gatekeeper from one early intervention service within the Health Service Executive in Ireland to select three child participants. The team nurse agreed to act as the gatekeeper. The author made phone and email contact with the gatekeeper and sent written information about the research and the recruitment process. The author asked her to select three children on the team's current EI caseload to include: range of severity: mild/moderate/severe global developmental delay; range for length of time involved in team: new (greater than 6 months), regularly involved, and ready for discharge; Range of Age: between two and five years. The gatekeeper was uncertain how to select the children based on the sampling strategy. Questions arose in relation to the range of severity and how it was defined. For example, were the child's difficulties defined quantitatively, in terms of cognitive scores on standarized tests? The gatekeeper highlighted that not all the children attending the EI service had quantitative measures of their difficulties. All children had qualitative measures of their strengths and weaknesses and some children had quantitative measures. In relation to the length of time a child was involved with the service, this data was not readily available to the gatekeeper. Subsequently, this led to uncertainty in the selection of the participants and following telephone and email contact with the gatekeeper over a six-month period, recruitment proved unsuccessful. Unfortunately, access to participants from this particular EI team proved lengthy and challenging. On reflection of the recruitment process, the author can only make assumptions as to why the process failed. Time pressures and lack of clarity in relation to the sampling strategy posed challenging for the gatekeeper. It could also be argued that this particular EI system did not have a framework in place to facilitate research with children. The learning, from this lengthy, unsuccessful recruitment process, facilitated the author to review the sampling strategy and recruitment process. Lewis and Porter (2004) argue that tensions can arise when sources of information and lines of communication are unclear. The view of children as being potentially vulnerable may be a stereotype that masks individual children's abilities, competencies and understandings (Hill, Davis, Prout, and Tisdall 2004). A new purposeful sampling strategy to support the recruitment process included: child with complex needs attending an early intervention team; range of age between two and five years. The new recruitment process involved: phone and email contact with the gatekeeper and where possible a face to face meeting. This was followed by a timeline of two months for the recruitment process with opportunity for reflection. The author acknowledged that in the event of difficulties arising the process should be abandoned in a timely fashion if no resolution was likely. Subsequently, the recruitment process with a different team was successful whereby young children with neurodevelopmental disorders were given the opportunity to take part in the study.

When entering the research field, it is important for researchers to be aware of their assumptions prior to recruitment. The author made the assumption that the EI team would want to participate in research in order to make their service better and would be willing to gain an understanding of the children's experiences of their service. When the gatekeeper selected and contacted families, parents were willing for their children to participate with some families very keen to participate. From an ethical perspective, I did not and could not directly approach the child and family without permission from the organisation. In the first recruitment process, the power of the gatekeeper was clearly exercised. Because the organization did not become involved the families and children did not get an opportunity to make a decision regarding their own involvement in the research study.

As discussed by Hood, Kelley and Mayall (1996) successful access to the children is only achieved by negotiating within the accepted framework of the 'hierarchy of gatekeeping'. Because research ethics committees and different levels of gatekeepers may stipulate so many safeguards, researchers often abandon their attempts to access children directly (Coyne 2010). Lewis and Porter (2004: 192) acknowledge that intermediaries have power to shape 'what is researched and whose voices are heard'. Nevertheless it is very important that researchers reflect, persevere and try again with a second recruitment process and uphold their resilient focus to facilitate children to have their voices heard (Christensen and James 2008; National Children's Bureau 2008; Office of the United Nations High Commisioner for Human Rights 1989).

Development of a protocol to facilitate children with disabilities in the research process

The pilot study checked the feasibility of the participation of children in the research and explored and evaluated the engagement of children with disabilities in the research process. The successful outcome of this feasibility study, which included three children with neurodevelopmental disorders, led to the development of a protocol to facilitate children in the research process based on Clarke and Moss's (2001) framework for listening. My objectives were to interact with the young children with disabilities in ways that respected their particular competence (Thomas and O'Kane 2000) and their unique and valued view of the world (Greene and Hill 2005); to view the children as active members of their EI team and to add the children's voices and engage them in the research process. The author needed to understand the context of the child's communication and the context of their early intervention service, the nature of the child's communication difficulties and style and how and why the child communicates in order to fulfill the aims of the pilot study. Given that this research was with children with a range of speech, language and communication needs, secondary to their primary diagnoses, the author used her skills as a speech and language therapist (SLT) and adopted an open, sensitive, flexible approach in her interactions with the children as is recommended when dealing with a heterogeneous sample of children with disabilities (Begley 2000; Kelly 2007; Watson, Abbott, and Townsley 2006).

Clark and Moss (2001; 2011) developed the Mosaic approach, which adopts an interpretivist approach for listening to children's perspectives, within a research context. There are six components to Clark and Moss (2011) framework for listening which is as follows: multi-method process, participatory, reflexive, adaptable, focused on children's lived experiences and embedded in practice. Methods of data collection with children with disabilities were in accordance with best practice guidelines (Whyte 2006) and how the children with disabilities were included in this study is discussed by Carroll and Sixsmith (2016a). The multi-method data collection process involved:

- at the outset discussions with the primary caregiver on how best to facilitate their child's participation and engage in the interaction;
- each interaction involved the child, researcher and one or both parents, was audio recorded and took place in the child's home;
- the use of a SenseCam, developed by Microsoft Research UK, facilitated auto photography and proved to be an innovative tool to collect observational data. The images facilitated a visual account of the experiences and contexts of the child's world. Vicon Motion Systems has now licensed the technology;
- Talking Mats (Murphy 1997) were used as a prop with the images and other pictures in my interactions with the children;
- informal observations;
- multiple interactions;
- a total communication approach was used, where non-verbal communication such as body language, facial expression, signing, gestures and pictures were valued as much as spoken language (Fargas-Malet, McSherry, Larkin, and Robinson, 2010).

The multi-method process facilitated the children's views to become embedded in the research process. An example from one of the three children will share more detail of how the child's voices was heard.

Noel: A case study example

At the time of the research, Noel was three years and ten months old and lived at home with his mother, father and three sisters. He was due to start preschool within three months. The author spoke with his mother prior to the first home visit. His mother described him as a friendly outgoing boy who was learning and developing all the time. The author visited the family on three occasions. On the first visit the author had a short interaction with Noel and his mother and gave the family the SenseCam. A SenseCam (as seen in figure 9.1) is a camera that can be worn around the neck and it takes photos automatically when the person wearing it moves.

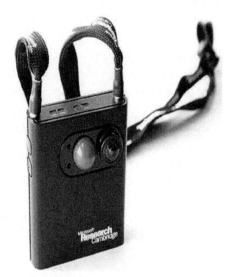

Figure 9.1: SenseCam

The second visit involved a short interaction with Noel and his mother and the author collected the SenseCam. For the third visit, the author had an opportunity to observe a home visit by the SLT that involved Noel, his mother and the SLT working together. The fourth visit involved Noel, his mother and the author using Talking Mats, SenseCam images, and pictures during the interaction.

SenseCam

Noel wore the SenseCam over four days for a total of 27.5 hrs (Average: 6.7 hrs per day). During these hours the contexts of his experiences were at home, most frequently in the back garden and in the kitchen, but there were also images in a bedroom, and in the sitting room. Other contexts included in the car, at an art class, at the shop, family, and visiting another house. His world involved people (mother, father, sisters, granddad) and objects (trike, TV, stacker, musical instruments, his bottle) and animals (rabbit, cats and dog). Activities involved sticking, gluing, making play-doh, making music, drinking, running, cycling, visiting, sitting, interacting with people. The SenseCam took photographs as Noel moved and was sensitive to light changes and movement. Because Noel was walking independently there were a lot of images. Some pictures were unclear and blurred. Examples of images include the following:

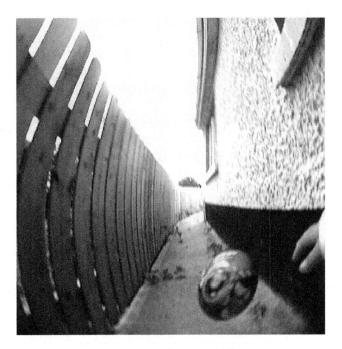

Figure 9.2: Chasing my ball

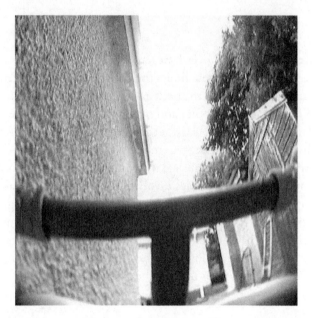

Figure 9.3: Outside on my trike

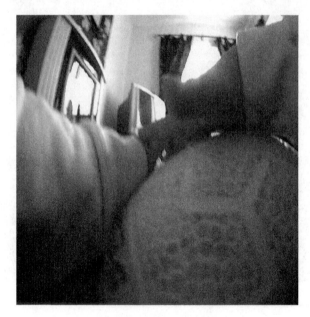

Figure 9.4: Holding my ball

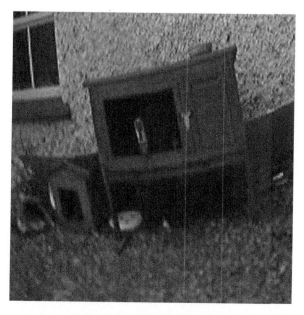

Figure 9.5: My rabbit's hutch

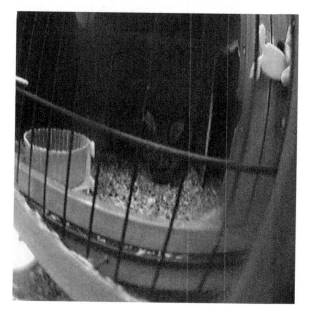

Figure 9.6: My rabbit

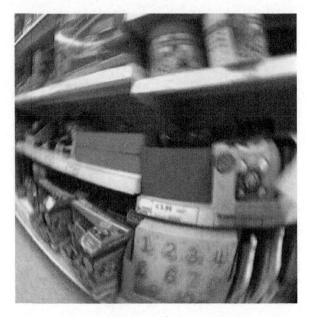

Figure 9.7: Shopping

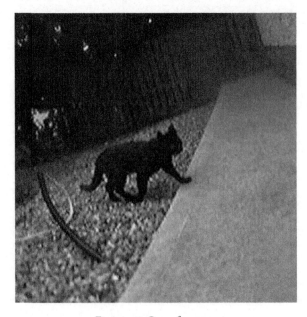

Figure 9.8: One of my cats

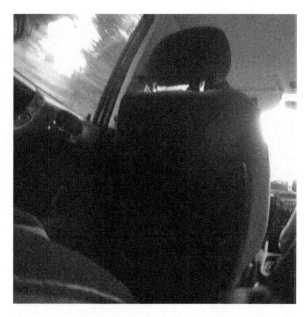

Figure 9.9: In the car

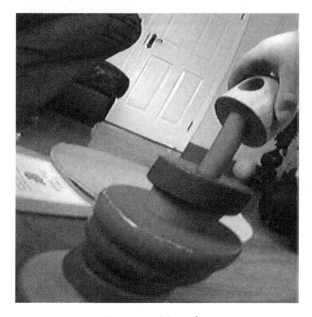

Figure 9.10: My stacker

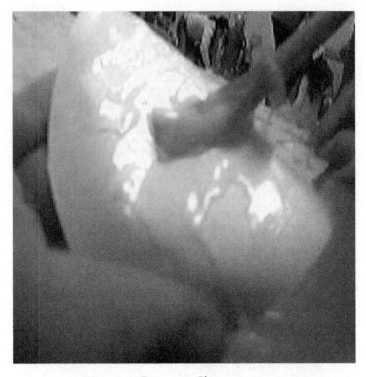

Figure 9.11: Gluing

Observation of SLT Home Visit

The SLT home visit lasted 45 minutes. The author sat in the corner of the room and the SLT interacted mainly with Noel. His mother interacted and helped although the interaction was mainly between Noel and SLT. The author took detailed notes of the session. Noel engaged in turn-taking, imitation, and communicated his needs and wants. He communicated using Lámh signs (Irish Manual Signing System) and his body together with word approximations. His word approximations contained different consonant and vowel structures, for example, vowels only (V), consonant plus vowel combinations (CV), and some consonant plus vowel plus consonant plus vowel combinations (CVCV). Noel sat for most of the session and smiled and engaged. The activities included listening to vehicle sounds and matching the sound to a picture (the sounds were animals vehicles); matching objects to pictures; matching pictures to pictures; matching objects in songs and then playing with bubbles at the end. The SLT gave the mother a worksheet of activities at the end and planned for the next session.

Following the observation the author discussed the session with his mother. His mother explained that it was great to have the services coming to the home and that the session was typical of how he would be in an SLT session. The author asked his mother if Noel knew what was going on and how his mother felt he was getting on. His mother responded by saying that she was sure he did know what was going on and that *once the speech therapist comes to the house there is a routine and he understands the routine.* When the author queried how he knew the routine she explained that listening is first and then matching a picture to a picture and so on. His mother reported that the SLT directs the activities for the most part and Noel would let her know when he was finished and had enough. The author observed Noel signing 'finished' when he wanted to move on to another activity. His mother also explained that when Noel can do something the activities change. The author explored with his mother regarding choices and she explained that *the SLT decides what we do and the OT comes with a big bag and he chooses.* The author observations were that the session was clinician directed and there was little conversation with the mother during the activities. There were no choices for Noel during the intervention. The animal activity observed did not include a horse, cat or rabbit, which are of particular interest to Noel. However, when the author asked his mother if she knew why the activities were being done and for most of them she did. This supports the view that the mother understood the rationale to support the choice of activities.

Interview with Noel

The interaction lasted 50 minutes. When using the SenseCam images Noel chose the pictures of his art class and the glue picture.

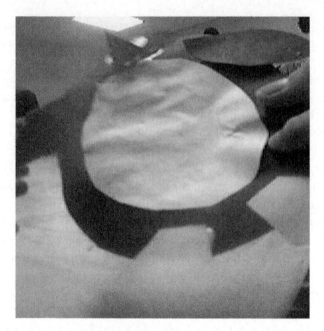

Figure 9.12: My penguin at art class

He also chose the group activity, his trike, baby, his cat, his stacker and his rabbit, mammy, two sisters, shop, paint, ball, and music. The interaction was child led and there was a lot of signing, word approximations and clapping hands, as well as pointing and looking at the author and his mother. He vocalized a lot and made attempts to name the objects/people when picking them up. He looked intently at the pictures. The author also used nursery rhyme pictures and Noel placed on the Talking Mat, under the smiley face, Baa Baa Black Sheep, Old McDonald, Twinkle Twinkle, Wheels on the Bus and Incy Wincy Spider.

He used a lot of signing as he sang the songs. The author made a story of Noel's preferences and contexts and experiences. Content analysis was used to make sense of the volume of material. Images were grouped into events by the author to form a pictorial diary of the child's experience. Noel decided that he didn't want to use the Talking Mat anymore and used his own coloured mats (one for likes and one for dislikes as he was very clear) another example of adapting and being flexible during the research process. Also an indication that Noel could communicate his wants.

Findings and conclusions

Following the interactions with the three children in the pilot study thematic analysis revealed four main themes which are listed below and interconnections between the themes are shown in Figure 9.13.

1. *Describing Child* included the child's personality, their development and their concentration.
2. *Communication* included how the child communicates (greeting, commenting, responding, requesting, understanding and why and their communication environment.
3. *Services* included needs, context and interactions in terms of how they interact with services and with whom and where.
4. *Activities* included the child's communication environment, their likes, and their choices, the child's interests in terms of what does he/she do? And where does he/she go?

This study represents a beginning in the realization of one of the National Framework (Government of Ireland, 2014) goals to achieve better outcomes. This is realized through an example of listening and involving children in a research process aiming to support evidence informed intervention. Research with children is difficult and is compounded by the complexity of their abilities and needs. Noel successfully communicated his experiences and contexts via pictures, his mother and via interviews with the author. His mother verified his communication skills during interactions and shared how he communicated, his personality, his routines and she aided the author's interpretation of Noel's communication attempts when they were unclear. The SenseCam images added and supported information and provided context to his experiences. His mother supported what

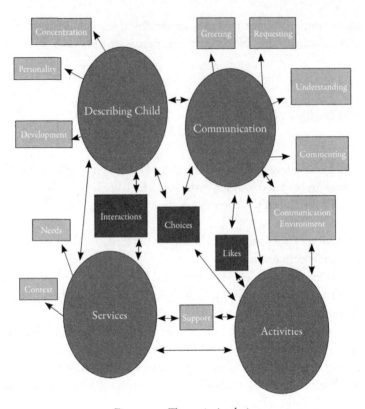

Figure 9.13: Thematic Analysis

was captured in his world, for example, people and animals by providing names and details. The author's awareness of strategies to promote effective interaction with children from a SLT perspective, for example, following the child's lead, eye contact, physically and verbally followed the child's lead, knowledge of sign language and interpretation of word approximations, also facilitated the research.

The discovery of the child's world through the use of the SenseCam is truly amazing. This tool allows us to get a real sense of the child's interests and a view of their microsystem. The amount of interactions that Noel had with his rabbit, his cats and his dog in the short period of time wearing the SenseCam allows us to get a sense of how important his animals are to him. It acknowledges the importance of animals in children's lives

(Sixsmith, Nic Gabhainn, Fleming and O'Higgins 2007). Although, Noel visited his rabbit's hutch and followed his cat a lot these activities did not feature in the early discussions with his mother. The use of the SenseCam images shaped subsequent interactions with Noel and his mother. We need to consider multiple methods to understand a child's interests and routines.

The findings relate to Bronfenbrenner's (2006) Process Person Context Time (PPCT) model as the child and parent created evidence related to child characteristics, contexts in which the child interacts at a particular time in the child's life. Knowledge of a child's world can add their perspective as a partner in EI intervention. Acknowledging their perspective will create new priorities for everyone involved in the intervention to allow the intervention to be both functional and inclusive. Key questions in relation to the child's micro and mesosystems will guide intervention. Rosenbaum and Gorter (2012) stress that goal identification is paramount. By including the child's perspective we can adjust the method to achieve the goal by incorporating the child's likes and interests. For Noel, methods used to achieve his goals during intervention could include the contexts of outside, in the car, in the kitchen, group activities and include the people important to him: his sisters, his mother, his father and his granddad.

Acknowledging Rosenbaum and Gorter's (2014) 'fun' concept would support the inclusion of Noel's interests in cats, dogs, rabbits, stacker, and musical instruments in his interventions which in turn would facilitate his motivation and engagement. The importance of refining interventions to suit the child and their family's individual needs, likes, interests would have benefits to all involved (Siller et al., 2014). Bjorck-Akesson et al. (2010) highlight that when considering a child's participation, component of the International Classification of Functioning – Child and Youth version (ICF-CY) (World Health Organization [WHO], 2007), their motivation and engagement also need to be considered. They also indicate that the ICF-CY could support interdisciplinary profiling of a child's functioning across diverse cultural contexts (Bjorck-Akesson et al. 2010). Simeonsson (2016) suggests that the UNCRC (1989) dimensional framework and the codes of the ICF-CY (WHO 2007) are applicable to document how a child's rights are realized in terms of a child's experience of limitations of functioning and access to their environment. He also suggests that EI practitioners can document the extent to which environments are responsive to a child's needs, document a child's limitations in performing activities or participation and document barriers to the environmental codes of the WHO's ICF-CY (2007) (Simeonsson 2016). Rosenbaum and Gorter (2011) propose that practitioners, researchers and advocates consider the concepts of function, family, fun, fitness, friends and future as a method to apply in childhood neurodevelopmental disorders. Family-centred practice is a social model for health, education and social care services that expands the focus of intervention beyond the child's level of functioning to view the child in the context of their family (Davies 2007). Including children's perspectives facilitates the participatory dimension of family-centred practice (Dunst, Trivette, and Hamby 2008), thus allowing a child's intervention to be individual, flexible, and responsive with informed choice. Interventions need to be relevant for the child and their families. Bruder (2010) stresses that the assessment process is the time to identify the child's and family's needs together with the services and supports required to meet these needs. Furthermore, by using a Routines Based Interview (RBI) (McWilliam 2005), families and professionals can combine their expertise to guide goals and to understand roles in the intervention planning process. RBI is recognized as a powerful tool to facilitate the development of functional goals and to establish positive relationships with the family (McWilliam 2010).

This pilot study example focused on the everyday lives, their microsystems and mesosystems, of these young children with neurodevelopmental disorders and supported their entitlement to share their voice about EI, a goal of the National Strategy on Children and Young People's Participation in Decision-making is to that children and young people have a voice in their individual and collective everyday lives (Department of Children and Youth Affairs 2015). Dockett and Perry (2007) state that we need to learn from the children themselves about their lives and experiences. Furthermore, by understanding their experiences EI services can be provided together with children. However in reality services are often provided 'to' children rather than 'for' them. 'The reasons for listening to young disabled children are the same as the reasons for listening to all children' (Dickins 2004: 1). We are listening and we need to keep doing it.

References

Adams, R. C., Tapia, C., and The Council on Children with Disabilities (2013). Early Intervention, IDEA Part C Services, and the Medical Home: Collaboration for Best Practice and Best Outcomes. *Paediatrics*, 132 (4). DOI: 10.1542/peds.2013-2305

Badham, B. (2000). *So Why Don't you Get Your Own House In Order? Towards Children and Governance in The Children's Society*. London: The Children's Society.

Bailey, D. B., Bruder, M. B., Hebbeler, K., Carta, J., Defosset, M., Greenwood, C., et al. (2006). Recommended outcomes for families of young children with disabilities. *Journal of Early Intervention*, 28, 227–251.

Begley, (2000). The educational self-perceptions of children with Down Syndrome. In A., Lewis and G. Lindsay (eds), *Researching Children's Perspectives*, pp. 98–112. Buckingham: Open University Press.

Beresford, B. (1997). *Personal Accounts: involving disabled children in research*. London: SPRU Papers, The Stationery Office.

Bjorck-Akesson, E., Wilder, J., Granlund, M., Pless, M., Simeonsson, R. J., Adolfsson, M., ... Lillvist, A. (2010). The International Classification of Functioning, Disability and Health and the version for Children and Youth as a tool in child habilitation/early childhood intervention – feasibility and usefulness as a common language and frame of reference for practice. *Disability and Society*, 32 (S1), S125–S138.

Bridle, L., and Mann, G. (2000). *Mixed feelings – a parental perspective on early intervention*. Paper presented at the Supporting not controlling: strategies for the new millennium, Australia.

Bruder, M. B. (2010). Coordinating services with families. In R. A. McWilliam (Ed.), *Working with families of young children with special needs*, pp. 93–126. New York: The Guilford Press

Carlhed, C. (2003). Defining dimensions of family-oriented services in early childhood intervention. *Scandinavian Journal of Disability Research*, 5 (2), 185–202. DOI: 10.1080/15017410309512621

Carroll, C., and Sixsmith, J. (2016a). Exploring the facilitation of young children with disabilities in research about their early intervention service. *Child Language Teaching and Therapy*, 32 (3), 313–325.

Carroll, C., and Sixsmith, J. (2016b). A Trajectory of Relationship Development for Early Intervention Practice for Children with Developmental Disabilities. *International Journal of Therapy and Rehabilitation*, 23 (2), 81–90.

Carter, B. (2009). Tick the box? The ethical positioning of children as vulnerable, researchers as barbarians and reviewers as overly cautious. *International Journal of Nursing Studies*, 46 (6), 858–864.

Christensen, P., and James, A. (2008). *Research With Children: Perspectives and Practices* (2nd edn). Abingdon, Oxon: Routledge.

Clark, A. (2005). Listening to and involving young children: a review of research and practice. *Early Child Development and Care*, 175 (6), 489–505. DOI: 10.1080/03004430500131288

Clark, A., and Moss, P. (2001). *Listening to Young Children: The Mosaic Approach* (1st ed.). London: National Children's Bureau.

Clark, A., and Moss, P. (2011). *Listening to young children: The Mosaic Approach* (2nd ed.). London: National Children's Bureau.

Coyne, Imelda (2010). Accessing children as research participants: examining the role of gatekeepers. *Child: care, health and development*, 36 (4), 452–454. DOI: 10.1111/j.1365-2214.2009.01012.x

Daly, L., Sharek, D., DeVries, J., Griffiths, C., Sheerin, F., McBennett, P., and Higgins, A. (2015). The impact of four family support programmes for people with a disability in Ireland. *Journal of Intellectual Disabilities*, 19 (1), 34–50.

Davies, S. (2007). *Team around the child: Working together in early childhood education*. Wagga Wagga, New South Wales, Australia: Kurrajong Early Intervention Service.

Davis, J. M. (2007). Analysing participation and social exclusion with children and young people: Lessons from practice. *International Journal of Children's Rights*, 15 (1), 121–146.

Davis, J. M., and Hogan, J. (2004). Research with children: ethnography, participation, disability and self-empowerment. In J. M. Barnes and G. Mercer (eds), *Implementing the Social Model of Disability: Theory and Practice*. Leeds: The Disability Press.

Department of Children and Youth Affairs (2015). *National Strategy on Children and Young People's Participation in Decision-making, 2015–2020*. Retrieved from <http://www.dcya.ie>.

Department of Health (2012). *Value for money and policy review of disability services in Ireland*. Dublin: Department of Health.

Department of Health and Children (2000). *National children's strategy: Our lives-their lives*. Dublin: Stationary Office.

Dickins, M. (2004). *Listening to Young Disabled Children*. London: National Children's Bureau.

Dockett, S., and Perry, B. (2007). Trusting children's accounts in research. *Journal of Early Childhood Research*, 5 (1), 47–63.

Dunst, C. J., Trivette, C. M., and Hamby, D. W. (2008). *Research synthesis and meta-analysis of studies of family centered practices*. Asheville, NC: Winterberry Press.

Franklin, A., and Sloper, P. (2006). Participation of disabled children and young people in decision making within social services departments: a survey of current and recent activities in England. *British Journal of Social Work*, 36 (5), 723–741.

Gallacher, L., and Gallagher, M. (2008). Methodological Immaturity in Childhood Research? *Childhood*, 15 (4), 499–516. DOI: 10.1177/0907568208091672

Government of Ireland (2014). *Better Outcomes Brighter Future: The National Policy Framework for Children and Young People 2014–2020*. Dublin: Stationery Office. Retrieved from <http://www.dcya.gov.ie/documents/cypp_framework/BetterOutcomesBetterFutureReport.pdf>.

Government of United Kingdom (2014). *The Children and Family Act*. London: The Stationery Office Limited. Retrieved from <http://www.familylaw.co.uk/system/uploads/attachments/0008/3981/Children_and_Families_Act_2014.pdf>.

Greene, S. M., and Hill, M. (2005). Researching Children's Experiences: Methods and Methodological Issues. In S. M. Greene and D. M. Hogan (eds), *Researching Children's Experience: Approaches and Methods: Methods and Approaches*, pp. 1–21. London: Sage.

Grover, S. (2004). Why don't they listen to us? On giving power and voice to children participating in social research. *Childhood*, 11 (1), 81–93.

Hayles, E., Harvey, D., Plummer, D., and Jones, A. (2015). Parents' experiences of health care for their children with cerebral palsy. *Qualitative Health Research*, 25 (8), 1139–1154.

Health Service Executive (2011). *Health Service Executive Corporate Plan 2011–2014*. Dublin: Stationery Office.

Health Service Executive (2012). *New directions: Review of HSE day services and implementation plan 2012–2016*. Dublin: Health Service Executive.

Hill, M., Davis, J, Prout, A., and Tisdall, K. (2004). Moving the participation agenda forward. *Children and Society*, 18 (2), 77.

James, A., and Prout, A. (1997). *Constructing and Reconstructing Childhood* (2nd ed.). Basingstoke: Falmer Press.

Kelly, B. (2007). Methodological Issues for Qualitative Research with Learning Disabled Children. *International Journal of Social Research Methodology*, 10 (1), 21–35.

Lewis, A., and Porter, J. (2004). Interviewing children and young people with learning disabilities: Guidelines for researchers and multi-professional practice. *British Journal of Learning Disabilities*, 32, 191–197.

McCormack, J., McLeod, S., McAllister, L., and Harrison, L. J. (2010). My speech problem, your listening problem, and my frustration: The experience of living with childhood speech impairment. *Language, Speech and Hearing Services in Schools*, 41 (4), 379–392. DOI: 10.1044/0161-1461(2009/08-0129)

McWilliam, R. A. (2010). Assessing families' needs with the Routines-Based Interview. In R. A. McWilliam (ed.), *Working with families of young children with special needs*, pp. 27–59. New York: The Guilford Press.

McWilliam, R. A. (2005). Assessing the resource needs of families in the context of early intervention. In M. J. Guralnick (ed.), *A developmental systems approach to early intervention*, pp. 215–234. Baltimore: Brookes.

Markham, C., and Dean, T. (2006). Parents' and professionals' perceptions of Quality of Life in children with speech and language difficulty. *International Journal of Language and Communication Disorders*, 41 (2), 189–212.

Markham, C., van Laar, D., Gibbard, D., and Dean, T. (2009). Children with speech, language and communication needs: their perceptions of their quality of life. *International Journal of Language and Communication Disorders*, 44 (5), 748–768.

Matthews, A., and Rix, J. (2013). Early intervention: parental involvement, child agency and participation in creative play. *Early Years: An International Research Journal*, 33 (3), 239–251.

Merrick, R. (2011). Ethics, consent and assent when listening to children with speech, language communication needs. In S. Roulstone and S. McLeod (eds), *Listening to children and young people with speech, language and communication needs*, pp. 63–72. Guildford: J&R Press Ltd.

National Children's Bureau (2008). How to involve children and young people with communication impairments in decision-making. In C. f. D. C. National Children's Bureau (ed.). London: Participation Works.

National Disability Authority (2004). *Towards Best Practice in Provision of Health Services for People with Disabilities in Ireland*.

National Economic and Social Council (NESC) (2012). *Quality and Standards in Human Services in Ireland: Disability Services*. Dublin: Economic and Social Council Office.

Office of the Minister for Children and Youth Affairs (2007). *The agenda for children's services: A policy handbook*. Dublin: Stationery Office.

Office of the United Nations High Commisioner for Human Rights (1989). *United Nations convention on the rights of the child*. Geneva, Switzerland: United Nations.

O'Kane, C. (2000). The Development of Participatory Techniques Facilitiating Children's Views about the Decisions which Affect Them. In P. Christensen and A. James (eds), *Research with Children: Perspectives and Practices*, pp. 136–159. London: Falmer Press.

O'Shaughnessy Carroll, C. (2016). *Understanding early intervention services in Ireland: a conceptual evaluation.* Doctoral dissertation. Health Promotion. National University of Ireland Galway. Galway, Ireland. Retrieved from <https://aran.library. nuigalway.ie/bitstream/handle/10379/6361/2016oshaughnessycarrollphd.pdf>.

Patton, M. Q. (2015). *Qualitative Research and Evaluation Methods* (4th edn). Thousand Oaks CA: Sage.

Press, F., Bradley, BS., Goodfellow, J., Harrison, LJ., McLeod, S., Sumsion, J., ... Stratigos, T. (2011). Listening to infants about what life is like in childcare: A mosaic approach. In S. Roulstone and S. McLeod (eds), *Listening to children and young people with speech, language and communication needs*, pp. 241–249. London: J&R Press.

Punch, S. (2002). Research with Children: The Same or Different from Research with Adults?. *Childhood*, 9 (3), 321–341.

Quortrup, J., Bardy, M., Sgritta, G., and Wintersberger, H. (eds). (1994). *Childhood Matters Social Theory, Practice and Politics.* Aldershot: Avebury.

Raghavendra, P. (2013). Participation of children with disabilities: Measuring subjective and objective outcomes. *Child: care, health and development*, 39 (4), 461–465. DOI: 10.1111/cch.12084

Rosenbaum, P., and Gorter, J. W. (2012). The 'F-words' in childhood disability: I swear this is how we should think! *Child:Care Health and Development*, 38 (4), 457–463.

Sameroff, A. J. (2009). *The Transactional Model of Development: How Children and Contexts Shape Each Other.* Washington, DC: American Psychological Association.

Siller, M., Morgan, L., Turner-Brown, L., Baggett, K. M., Baranek, G. T., Brian, J., and Zwaigenbaum, L. (2014). Designing Studies to Evaluate Parent-Mediated Interventions for Toddlers With Autism Spectrum Disorder. *Journal of Early Intervention*, 35, 355–377.

Simeonsson, R. J. (9 June 2016). *UNCRC and ICF-CY: Defining and documenting universal rights of children.* Paper presented at the International Society on Early Intervention Conference: Children's Rights and Early Intervention, University of Stockholm, Sweden.

Sixsmith, J., Nic Gabhainn, S., Fleming, C., and O'Higgins, S. (2007). 'Children's, parents' and teachers' perceptions of child wellbeing', *Health Education*, 107 (6), 511–523.

Sloper, P., and Beresford, B. (2006). Families with disabled children: Editorial. *BMJ*, 333, 928–929.

Thomas, N., and O'Kane, C. (2000). Discovering what children think: Connections between research and practice. *British Journal of Social Work*, 30 (6), 817–833.

Tisdall, E. K. M. (2012). The Challenge and Challenging of Childhood Studies. *Children and Society*, 26, 181–191.

Uprichard, E. (2010). Questioning Research with Children: Discrepancy between Theory and Practice? *Children and Society*, 24, 3–13. DOI: 10.1111/j.1099-0860. 2008.00187.x.

Watson, N., Abbott, D., and Townsley, R. (2006). Listen to me, too! Lessons from involving children with complex healthcare needs in research about multi-agency services. *Child: Care, Health and Development*, 33(1), 90–95.

Whitehurst, T. (2006). Liberating silent voices – perspectives of children with profound and complex learning needs on inclusion. *Brtish Journal of Learning Disabilities*, 35(1), 55–61.

Whyte, J. (2006). *Research with children with disabilities: Guidelines for good practice.* National Disability Authority. Retrieved from: <http://nda.ie/File-upload/ Research-with-Children-with-Disabilities.pdf>.

World Health Organization (2001). *International Classification of Functioning, Disability and Health*. Geneva: World Health Organization.

Yung, L. E. (2010). Identifying families' supports and other resources. In R. A. McWilliam (ed.), *Working with families of young children with special needs*, pp. 9–26. New York: The Guilford Press.

Exploring the facilitation of young children with disabilities in research about their early intervention service

Provided by the authors with permission from SAGE Publishers.
Carroll, C. and Sixsmith, J. (2016). Exploring the facilitation of young children with disabilities in research about their early intervention service. *Child Language Teaching and Therapy*, 32(3), 313–325. doi: 10.1177/0265659016638394.

Abstract

While participatory research approaches are being developed and applied within speech and language therapy practice it is not clear that all children are afforded the opportunity to participate in such activities. This study aimed to explore the involvement of young children, aged between two and four years, with developmental disabilities in the research process, focusing on early intervention disability services. Eight young children took part in this qualitative research. Clark and Moss's (2011) framework for listening was used to structure the multi-method data collection process. The design was iterative; the collection of data from each participant was followed by a review of theoretical ideas to support the emerging data. Findings suggest that the use of an asset based approach to participation in research, focusing on participants strengths through a variety of data collection tools, used by a skilled facilitator, supported by parental expertise enabled the children to be part of the data collection process. The research highlights that speech and language therapists can facilitate the inclusion of children with disabilities in research activities about their early intervention service they receive. As members of early intervention teams speech and language therapists need to promote their skills in facilitating the active engagement of children with developmental disabilities in research. Thus making their participation in early intervention research, a reality with potential to promote holistic practice.

Keywords

Participation, qualitative research, early intervention team, young children, disabilities.

Introduction

Article 3 of the United Nations Convention on the Rights of the Child established the principle that all children should enjoy the 'freedom to seek, receive and impart information and ideas of all kinds' (Office of the United Nations High Commissioner for Human Rights, 1989). Nevertheless, children, including those with developmental disabilities, were virtually excluded as active participants in the research process and were rarely asked to tell their own stories (Grover, 2004). While, the National Federation of Voluntary Bodies (2008) states that the presumption should be of capacity rather than incapacity when involving a person with disabilities in a research process, children with disabilities may experience a double disadvantage because they are young and they have a disability (Dickins, 2004). Gallacher and Gallagher (2008) argue that it is not sufficient to carry out research *on* or *about* children and that it is no longer enough to simply reposition children as subjects – rather than objects – of research. Researchers must research *for* and *with* children and engage them as participants in the research process (Punch, 2002). It is recognized that children have different experiences and knowledge to adults (Christensen and James, 2008; James and Prout, 1997) and that we cannot rely on adult proxies to give valid accounts of children's experiences (Beresford, 1997; Markham and Dean, 2006; Markham et al., 2009). Hence, participation of children in research is essential, supporting the view of children as competent social actors, with their own agency and voice, acknowledging children as experts of their childhood (Carter, 2009).

By promoting and facilitating children's participation in research we are advancing childhood research, adding to research generally (Tisdall, 2012) and responding to our ethical responsibility to explore ways to make children's participation a reality (Merrick, 2011). In this article, the authors share the results of a research study, which explored the involvement of young children with developmental disabilities in research through the application of a variety of tools. We argue that the SLT as a member of an early intervention (EI) team has a unique role and skill set to facilitate children with disabilities to participate together with their parents, in research.

1. Involving Children with Disabilities in Research

Research is gradually emerging involving school-aged children with speech, language and communication needs (SLCN), (Lyons et al., 2013; Markham, 2011; Merrick and Roulstone, 2011) and young children with SLCN (Press et al., 2011; Roulstone et al., 2013). Although, leading researchers in the field promote the facilitation of children with disabilities in research (Franklin and Sloper, 2006; Sloper and Beresford, 2006; Tisdall, 2012; Whitehurst, 2006), there is a scarcity of research involving young children and school-aged children with developmental disabilities. Within the field of disabilities, research is also developing to facilitate the participation of school-aged children with disabilities (Beresford et al., 2004; Mitchell and Sloper, 2011; Porter et al., 2011) with one research study involving young children with developmental disabilities (Paige-Smith and Rix, 2011). Rabiee et al. (2005) suggest that the exclusion of children with developmental disabilities, in research, may be related to the lack of appropriate data collection methods to facilitate their inclusion. In studies to date, multiple data sources have been used to record and represent the children's everyday lives, including Baby Cam (Press et al., 2011), observations, interviews and KiddyCam (Roulstone et al., 2013), narrative observations and photographs of daily events (Paige-Smith and Rix, 2011). Research including young children with developmental disabilities is warranted both internationally and in the country where the research took place. Research focusing on data collection methods to support their inclusion is necessary to progress this agenda forward.

Dickins (2004) recognises that listening to and consulting with young disabled children, with complex needs, requires the listener to use communication techniques and interpretation skills. Participation of a heterogeneous group of young children with developmental disabilities requires the researcher to use an open and flexible approach in the use of different research tools to aid communication (Franklin and Sloper, 2009; Kelly, 2007; Mitchell and Sloper, 2011; Paige-Smith and Rix, 2011).Although we cannot rely on adult proxy reports of children's experiences alone (Markham et al., 2009), it is important to recognise that parents are adept interpreters of their child's signals (Press et al., 2011) and that the skills of speakers and listeners influence successful communication (McCormack et al., 2010). In family centred practices, the family is recognised as the expert on the needs of the child (Trute, 2007). Recognising parents' expertise in early intervention and responding to parents' needs and wishes is important for building relationships with parents (King et al., 1998; McWilliam et al., 1998; O'Neil and Palisano, 2000). Therefore, the roles played by the parents and the researcher, in the research process, need to be valued and supported.

2. Context of Study

Designed to support family patterns of interaction that best promote children's development, EI services have long-term benefits for children and their families (Guralnick, 2005). For children with disabilities and their families, access to effective EI services, within the first five years of life, is critical to the child's development (Guralnick, 2011). Within the context of the current study, EI services for children with disabilities are provided by multidisciplinary teams to children from birth to five years who are experiencing significant difficulties in two or more areas of their development (Carrroll, Murphy and Sixsmith, 2013). The way that teams function varies across the country. Teams typically comprise of families, parents and children with disabilities, and a variety of professionals, including Occupational Therapists, Physiotherapists, Speech and Language Therapists (SLT), Nurses, Psychologists, Social Workers, Family Support Workers and in some teams, a Team Leader.

The country's EI services, underpinned by the bio psychosocial model, must be family centred, integrated and inclusive (Health Service Executive, 2011). The bio psychosocial model proposes that health and wellness are caused by a complex interaction of biological, psychological, and sociocultural factors. This model provides a framework for EI team interventions. The focus of integrated EI services is on the child in the context of their family and considers the influence of the family on the child's development (Dunst et al., 2007). This family-centred approach is also advocated in SLT service delivery (McLeod and Threats, 2008). An approach to intervention that is both family-centred and strengths-based helps families feel more confident and comfortable in supporting their children's development (Wilcox, 2001). The American Speech-Language-Hearing Association (ASHA) (2008) highlight that EI services should be 'developmentally supportive and promote children's participation in their natural environments' (p.3). For children with disabilities, participation in these activities is dependent on their skills within communication, motor, social and emotional developmental domains (Wilcox and Woods, 2011).

Blackman (2003) emphasises the key role played by families as a success factor of interventions. The Health Service (2011) stress that services must be accountable, evidence based and evaluate outcomes. Facilitating a level of independent participation is an important outcome for children receiving EI (Wilcox and Woods, 2011). In keeping with EI philosophy, research is shifting to focus on enhancing young children's participation and notably their communicative participation (Ragavendra, 2013). Hearing the voice of children is vital in order to understand their experiences (Department of Health and Children, 2000; Government of United Kingdom, 2014) and their voices must inform practice (Whitehurst, 2006).

3. Aims of the Study

This research study aimed to answer two research questions.

1. Can young children with developmental disabilities be facilitated to engage in research?
2. If so, how can their engagement in research be supported?

Methods

An asset based methodological approach was used in this study. The researcher's objectives were to interact with young children with disabilities in ways that respected their particular competence (Thomas and O'Kane, 2000) and their unique and valued view of the world (Greene and Hill, 2005); to view the children as active members of their early intervention team and to add the children's voices and engage them in the research process. Initially, the researcher took a leadership role and following a process of co-construction (Mason and Urquhart, 2001), the children's interactions led the data collection activities. The researcher was a SLT by profession and at the time of research had over thirteen years of clinical experience working in EI and with children with disabilities, was a sign language user and skilled in the nuances of communication facilitation. These skills included active listening, being resourceful, respectful of the child and their style of communication, open, sensitive, and flexible.

1. Participants

A purposeful sampling strategy was used to select potential child participants from two non-government organisations (NGO) who were receiving EI services. The gatekeepers, who were managers within the organisations were asked to select: children with complex needs attending an EI team, and ranging in age from two to five years. Eight children were recruited; all attended EI team services for children with developmental disabilities in their local areas. The details of each participant are outlined in Table 1. Following the selection and recruitment procedure:

1. The researcher contacted the parents of the children identified through the selection process.
2. The parent provided consent for the researcher to meet with their child for the research.
3. The child assented to participate in an interaction with the researcher. The approach to the interaction was based on the child's level of ability.

Table 1: Child Sample

Child	Gender	Age (yrs)	Yrs with Team	Diagnosis	Education	No. of siblings	No. of interviews	Use of Sense Cam
Child 1	Male	3	3	Down Syndrome	Mainstream preschool	3	2	No
Child 2	Male	3	3	Down Syndrome	Mainstream preschool	0	2	Yes
Child 3	Male	4	4	Physical and intellectual disability	Special Preschool	2	2	No
Child 4	Male	3	3	Down Syndrome	Mainstream preschool	2	1	No
Child 5	Male	3	3	Down Syndrome	Not yet	2	2	Yes
Child 6	Female	4	3.5	Down Syndrome	Mainstream preschool	2	2	Yes
Child 7	Male	3	2.5	Down Syndrome	Not yet	2	3	Yes
Child 8	Male	2	1.5	Down Syndrome	Not yet	0	2	Yes

2. Data Collection

Clark and Moss's (2011) Framework for Listening was used to guide the data collection process because it views children as 'beings not becomings' (Quortrup et al., 1994), and listens to children's voices. The multi-method process involved interactions with each child, use of a Microsoft SenseCam (Hodges et al., 2006), SenseCam images, pictures, Talking Mats (Murphy, 1997), and observations. Multiple interactions also allowed the needs of the child to be respected (Irwin and Johnson, 2005) and strengthened the trustworthiness of the data (Dockett and Perry, 2007). The participants were all individuals with heterogeneous experiences and diverse interests and needs. Prior to the initial interaction, the researcher and the primary caregiver had a telephone conversation, on how best to facilitate their child's participation to engage in the interaction. Each interaction involved the child, researcher and one or both parents, was audio recorded and took place in the child's home. The parents' role was one to support the child and the researcher during their interactions. Thus, supporting the view that the parent and researcher worked in partnership and also to ensure that the research was carried out to the appropriate ethical standards. The researcher engaged in active listening, and took field notes following each interview. A Total Communication approach was used, where non- verbal communication such as body language, facial expression, signing, gestures and pictures were valued as much as spoken language (Fargas-Malet et al., 2010).

At the end of the first interaction, the researcher gave the parent/s a SenseCam for the child to wear over the subsequent few days. There was one SenseCam available for the study; subsequently five children were selected, based on nearest travel distance from the researcher, to use the SenseCam. The SenseCam, developed by Microsoft Research UK, is a passive wearable camera, fitted with a wide-angle (fish-eye) lens, which results in nearly everything in front of the camera being photographed. It takes photographs automatically and the images provide a visual account of daily tasks and activities from the child's perspective. It offers a novel route to the collection of observational data. The use of the SenseCam provided the children with a means to share their lives from their perspective (Wang, 2006). The researcher collected the camera and a record sheet (noting the date and length of time the child wore the camera) prior to the second interaction. SenseCam Image software was used to process all the SenseCam images and the images of toys, people, places, and activities from the child's world were printed. During the second interaction, with the five children who used the SenseCam, the researcher used Talking Mats (Murphy, 1997), along with the print outs of SenseCam images and other pictures based on the child's preferences. The tools were varied and reflective in accordance with the research question and the individual abilities and preferences of the children.

3. Data Analysis

An interpretative framework shaped the interpretation of the data (Grover, 2004). The interactions were analysed using a constant comparative approach. Transcripts were coded to identify themes directly from the interactions. The SenseCam images were analysed using content analysis in order to reduce and make sense of the volume of qualitative material (Patton, 2002). The images were grouped into events, for example, mealtime, playtime, watching TV, people, by the researcher to form a pictorial diary of the child's experiences. This analytical method involved the researcher adopting an outsider perspective by personally interpreting the photographs, examining and describing them as thoroughly as possible. Punch (2002) suggests that the researcher needs to be critically reflective in analysing different types of data. An interpretative framework facilitated the identification of themes in the data.

4. Rigour

The design was iterative; the collection of data from each participant was followed by a review of theoretical ideas to support the emerging themes. In flexible designs such as this Patton (2002) advocates the use of an audit trail, therefore the researcher kept a reflective diary which included thoughts, feelings, biases that may have influenced all aspects of the research process and attempts made to manage them (Davis et al., 2000; Driessnack, 2006). The parents were present during all interactions with their children (as a requirement of the research) and facilitated the researcher in her interactions with the children and verified the accuracy of the researcher's observations and interpretations. The second author acted as peer checker of the data, by viewing the images, which supported the trustworthiness of the data collection process and data analysis.

5. Ethical Considerations

The research underwent two independent reviews and received full ethical approval from two University research ethics committees. The parents were fully informed of the research and knew that they had the right to withdraw their child at any stage. Their confidentiality was assured and pseudonyms were used to provide confidentiality. The researcher wanted to facilitate the participation of the children who attended the EI services in this research and allow them to have a voice and to include those for whom obstacles may make participation difficult. Stancliffe (1999) argued that when someone is unable to communictate their own views, a well-infomred guess may be preferable than no information. The National Federation of Voluntary Bodies (2008) states that where children do not have the capacity to consent a guardian (usually parent) appointed must give consent. All parents provided their written consent for their child to take part in the research. The parents knew that they might be probed to give supportive evidence to statements made by their child during the interviews. However, there should also be an opportunity for the child to express assent. In accordance with (Ireland and Holloway, 1996; Scott, Wishart and Bowyer, 2006), the agreement of the children to take part in the research was also requested. The researcher checked at the beginning of each interaction that the child was willing to participate. The age and level of ability of the child dictated how the child's own assent and participation could be achieved (Ireland and Holloway, 1996; Scott et al., 2006). The researcher looked for verbal and non-verbal signals of the child's willingness to partake or withdraw.

Findings

The research demonstrated that the young children with disabilities could participate in the research process about their early intervention service. The children's engagement was facilitated successfully through the use of a number of strategies during the process of data collection. It emerged that a variety of data collection tools were needed, together with parent knowledge and skills and researcher knowledge and skills. The findings are reported under these headings.

1. Variety of Data Collection Tools

The tools that supported the children in this study were the use of the SenseCam and Talking Mats. The SenesCam was used as a recorder of the child's everyday experiences and the contexts they experienced. Five children wore the SenseCam for an average of five hours over a three-day period. During the study, Child 6 did not want to wear the SenseCam around her neck, and used it as a 'handbag' and wanted to take pictures herself. Her mother responded to her communicative signals and facilitated her to wear the camera by stitching the camera to her vest. She wore the camera and communicated to her mother when she did not want to wear it and her mother responded by taking the vest off. Child 6 moved outside during the first interaction and the researcher followed the child's lead and the interaction continued outside. Thereby allowing her to be an active participant in the research process.

Child 7 wore the SenseCam during an EI therapy session and also during his EI group interventions. This provided images and observations of his interactions with his therapists and demonstrated his participation during intervention. The SenseCam images included a playdoh activity showing him rolling playdoh with his hands, then rolling playdoh with a roller and then placing a shape in the playdoh and then the final product. For Child 7, the SenseCam allowed us view his interest in the outside world with images of his pets consistently being captured on his visits outside. His siblings and his mother were also very important people in his life. For Child 8, the images showed us his interest in Thomas the Tank Engine programmes on TV.

When using Talking Mats (Murphy, 1997), the children chose the images of their world and used non-verbal expressions such as smiling or verbally commented. The child and their parent viewed them and validated their importance in the child's life. Of the five children who used the SenseCam, Talking Mats were used as a tool with three of the children when looking at the photos. Child 5 looked at the SenseCam images on the researcher's laptop and named and pointed to the ones he liked. Child 2 looked, and pointed and named the pictures.

2. Parents' Knowledge and Skills to Support Engagement

The child interacted with the researcher and participated in the research. The parents supported their child's interactions when it was needed, between the researcher and the child, and the parents on occasion directed the interactions.

> I am going to do music with him now. I have a few cds that get him up. There is an Irish dancing cd and he goes mad for that. (Mother of Child 1 interaction 1)

Child 5's mother showed the researcher his activities and carried out their therapy routine and involved the researcher to take turns in the Mr Potato Head activity.

> Here are some of his routines, that's kind of a list of all the ones we've built up and then I kind of have them in pockets so we might do a song, ... we've Mr Potato head and the new thing then is the pictures with the words. (Mother of Child 5 Interaction 1)

Parents influenced the interactions in EI by contributing knowledge about their child. The parents shared how their child interacted in EI.

> He would push away or wriggle off my lap or turn away. If he really doesn't want something done he would let you know alright. (Parent of Child 1 Interaction 1)

> People who will actually play with him and sit down with him. He responds to them much more. (Parent of Child 2 Interaction 1)

Within the interactions in the home it was clear that a parent influenced and effected change in their child particularly in relation to using home opportunities to include treatment goals. When an investment in structure and routine was attached to EI, it facilitated interaction.

> Looking back it was great they (professionals) really got them into the routine. It (therapy sessions) became very familiar to them. The hello song at the beginning. (Mother of Child 4 Interaction 1)

When the researcher and his mother were observing Child 5 holding on to a toy, his mother commented that 'he wouldn't have done that a year ago' (Child 5 Interaction 1). Accordingly, involvement in EI enabled developmental progress.

> The words are coming great. The last time then she (SLT) gave me these ones (mother showed the researcher cards) with just the words and he is getting it. He has strengthened no end. (Child 4 Interaction 1)

> He is completely different (to when he was two). Even in the last 2 months he has come on. (Child 1 Interaction 1)

3. Researcher Knowledge and Skills to Support Engagement

During the interactions the researcher verbalised what the child was doing and how they responded when the response was not verbal, for example, when the child signed and/or vocalised the researcher said 'signed car and said da'. This allowed for more accurate transcription of the audio recording. The researcher, being a SLT and using a Total Communication approach, could read a lot of the children's signals and signs. The researcher also asked the parents during the interactions to verify the accuracy of her interpretations of unclear signs, signals, gestures, vocalizations and words. The researcher followed the child's lead in all the interactions. During the interviews, all forms of communication were viewed as equal.

The researcher observed Child 2, during interaction 1, playing a game with marbles and he allowed the researcher to take turns and play hide and seek with them. Marbles were of interest to this child. The child's motivation also influenced activities, and the materials used made a difference.

The researcher read the child's non-verbal communication to alert her as to when she had how to take her next turn. The researcher and Child 1, during interaction 2, played with playdoh. The child opened the playdoh boxes, squeezed the playdoh and rolled it out into a snake. The task was completed under the direction of his mother. Also during this interaction, the researcher noted that his mother commented on good sitting, commented saying 'open', 'squeeze' and made noises to go with the activity, named colours, named verbs 'pull', 'push', and used short phrases 'good open', 'take some out', 'lid off', 'we scoop', 'in the box', 'lid on', 's', 'small snake', 'big snake', and changed her intonation patterns and stressed different words. His mother noted that:

> 'You have to be patient. You have to go slowly. Face to face contact. (Child 1 Interaction 2)

All eight children involved in the study communicated non-verbally when, they did not want to take part, were no longer interested in an activity and when they were finished interacting. They interacted by moving away or turning away from the researcher, pushing a toy or pictures away, not wanting to wear the SenseCam or wanting to leave the room. The researcher responded to the children's communicative attempts by following the child's lead and either changing the activity or stopping the interview. Initially the process was researcher led, followed by a period of co construction and finally child led. The researcher adapted the data collection methods according to each child.

Discussion

This research demonstrated that young children with disabilities could participate in research about their EI service. The research demonstrated that, although engaging these children with developmental disabilities in the research is difficult and complex, it is possible. EI services strive for inclusion and to be accountable (Health Service Executive, 2011). This research shows that the young children involved in these services were included in adding to research about EI services. Young children with disabilities are central to EI services. The ideology of EI services is participation of all children with diabilities in their everyday activities. Within this research, the children were viewed as competent social actors and given the opportunity to take part in research about EI. Similar to other research findings (Beresford et al., 2004; Franklin and Sloper, 2009; Kelly, 2007), a range of data collection techniques, skills and support was required to engage this heterogeneous group of young children to participate in the research. Research with children with developmental disabilities is difficult and is compounded by the complexity of impairment and by the complex variety of children. Hence, for the children in the study, their level of participation in activities varied and was dependent on their abilities and on the context of the activity, a finding similar to those found by Paige- Smith and Rix (2011). This research also found that the people, that is, parents and the researcher were key factors in the children's engagement. This study provides evidence that a multi-method process allowed the children in this study to give a picture of their skills, needs and interests, identified what motivated them, identified their capacity to make decisions and how they interacted in their home context.

Within the research, the parents played an important role in their child's participation. The children in the study were engaged in the process with the support of their parents. Firstly, the parents consented to their children being involved in the study. The parents acknowledged their child's capacity to take part (Federation of Voluntary Bodies, 2008). Secondly, the parents were a factor in the success of their child's engagement in the research process. This is similar to the opinion that parent involvement in EI is a key factor to successful intervention (Blackman, 2003). Similar to Trute's (2007) view that parents should be regarded as partners with professionals in family centred practices, the parents and the researcher were partners in the research process. The researcher perceived the parents from a position of equal expertise (Carpenter et al., 2004) and did not rely on them to act as proxies for the children (Markham et al., 2009). Rather than acting as proxies, they enabled their child's inclusion and their participation in the research. Without the active commitment of the parents in the research process the use of the SenseCam (Hodges et al., 2006) as a tool for data collection would not have been positive. The parents provided the opportunities for their children to wear the SenseCam in their home settings. Thirdly, during the interactions with the children in their homes, the parents verified their child's communication skills, their interests and demonstrated how interventions were supported within the home context. The parents made activities available to their child and integrated therapy interventions into home activities. Thus supporting Axelsson et al. (2013) suggestion that child-focused activities are more involving than routines. Lastly, the parents acted as interpreters when it was required, verifying the accuracy of the researcher's interpretations of their child's communicative signals. Thus supporting the reliability of the researcher's interpretations.

The data collection tools used in the study facilitated the young children to participate in the research process. At the time of the research, the SenseCam (Hodges et al., 2006) had not been previously used with young children with disabilities. This research demonstrates that it is a useful research tool to use with this heterogeneous group of children. The SenseCam facilitated auto photography, where the world inhabited by the children was captured while, at the same time, reflecting the worlds they live in (Erdner and Magnusson, 2011). The SenseCam allowed the researcher to gain a more comprehensive picture of the children's worlds obtaining data that traditional interactions could never have provided. The use of photography is supported by previous research (Press et al., 2011; Roulstone et al., 2013) and this research adds to the evidence base to include young children with disabilities. The use of Talking Mats (Murphy, 1997) also facilitated the children's engagement in the research and provided a prop to use pictures and images taken by the SenseCam in the interactions. In order to engage these children in research activities, the researcher and the parents needed to be flexible and respond to the child's individual capabilities.

Consulting with young children with disabilities requires the listener to use communicative techniques and interpretative skills (Dickins, 2004), which can have a substantial influence on communication (McCormack et al., 2010). This research suggests that the techniques and the skills of the researcher were an integral factor in the successful engagement of the children with disabilities in this research. The researcher was a speech and language therapist, with a professional qualification in the nuances of communication facilitation (ASHA, 2008). The authors argue that the researcher was not only a competent researcher but also had clinical competence to actively engage with the children in ways that another researcher may not. The researcher's specialist expertise and experience in working with children with disabilities facilitated the interactions and allowed the interactions to flow as the researcher understood sign language and made consistent attempts to interpret the child's communicative intentions, which is supported by McCormack et al. (2010) and Dickins (2004).

An important outcome of EI for a child with a disability is independent participation (Wilcox and Woods, 2011). This independence to participate in research can be hindered by a number of factors such as communicative competence. This research provides an example of children with disabilities displaying communicative participation in research. Speech and language therapists have a role to ensure that communication is conceptualised as a skill that is central to participation across all activities and routines in EI (Wilcox and Woods, 2011). While all professionals within EI have skills to work with these children, SLTs have clinical competencies to help interpret and report children's views (Wilcox and Woods, 2011). SLTs can facilitate children in research and support researcher colleagues, in research about EI. SLTs can help colleagues to understand how each child communicates, shows their likes and dislikes, makes choices and to interpret a child's communicative signals. This knowledge is also important for planning family-based interventions (Dunst, 2001; McWilliam, 2010). SLTs together with their EI colleagues need to consider the young children, with whom they are working, as potential research participants and need to consider ways to facilitate participation.

The strengths of the study are that it involved multiple interactions allowing the needs of the child to be respected (Irwin and Johnson, 2005) and strengthened the trustworthiness of the data (Dockett and Perry, 2007). The researcher was reflexive by considering her role as a researcher and the power relations in the research process (Davis et al., 2000; Edmond, 2006). The researcher's clinical qualifications and clinical experience together with the parents' expertise helped ensure reliability of the data. The second author also facilitated peer checking of the data adding to the rigour of the research process (Patton, 2002). However, the research could be criticised for being non standardised and that the analysis of the findings are the researcher's interpretations and may not take account the child's own insights. The study was limited by the time that was allotted to collect the data with only eight children taking part in the study, and five wearing the SenseCam. The practice of auto photography could be seen as passive participation, however in this research the photographs were used to facilitate active participation. There is opportunity to extend the use of the SenseCam to ensure that the images are representative of the child's life. The positive outcome of the study may have also been attributable to the children's motivation and that of their parents to facilitate their child in the research.

In conclusion, the importance of facilitating research *with* children rather than *on* children is increasingly recognised and promoted. Systems can make this participation in research activities a reality through the use of; an asset based methodological approach, a variety of data collection tools, with the support of parents and an interviewer skilled in the nuances of communication facilitation.

Enabling young children with disabilities to have a voice in research has the potential to positively influence the services they receive facilitating a more truly holistic approach to EI practice.

References

American Speech-Language-Hearing Association (2008). Roles and responsibilities of speech-language pathologists in early intervention: Guidelines. Retrieved from <http://www.asha.org/policy/GL2008-00293/>.

Axelsson, A. K., Granlund, M., and Wilder, J. (2013). Engagement in family activities: a quantitative, comparative study of children with profound intellectual and multiple disabilities and children with typical development. *Child: care, health and development*, 39, 523–534.

Carroll, C., Murphy, G., and Sixsmith, J. (2013). The progression of early intervention disability services in Ireland. *Infants and Young Children*, 26, 17–27.

Beresford, B. (1997). *Personal Accounts: involving disabled children in research*, London: SPRU Papers, The Stationery Office.

Beresford, B., Tozer, R., Rabiee, P., et al. (2004). Developing an approach to involving children with autistic spectrum disorders in a social care research project. *British Journal of Learning Disabilities*, 32, 180–185.

Blackman, J. A. (2003). Early intervention: An overview. In S. L. Odom, M. J. Hanson, J. A. Blackman, and S. Kaul (eds), *Early intervention practices around the world*, pp. 1–84. Baltimore, MD: Brookes Publishing.

Carpenter, B., Addenbrooke, M., Attfield, E., et al. (2004). 'Celebrating Families': an Inclusive Model of Family-Centred Training. *British Journal of Special Education*, 31, 75–80.

Carter, B. (2009). Tick box for child? The ethical positioning of children as vulnerable, researchers as barbarians and reviewers as overly cautious. *International Journal of Nursing Studies*, 46, 858–864.

Christensen, P., and James, A. (2008). *Research With Children: Perspectives and Practices*. Abingdon, Oxon: Routledge.

Clark, A., and Moss, P. (2011). *Listening to Young Children: The Mosaic Approach* (2nd edn), London: National Children's Bureau.

Davis, J., Watson, N., and Cunningham-Burley, S. (2000). Learning the lives of disabled children: developing a reflexive approach. In P. Christensen and A. James (eds), *Research with children – perspectives and practices*. London: RoutledgeFalmer.

Department of Health and Children (2000). *National children's strategy: Our lives – their lives*. Dublin, Ireland: Stationery Office.

Dickins, M. (2004). *Listening to Young Disabled Children*. London: National Children's Bureau.

Dockett, S., and Perry, B. (2007). Trusting children's accounts in research. *Journal of Early Childhood Research*, 5, 47–63.

Driessnack, M. (2006). Draw-and-tell conversations with children about fear. *Qualitative Health Research*, 16, 1414–1435.

Dunst, C. J. (2001). Participation of young children with disabilities in community learning activities. In: Guralnick M. J. (ed.), *Early childhood inclusion: Focus on change*, pp. 307–333. Baltimore, MD: Paul H. Brookes.

Dunst, C. J., Trivette, C. M., and Hamby, D. W. (2007). Meta-analysis of family-centered help giving practices research. *Mental Retardation and Developmental Disabilities Research Reviews*, 13, 370–378.

Edmond, R. (2006). Reflections of a researcher on the use of a child-centred approach. *The Irish Journal of Psychology*, 27, 97–104.

Erdner, A., and Magnusson, A. (2011). Perspectives in Photography as a Method of Data Collection: Helping People With Long-Term Mental Illness to Convey Their Life World. *Perspectives in Psychiatric Care*, 47, 145–150.

Fargas-Malet, M., McSherry, D., Larkin, E., et al. (2010). Research with children: methodological issues and innovative techniques. *Journal of Early Childhood Research*, 8, 175–191.

Franklin, A., and Sloper, P. (2006). Participation of disabled children and young people in decision making within social services departments: a survey of current and recent activities in England. *British Journal of Social Work*, 36, 723–741.

Franklin, A., and Sloper, P. (2009). Supporting the participation of disabled children and young people in decision-making. *Children and Society*, 23, 3–15.

Gallacher, L., and Gallagher, M. (2008). Methodological Immaturity in Childhood Research? *Childhood*, 15, 499–516.

Government of United Kingdom (2014). *The Children and Family Act*. London: The Stationery Office.

Greene, S., and Hill, M. (2005). Researching children's experiences: methods and methodological issues. In S. Greene and D. Hogan (eds), *Researching Children's Experiences: Approaches and Methods*. London: Sage Publications.

Grover, S. (2004). Why don't they listen to us? On giving power and voice to children participating in social research. *Childhood*, 11, 81–93.

Guralnick, M. J. (2005). Early intervention for children with intellectual disabilities: Current knowledge and future prospects. *Journal of Applied research in Intellectual Disabilities*, 18, 313–324.

Guralnick, M. J. (2011). Why early intervention works: A systems perspective. *Infants and Young Children*, 24, 6–28.

Health Service Executive (2011). *Health Service Executive Corporate Plan 2011–2014*. Dublin: Stationery Office.

Hodges, S., Williams, L., Berry, E., et al. (2006). SenseCam: A Retrospective Memory Aid. In P. Dourish and A. Friday (eds), *UbiComp 2006: Ubiquitous Computing*, pp. 177–193. Berlin, Heidelberg: Springer.

Ireland, L., and Holloway, I. (1996). Qualitative health research with children. *Children and Society*, 155–164.

Irwin, L. G., and Johnson, J. (2005). Interviewing young children: explicating our practices and dilemmas. *Qualitative Health Research*, 15, 821–831.

James, A., and Prout, A. (1997). *Constructing and Reconstructing Childhood*. Basingstoke: Falmer Press.

Kelly, B. (2007). Methodological Issues for Qualitative Research with Learning Disabled Children. *International Journal of Social Research Methodology*, 10, 21–35.

King, G., Law, M., King, S., and Rosenbaum, P. (1998). Parents' and service providers' perceptions of the family-centredness of children's rehabilitation services. *Physical & Occupational Therapy in Paediatrics*, 18, 21–40.

Lyons, R., Jones, M., and Roulstone, S. (2013). Identity and meaning-making in children with primary speech and language impairments. *Speech & Language Therapy Research Unit*. Unpublished Thesis. University of Bristol.

McCormack, J., McLeod, S., McAllister, L., et al. (2010). My speech problem, your listening problem, and my frustration: The experience of living with childhood speech impairment. *Language, Speech and Hearing Services in Schools*, 41, 379–392.

McLeod, S., and Threats, T. T. (2008). The ICF-CY and children with communication disabilities. *International Journal of Speech-Language Pathology*, 10: 92–109.

McWilliam, R. A., Ferguson, A., Harbin, G. L., Porter, P., Munn, D., and Vandiviere, P. (1998). The family-centeredness of Individualized Family Service Plans. *Topics in Early Childhood Special Education*, 18, 69–82.

McWilliam R. A. (2010). *Working with families of young children with special needs*. New York: The Guilford Press.

Markham, C. (2011). Designing a measure to explore the quality of life for children with speech, language and communication needs. In S. Roulstone and S. McLeod (eds), *Listening to children and young people with speech, language and communication needs*. London: J&R Press.

Markham, C., and Dean, T. (2006). Parents' and professionals' perceptions of Quality of Life in children with speech and language difficulty. *International Journal of Language and Communication Disorders*, 41, 189–212.

Markham, C., van Laar, D., Gibbard, D., et al. (2009). Children with speech, language and communication needs: their perceptions of their quality of life. *International Journal of Language and Communication Disorders*, 44, 748–768.

Mason, J., and Urquhart, R. (2001). Developing a model for participation by children in research on decision making. *Children Australia*, 26, 16–21.

Merrick R. (2011). Ethics, consent and assent when listening to children with speech, language communication needs. In S. Roulstone and S. McLeod (eds), *Listening to children and young people with speech, language and communication needs*, pp. 63–72. Guildford: J&R Press.

Merrick, R., and Roulstone, S. (2011). Children's views of communication and speech-language pathology. *International Journal of Speech and language Pathology*, 13, 281–290.

Mitchell, W., and Sloper, P. (2011). Making choices in my life: Listening to the ideas and experiences of young people in the UK who communicate non-verbally. *Children and Youth Services Review*, 33, 521–527.

Murphy, J. (1997). Talking Mats: a low-tech framework to help people with severe communication difficulties express their views. Stirling: University of Stirling.

National Federation of Voluntary Bodies (2008) *Research strategy 2008–2013*. Galway, Ireland: National Federation of Voluntary Bodies Providing Services to People with Intellectual Disabilities.

Office of the United Nations High Commissioner for Human Rights (1989). United Nations convention on the rights of the child. Geneva, Switzerland: United Nations.

Paige-Smith, A., and Rix, J. (2011). Researching early intervention and young children's perspectives – developing and using a 'listening to children approach'. *British Journal of Special Education*, 38, 28–36.

Patton, M. Q. (2002). *Qualitative Research and Evaluation Methods*, Thousand Oaks: Sage.

Porter, J., Daniels, H., Feiler, A., et al. (2011). Recognising the needs of every disabled child: the development of tools for a disability census. *British Journal of Special Education*, 38, 120–125.

Press, F., Bradley, B., Goodfellow, J., et al. (2011). Listening to infants about what life is like in childcare: A mosaic approach. In S. Roulstone and S. McLeod (eds), *Listening to children and young people with speech, language and communication needs*. London: J&R Press, 241–249.

Punch, S. (2002). Research with Children: The Same or Different from Research with Adults? *Childhood*, 9, 321–341.

Quortrup, J., Bardy, M., Sgritta, G., et al. (1994). *Childhood Matters Social Theory, Practice and Politics*. Aldershot: Avebury.

Rabiee, P., Sloper, P., and Beresford, B. (2005). Doing research with children and young people who do not use speech for communication. *Children & Society*, 19, 385–396.

Raghavendra, P. (2013) Participation of children with disabilities: Measuring subjective and objective outcomes. *Child: Care, Health and Development* 39, 461–465.

Roulstone, S., Harding, S., Coad, J., et al. (2013). Preschool Children's engagement in Speech and Language Therapy. *Child language Seminar.* University of Manchester.

Scott, J., Wishart, J., and Bowyer, D. (2006). Do current consent and confidentiality requirements impede or enhance research with children with learning disabilities? *Disability & Society*, 21, 373–287.

Sloper, P., and Beresford, B. (2006). Families with disabled children: Editorial. *BMJ*, 333, 928–929.

Stancliffe, R. J. (1999). Proxy respondents and the reliability of the Quality of Life Questionnaire Empowerment factor. *Journal of Intellectual Disability Research*, 23 (3), 185–193.

Thomas, N., and O'Kane, C. (2000). Discovering what children think: connections between researchand practice. *British Journal of Social Work*, 31, 819–835

Tisdall, E. K. M. (2012). The Challenge and Challenging of Childhood Studies. *Children & Society*, 26, 181–191.

Wang, C. C. (2006). Youth Participation in Photovoice as a Strategy for Community Change. *Journal of Community Practice*, 4, 147–161.

Whitehurst, T. (2006). Liberating silent voices – perspectives of children with profound and complex learning needs on inclusion. *British Journal of Learning Disabilities*, 35, 55–61.

Wilcox, M. J., and Shannon, M. S. (1996). Integrated early intervention practices in speech-language pathology. In R. A. McWilliam (ed.), *Rethinking pull-out services in early intervention: A professional resource*, pp. 217–242. Baltimore, MD: Brookes.

Wilcox, M. J., and Woods, J. (2011). Participation as a basis for developing early intervention outcomes. *Language, Speech and Hearing Services in Schools*, 42, 365–378.

PART III

Disciplinary illustrations and explorations around voice

HELEN LYNCH

10 Beyond voice: An occupational science perspective on researching through doing

Researching with children: A rights-based approach and the International Classification of Function, Disability and Health (ICF): Issues of participation

Researching children's lives is both a challenge and an opportunity. At times, it feels like going on a mystery tour, with no clear road-map, and few signposts to follow. From ethics boards who may not understand the nature of children's research, to text books and training courses that do not include consideration of the different nature of children's research, researchers can end up feeling lost. Therefore, implementing a study with children (especially children with disability) can be a journey down an unexpected route. No matter how carefully it is planned, you may need to amend your methods or change approaches: there is a fundamental need to approach the research project with flexibility, patience, reflexivity, and creativity. Despite these challenges, there is an opportunity to explore this difficult terrain and trust that the efforts you implement will achieve the required result: of illuminating the child's world by experiencing what it might be like being in the child's shoes. This chapter is underpinned by a rights-based approach: it aims to share insights from occupational science studies that draw from theories of agency, purposefulness, and participation. Furthermore, through presenting a background in occupational science, participation in research through doing will be presented as offering a powerful way to strengthen research with children.

A children's rights-based approach is driven significantly by the United Nations Convention on the Rights of the Child (UNCRC) (1989) and furthermore by the United Nations Convention on the Rights of Persons with Disabilities (UNCRPD) (United Nations 2006). In both the UNCRC and the UNCRPD, children's rights to participate are clearly stated: Article 12 (UNCRC) and Article 7 (UNCRPD) are concerned with providing for the child's right to have a say, to participate in decisions that affect them, irrespective of their carers. This is set out in the context of allowing for age, maturity, and ability, with the onus on the States Parties to ensure all efforts are made to give assistance to the child to achieve this:

> States Parties shall ensure that children with disabilities have the right to express their views freely on all matters affecting them, their views being given due weight in accordance with their age and maturity, on an equal basis with other children, and to be provided with disability and age-appropriate assistance to realize that right. (UNCRPD 2008: 10)

In occupational therapy, participation has also come to the fore in a significant way through the influence of the World Health Organization's (WHO) framework: The *International Classification of Function, Disability, and Health (ICF)*. This model of health, function and disability was developed and ratified by the WHO in 2001 and aims to standardize language, and conceptual approaches in researching and working in the health sector. It aims to combine a biopsychosocial approach, which is an integration of biological, psychological, and social science knowledge, at an individual and community level. The ICF-CY (WHO 2007) was subsequently developed to apply specifically to children.

The ICF-CY framework consists of core categories of concern: body function/structure, *activity, participation*, personal factors and the environment. Consequently, in research with children with disabilities, there has been a significant expansion towards researching *activity and participation* (e.g. Law, Petrenchik, King and Hurley 2007; Poulsen, Ziviani and Cuskelly 2007; Harding et al. 2009; Coster et al. 2012; Anaby et al. 2013; Dunford, Bannigan and Wales 2013; King, Law, Petrenchik and Hurley 2013). In this context, participation relates to involvement in a life situation, and is usually integrated with activity. So, from a rights-based, disability perspective, participation signifies not just having a say in matters that effect you, but also being able to be actively participating in home, school and community life.

An occupational science perspective

The discipline of occupational science emerged in the late 1980s in Southern California and is a science that is concerned with understanding the relationship between daily activity (occupations), and health, well-being and development (Pierce 2001; Hocking 2009). Although it has strong roots in occupational therapy, occupational science draws significantly from anthropology, architecture, human geography, psychology, and social sciences. Occupational science is the study of occupations, which are considered to be transactional engagements that occur between the person, and the environment. As such, occupational science underpins occupational therapy practice, which is concerned with the health and wellbeing of individuals, through doing in the world. Occupations are defined as *'chunks of daily activity that can be named in the lexicon of the culture'* (Zemke and Clark 1996: vii). An occupational science approach is based on key assumptions of occupation:

• humans have a basic drive to engage in occupation;
• occupations and environmental contexts are inseparable;
• occupations are fundamental to health, wellbeing, and development;
• occupations are contextual-and include the temporal, socio-cultural; political contexts of occupation, and the physical and biological factors that influence such occupations;
• occupations hold meaning for the individual.

Therefore, occupations are typically considered to be complex and multidimensional.

It is clear from the outline of occupational science, that meaning and context are fundamentally important. This includes more recently, the development of a human rights perspective to the study of occupation, with a focus on societal contexts and occupational justice (Durocher, Gibson and Rappolt 2014). Emerging from this work, is the commitment to a child's rights-based approach, with the shared belief in the child's agency, autonomy and as rights holders and citizens. This reflects a social constructivist perspective, which includes consideration of children as meaning-makers, who have an active role in constructing their social lives (Rogoff 2003). Although occupational science speaks of doing, being and becoming (Wilcock 1998), this does not reflect an emphasis on the future adult, but gives equal recognition to childhood as a time of being, of well-being or more accurately, well-doing.

Within occupational science, play is considered to be the main occupation of childhood (Reilly 1974) and is 'characterized as intrinsic, spontaneous, fun, flexible, totally absorbing, vitalising, challenging, nonliteral, and an end in and of itself' (Knox 2008: 55). Play occupation is noted to encompass playfulness which is the expression of the play experience (Skard and Bundy 2008) and involves intrinsic motivation, internal control and suspension of reality. Play occupation has more recently been compared to 'play for play sake' or free-play to distinguish it from the therapeutic use of play in developing or teaching skills (Lynch and Moore 2016; Ray-Kaeser and Lynch 2016). Overall, an occupational science perspective of play is that it can be both productive as well as pleasurable: that it can be embedded in obligatory tasks and require effort (Humphry 2002). Although occupational science values the functional contribution of play to child development, it also values the meaning for the child: 'play is a vehicle for meaning' (Parham 1996: 78). The study of play occupation therefore requires attending to socio-cultural and physical contexts to gain insight into the unfolding transactional events as they occur in daily life (Lynch, Hayes and Ryan 2015). Overall, from an occupational science perspective, the focus is on 'being at play' as a process, more than the skill involved or the outcome. Hence, a rights-based, occupational science approach reflects a fundamental valuing of the centrality of children's participation, that goes beyond voice.

Researching childhood occupations

From a rights-based approach to research, eliciting the child's views requires 'an active process of communication involving hearing, interpreting, and constructing meaning ... not limited to the spoken word' (Clark 2005: 491).

Thus, a child rights-based approach requires researchers to develop suitable methods that elicits children's views. This needs to involve careful consideration to designing 'safe, inclusive and engaging opportunities for children' (Lundy and McEvoy 2012: 1) through the design of methods that appeal to children's developmental abilities and interests (Lynch and Lynch 2013). It is about exploring methods that enable an adult researcher to understand a child's communication style: from voice, expression, non-verbal communication, emotional response and behaviour, and from observing the child's actions. Thus, there is a need to go beyond voice.

Within this context, an occupational science researcher begins from the position of valuing 'doing'. This has a strong position for any researchers of children's worlds however, and not just from an occupational science perspective. Children communicate through what they do, and in some cases more effectively. For example, young children are more reliant on non-verbal communication, and frequently communicate through silence (Curtin 2001). Many researchers of young children have designed research by interacting through occupation or through naturalistic observation of occupation (Corsaro and Eder 1990; Haight and Miller 1993; Pellegrini, Kato, Blatchford and Baines 2002; Clark 2007). In some cases, children are engaged as co-researchers, where they generate data through photography, map-making, drawing, walking (Clark 2005; Waller 2007; Clark 2010; Kilkelly, Lynch, O'Connell, Moore and Field 2016). These participatory approaches aim to empower children as knowledge producers, and involve a *continuum of participation* from being research participants, to co-researchers (Lundy and McEvoy 2012).

For researchers who are concerned with gaining insight into the 'doing' of everyday occupations, these methods of data generation can be further extended. For example, in occupational science, one method that has been employed to good effect with children as research participants, is the use of time-diaries to map daily events and routines (e.g. Kellegrew 2000; Lynch 2009; Minkoff and Riley 2011; Orban, Edberg, Thorngren-Jerneck, Onnerfalt and Erlandsson 2013). This method has helped illuminate how children name their occupations differently to adults (Lynch 2009). In a study of children's play occupations in a city in Ireland Lynch (2009) identified 'non-conventional' occupations of children in middle childhood that children named as: catching ladybirds, lying in the grass, or playing with friends on the green. Instead parents named the same play occupations as playing outside or playing soccer. From the child's perspective lying in the grass was a 'valid' play activity, yet was named differently by the adults. From an occupational therapist's perspective, lying in the grass is an occupation that is not typically named in activity checklists. One explanation is that the parent did not know exactly what the child was doing. However, another explanation is that adults do not have the same perspective as children, when it comes to naming meaningful occupations. Adults may consider lying in the grass to be a passive activity of little value, but from a child's viewpoint this may be a special activity. So, it is a matter of gaining insight into occupations from a child's perspective: to aim to understand the significance of occupation for the child.

Another key method in the study of children's occupational lives has been achieved through multiple means that typically includes observation, so the there is an 'intimate familiarity' with the social world being explored (Brewer 2000: 11). This research methdology is frequently named as participant observation but comes from an ethnographic tradition. In ethnography, data is gathered from multiple sources but with observation (and specifically participant observation) being a core feature (Hammersley and Atkinson 2007). The result is an interpretive account that details the physical, social, and cultural lives of children. Ethnographic studies of childhood occupations have been carried out with typically developing children and families in naturalistic environmental contexts (Primeau 1998; Pierce 2000; Bazyk, Stalnaker, Llerena, Ekelman and Bazyk 2003; Lynch 2012). The common threads throughout these studies include the extensive use of observation and interview in the home or community environments being researched, with the emphasis on identifying and exploring the experiences of children as occupational beings.

To summarize, when researching childhood occupations, a researcher needs to be ready to design methods that are designed for appeal, are appropriate to the competencies and interests of the child, and that maximize the potential to gain insight into a child's perspective. For many research questions, this may also include the need to adopt methods that include 'doing'- either to engage a child in activity, or to use observational methods to study the child's occupational behaviour (Reilly 1974) as the unit of analysis.

Researching with children with disabilities

When researching with children with disabilities, similar concerns about methods that capture the meaning of occupation need to be considered. It is likely that their world is equally different to an adult world, in terms of meaning and occupation, as has been noted in other studies of childhood occupation. Importantly, their occupations may have no name (Hocking 2009) and may appear to be merely *less complex* versions of known adult occupations (Humphry 2005). However, within the occupational science community, the issue of complexity has been challenged, particularly when exploring the occupational lives of children or those who have disabilities (Humphry 2002, 2009; Spitzer 2003a; Humphry and Wakeford 2006). For example, if an infant swipes at a mobile, is it a complex or a simple occupation? These early play behaviours are unskilled from an adult's perspective, and to many may seem purposeless. Yet, when one considers the competencies and interests of a young infant, this may represent the most complex play event in their lives to date. So, when researching children's occupations, a researcher should avoid judging occupation in relation to complexity:

> A definition of occupation that does not acknowledge the occupations of children with developmental disabilities because of the requirement of skill and complexity essentially dehumanises those who engage in 'less skilled' or 'simple' activities. (Spitzer 2003a: 71)

In addition, understanding the nature and context of how children engage in their environments is fundamental. Children can be engaged by simply 'being in the atmosphere of doing' (Jonsson 2007), which is a common form of engagement for young infants or for children with severe disabilities (Lynch 2010). For example, in a study of children with autism in a classroom context, Bagatell established that onlooker participation is a common mode of engagement (2011). In her study, she identified that although one child looked disengaged, he still showed signs of listening and attending to what was happening about him, by answering the teachers question correctly. The researcher asserts that this appeared to demonstrate the pattern of onlooker participation that has been noted in other studies (e.g. Humphry 2009; Pereira, laCour, Jonsson and Hemmingsson 2010) and has been noted as an important distinction from considering onlooker participation to be merely passive (Lynch and Moore 2016). In another study, Lynch (2012) also notes this play style among young infants: some infants chose to observe occupations before engaging in them, while others enter the play event without pausing. Engagement needs to be considered as a continuum from onlooker to full participation.

However, once the nature of childhood occupations is considered, there is still the need to determine methods that enable a child with disabilities to participate in research. Although, few studies have been conducted to date with children with disabilities, there is an emergent area of occupational research that reflects the move towards the use of more visual methods (Lynch and Stanley 2017). For example, Phelan and Kinsella (2014) conducted a study with eleven participants, aged ten to twelve years, who had physical impairments. In their study of occupation and identity, multiple methods were used that included photographic logs (developed by participants), alongside photo elicitation interviews. These participants were able to both contribute as co-researchers, and engage in language communication to explain subjective experiences. However, not all children are able to be active data generators or contributors: a young infant or a child with varied forms of disabilities may not be able to engage in active photography or other visual methods, such as drawing. In this case, the researcher is required to consider how the child can be a research participant, through 'doing-in-context', that is, through carrying out daily play occupations while in the company of the researcher (who acts as a participant observer) or using video (videography). From a social constructivist perspective, this approach is one that centralizes childhood occupations in context as an important way to respect the child's agency. Participant observation might reflect for that child, the greatest level of participation that he or she can achieve, and may be the most child-centred method of choice.

Study One: Participant observation to explore 'being at play'

Spitzer's work is one study that serves as an exemplar participant observation in researching with children with disabilities. Spitzer's qualitative study explored the daily play occupations of five children with autism aged from three to four years. Her challenge was that these children were predominantly non-verbal and rarely used spontaneous language; hence her methodology relied heavily on participant observation, in multiple contexts, over several months. Spitzer's approach was to take part in the occupations when appropriate, and to make detailed notes about what each child did, and how and where the occupations were completed, without using pre-set codes or checklists of activities. This was accompanied by interviews with family members and carers. The result was the identification and description of important play occupations in which her participants engaged (see Table 10.1). By giving words to these occupations, Spitzer's work reflects her efforts to illuminate the personally meaningful occupations enjoyed by these children.

In her study of these 'uncommon' play occupations, Spitzer is informed by the underlying knowledge that individuals engage in occupations that are meaningful to them; and that the purpose of this engagement is to meet a biological need perhaps, or social need for identity and belonging, for pleasure and enjoyment, to explore, learn and master some new skills (Humphry 2002; Spitzer 2004). Some occupations are driven by internal, subjective motivations, such as play (Bundy 1997). Others are driven by external factors, such as social expectations to complete chores set by adults (Humphry 2009), and so are not so freely chosen. Hence the purpose may be different but each engagement in occupation contains underlying meaning and motivation.

However, Spitzer notes that the meaning of these occupations is difficult to determine, especially when individuals cannot express themselves

Table 10.1: Examples of Common and Uncommon Occupations:
Three Vignettes (Spitzer 2003b: 69)

Vignette 1: Drumming with dolls occupation
Britany would sit in the kitchen doorway, which was the centre of all the household activities. She banged her dolls on the floor one at a time with a flick of the wrist. The dolls clicked softly on the linoleum floor as they hit it lightly in a steady, rhythmical pattern. With her mother, Britany would alter the speed/tempo of banging her dolls and look at her mother, who makes 'ow' sounds with each bang, speeding up or slowing down her 'ows' to correspond with Britany's banging.
Interpreted meaning: Rhythm; restoration (comfort); interpersonal interaction
Vignette 2: Dropping dirt occupation
Mike would drop one handful of dirt at a time in partial shade, where the dust would glisten in the sunlight. With his mother, would hold the handful in front of him, Drop the dirt. She would blow the dirt as it fell, creating a bigger and longer-lasting cloud of dirt. They would both laugh
Interpreted meaning: visual aesthetics
Vignette 3: Gotcha game occupation
Justin would move away from an adult slightly, just out of arms reach. As the adult reached he would continue to move just slightly out of reach, smiling:
Interpreted meaning: Social interactions; 'playing with' experiences of security and safety

through language. It is difficult to establish the significance of any occupation for another individual; for example, the child who chose to bang the doll appeared to enjoy the rhythm of the banging activity, whereas the doll itself may not have had any symbolic significance as a miniature human figure (which may be the adult assumption). Spitzer notes that observation alone is not enough, but that through repeated observation, supplemented by parent and carer interviews, signs of subjective meaning can be ascertained, by observing play preferences, and engagement when free choice is involved. Furthermore, by including multiple observations of self-selected occupations compared to those that a child refuses or reluctantly engages in, there are multiple points of comparison to clarify subjective meaning. Researchers can also be informed by insights from adults with autism, who write of their subjective experiences of growing up with autism (see for example, Grandin and Scariano 1986; Williams 1992). All contribute to a shared subjectivity that can strengthen qualitative research with children with disabilities.

Study Two: Beyond participant observation: using videography to explore 'being at play'

In some circumstances, participant observation is not enough, and additional methods need to be considered to answer a research question, for example when a more microanalytical approach is needed. This issue arose for the author in the outset of her journey to explore the role of the physical environment in the emergence of early play occupation in home settings (Infant Study). Although participant observation was considered suitable, it soon became apparent that infants engage in different forms of early play occupation than older children; they can be brief and fleeting, and can be easily missed by the observer, and may not be repeated within the same hour or time of day. Consequently, the researcher began to explore the use of video as a qualitative method for researching play occupations in naturalistic settings. Although the infants in this study were developing typically, the same issues arise around identifying methods that enable research with children who are non-verbal, or who have different communication styles.

Video methods have advanced significantly in recent years and have slowly been emerging out of quantitative tradition, where they have been used to quantify behaviour or represent a view of objective reality (Pink 2013). Instead, from a qualitative perspective, video methods record events in naturalistic settings that can then be interpreted socially and framed within their contexts (Knoblauch and Tuma 2011). Hence, Knoblauch and Tuma propose the term *videography* to represent the use of video from an interpretive perspective. Video data can be used in multiple ways to add depth and breadth to a study: for example, *video stills* can capture key moments, while specific videoed events can be used for *video elicitation* (where participants view the event together with the researcher to co-construct meaning). Videography can support detailed, repeated analysis of multiple events, or influences within the environment, that shape the evolving event, while multiple researchers can analyse the same event collaboratively to strengthen the analytical process. Furthermore, video supports a detailed analysis of spaces, objects, and artefacts, including what is used and valued by the family in the home. This aspect of ethnographic study is noted to be underexplored to date (Hammersley and Atkinson 2007).

Hence, for a study that aimed to explore the influences of the physical and social environment on an infant's play, video provided one means to support in-depth, micro-analysis.

The challenge with a videography study is to determine clear methods of analysis. To date, there is little consensus on how video data should be analysed in videography, with some recommending full transcription of video while others recommend selection of key events for transcription (Ratcliff 2003; Knoblauch and Tuma 2011). Although it is typical to convert some or all of the video into words for analysis of text, there are many challenges: there is a danger that we impose words on events that do not accurately capture what occurred, or that words are not carefully chosen to ensure rigour. Video data does not come ready-made with words. Video analysis will depend on the research question and purpose of the study, so naturally the choices about what words to use for transcription will be led by the focus of the research. For example, it may be a study of micro processes such as facial expressions or gestures to support interpretation of meaning, or it may be a more meso level of research that explores whole events such as a birthday party. Finding the important words that capture what is being researched is a vital step: as 'experience, action, artefact, image or idea is never just one thing but may be redefined differently in different situations, by different individuals and in terms of different discourses' (Pink 2013: 19). So, in videography, careful attention to translating the video into text format, is required. The researcher must carefully identify the initial words and then the interpretive words through co-construction of meaning ideally with the participants and if not, with a co-researcher to support reflexivity and rigour (Lynch and Stanley 2017).

In the Infant Study, five families were recruited from varied urban and rural environments in Ireland, to participate in a longitudinal study over twelve months (Lynch 2012). These were families of infants that were newborn (two families) or one year old (3 families) at the outset of the study. Families were visited each month and video used to record the infants play occupation in the natural environment, that sometimes included the back garden, the grandmother's house, as well as multiple rooms and spaces in each home where the infant typically played. Similar to Spitzer's study, observations were supplemented by monthly interviews with adults who knew the infant. Video data were generated that supported the video elicitation approach, while key events captured on video enabled the researcher to produce video stills. This form of data supported further detailed microanalysis of important moments (see vignette).

Vignette: In one play event, Karen (aged ten months) was observed playing with a small, lightweight toy that seemed to be motivating her play. The still below shows her engagement in the play event, which involved her reaching for the small toy. The video still captures the moment she tries to reach and successfully get to the toy. However, the video data shows that her play involves 'chasing the toy' – once she has it in her hands, she does not play with it but instead continues to throw it and challenge herself to regain it.

In the Infant Study, infants were observed being at play, and video added further insights to how to describe play interactions in the social and physical environment: by describing *how* the infant played with spaces and objects in the environment, rather than simply *naming* play items or frequency of use. The challenge in adopting this approach, is to find ways to analyse occupational behaviour of young infants, who may have a very limited repertoire of movements. So, one solution to this dilemma was to draw from other studies that identify occupational behaviour as involving intentionality and purposiveness and observable through environmental transactions (Wood, Towers and Malchow 2000). Intentionality is evident when a child is observed focusing on things deliberately, while purposiveness refers to behaviours that appear to have some aim (that is, not unintentional or aimless behaviour). When researching with children with severe disabilities, these ways of thinking about what the child is doing can support the development of insight into their occupational worlds. Finally, through this analytical framework, a researcher can explore the agency and adaptedness of infant engagement in occupation, which is known to be evident in typically developing infants in the earliest ages (Nagy 2011; Trevarthen 2011). Hence, from a rights-based, occupational science perspective, this concept of agency at the micro-level, can equally be considered for children with severe disability.

Analysis of the play transactions in this study required the researcher to consider to the role of the physical environment in influencing play occupation. This was a further challenge that was resolved by adopting the theory of affordances. Affordance theory considers how individuals develop an understanding of the world based on the functional use of spaces and objects (Gibson 1977). Affordances are intrinsic to the person-environment relationship as they are based on the person's ability to perceive the potential affordances or functional properties of the environment (for example, instead of naming an object a foot stool, it can be described by how it is used: a place to play for an infant or a place to rest your leg if you are an adult). More importantly, an affordance approach reflects a child's perspective, where there is 'the tendency of children to name places in terms of their functional significance' (Heft 1988: 35). In affordance theory, the person and the physical environment are both considered to have agency (Clark and Uzzell 2002). From the initial analysis of affordances in the home, video contributed to an understanding that places need to be named by their occupational use (see Table 10.2).

Videography in the Infant Study enabled the researcher to consider play in context. For example, no one type of play was observed in isolation, with object play being part of space or social play at one time, thus demonstrating that play is a dynamic, inter-related transaction with the social and physical environment. Physical activity play (Pellegrini and Smith 1998) was observed as being frequently social. Equally, social play was observed primarily through family play and interaction games led by more mature players. It would seem that arguments against the need for categorization of play are supported here in an ecological study, where play is observed as a contextual, holistic transaction (Sutton-Smith 1986). Consequently, play was described in this study as *infant play*, which encompasses all the different characteristics of play observed in infants under two, rather than attempting to name the play form (for example, exercise play) or on the nature of interaction (for example, object play or social play) (see Lynch and Stanley 2017 for further insights).

Table 10.2: Example of Occupational Use of Places in the Home

Affordances: Functional use of places	*Formal places: Purpose-built/ designed for infants*	*Family places/adapted; use of existing furniture or spaces for infants' needs*	*Informal: use of social and physical setting*
Place for sleeping	Moses basket Cot	Bed with cushions to protect from falling	Corner of the couch
Place for grooming	Changing table Baby bath	Bath with insert	On mother's lap
Place for feeding	Baby-bouncers High-chair at table Booster seat at table	Family kitchen chair with cushioning	On mother's lap Designated floor space for infants who can sit independently
Place for toileting	Changing table Potty	Toilet not used until toilet training at later stage	On bed On mother's lap
Place for personal space	Baby room	Shared bedroom- with parents or siblings	Within Moses basket, buggy, playpen
Place for play	Play-pen	Play room or designated play area	Anywhere in the home/ use of toy boxes
Place for socialising	Baby bouncers, baby standers and walkers placed centrally in family activity	Use of arm-chairs, couches to enable infant to be in the middle of the social environment	On floor On mother's lap

Considerations for researching through an occupational lens: strengthening strategies

In this chapter, two studies have been presented that represent two different approaches to researching with children who engage in uncommon or early occupational behaviour. Both examples are used to illuminate the different ways to approach researching through occupation: through doing. While both examples draw from an ethnographic tradition with participant observation as a central approach to data generation, one study includes the addition of videography for further consideration. Before concluding, some specific strategies can be highlighted that may help strengthen researching occupational behaviour. Researchers need to develop a range of strategies to strengthen their skills in effective participant observation (Spitzer 2003a, 2004). Observations alone are not enough to inform the meaning of an occupation (Coster and Khetani 2008), yet observing occupation enables the researcher to identify what activity is meaningful for the individual. Spitzer proposes some important ways to help the process:

1.   to suspend adult assumptions;
2.   assume all actions are potentially communicative;
3.   attend to communication through occupational engagement;
4.   develop a shared history with the child;
5.   interview adults knowledgeable about the child;
6.   scrutinize data and interpretations for effect of adult presence (Spitzer 2003a: 71).

Suspending adult assumptions comes from the dilemma of interpretation, when an adult perspective of meaning can be problematic:

> Adults often have trouble interpreting children's actions from the child's perspective rather than from their own adult standards, needs and wants. (Spitzer 2003b:70)

To be effective in this form of research, *adults need to readjust their lens* and aim to understand experiences from a child's perspective. Adult habits of communication are different to that of the child who engages in other ways to communicate (Curtin 2001; Spitzer 2003b). So, to establish a better understanding from a child's perspective, the researcher might consider engaging in the same occupation with the child, and follow his or her lead. By sharing in the experiences of the occupation, *the experience is felt by both participants* (the child and the researcher). Furthermore, the researcher follows the child's lead rather than presenting him or herself as the authoritative adult. When researching with children with autism,

Spitzer adds the strategy of consciously sharpening the senses- to attune more to the child's experience, which for a child with autism maybe highly related to features in the sensory environment (Spitzer 2003a)

Conclusion

Observing children play can be a powerful way to research children's lives. However, observation can also be problematic as in traditional approaches, modes of observation were frequently considered to be an objectification of children (Gallacher and Gallagher 2008). But observation can be a qualitative method once the aim of the researcher is to understand meaning, and once the approach is to analyse action from a subjective perspective, that goes beyond counting behaviours. Indeed, Rogoff reflected that observational studies are more likely to be interpretive than not: 'researchers cannot avoid interpretation in any kind of research because they must rely on knowledge of the context and of norms of behaviour in order to recognize the relevance of the observed behaviour for the theory being tested' (Rogoff, Mistry, Goncu and Mosier 1993: 32). Observation can be augmented by the use of videography, as video can capture the spatial, temporal, and interactive elements of any activity and therefore has a close connection to researching processes of transactions over time. Thus, videos can be used to generate data that cannot be adequately expressed through words or texts, usually where there is a need to interpret data in relation to the context from which it originated (Mason 2002).

Both observation and video methods require the adult to 'listen' to the child. Fundamental to these interpretive approaches is that the researcher is required to understand the nature of childhood and how it differs from adulthood. This includes understanding child development, including communication, sociocultural influences, agency, autonomy, power relations and ethical practice. Specifically, when engaging with children, there is a need to address power issues is an essential feature of effective research. The researcher is challenged to consider which methods to choose to reduce power imbalances and to maximize the child's potential to communicate and participate (Curtin 2001). In addition, when the child has a disability, there is a need to consider developmental difficulties and differences in cognitive, linguistic and perceptual abilities (Spitzer 2003a).

Overall, from an occupational child rights perspective, we need to ensure that children (including infants and children with disabilities) inform our understanding of their occupational lives and their occupations in the same way as adults have informed occupational research to date. Children's occupations are not an issue of less complexity but simply of difference. Children do not just reproduce their cultural worlds, they also create them. Furthermore, their cultural worlds are not only social, they include material culture of childhood: with places and objects for play that are known (for example, playgrounds or toys) or 'unknown' (for example, derelict sites or empty boxes). Hence the use of video and participant observation can be seen to have great potential to contribute to a greater understanding of children's worlds.

References

Anaby, D., Hand, C., Bradley, L., DiRezze, B., Forhan, M., DiGiacomo, A., and Law, M. (2013). The Effect of the Environment on Participation of Children and Youth with Disabilities: A Scoping Review. *Disability and Rehabilitation*, 1–10. DOI: 10.3109/09638288.2012.748840

Bagatell, N. (2011). 'Engaged Moments: Mediated Action and Children with Autism in the Classroom Setting. *OTJR: Occupation, Participation and Health*, 32 (1), 258–265. DOI:10.3928/15394492-20110722-01

Bazyk, S., Stalnaker, D., Llerena, M., Ekelman, B., and Bazyk, J. (2003). Play in Mayan Children. *American Journal of Occupational Therapy*, 57 (3), 273–283.

Brewer, J. (2000). *Ethnography: understanding social research*. Maidenhead: Open University Press.

Bundy, A. (1997). Play and Playfulness: What to Look For. In L. D. Parham and L. Fazio (eds), *Play in occupational therapy for children*, pp. 52–66. St Louis, MO: Mosby.

Clark, A. (2005). Ways of Seeing: Using the Mosaic Approach to Listen to Young Children's Perspectives. In A. Clark, P. Moss and A. Kjorholt (eds), *Beyond listening: children's perspectives on early childhood services*, pp. 29–49. Bristol: Policy Press.

Clark, A. (2007). Views from Inside the Shed: Young Children's Perspectives of the Outdoor Environment. *Education 3–13*, 35 (4), 349–363.

Clark, A. (2010). Young Children as Protagonists and the Role of Participatory, Visual Methods in Engaging Multiple Perspectives. *American Journal of Community Psychology*, 46, 115–123.

Clark, C., and Uzzell, D. (2002). The Affordances of the Home, Neighbourhood, School and Town Centre for Adolescents. *Journal of Environmental Psychology*, 22, 95–108.

Corsaro, W., and Eder, D. (1990). Children's Peer Cultures. *Annual Review of Sociology*, 16, 197–220.

Coster, W., and Khetani, M. (2008). Measuring Participation of Children with Disabilities: Issues and Challenges. *Disability and Rehabilitation*, 30 (8), 639–648.

Coster, W., Law, M., Bedell, G., Khetani, M., Cousins, M., and Teplicky, R. (2012). Development of the Participation and Environment Measure for Children and Youth: Conceptual Basis. *Disability and Rehabilitation*, 34, 238–246.

Curtin, C. (2001). Eliciting Children's Voices in Qualitative Research. *American Journal of Occupational Therapy*, 55 (3), 295–302.

Dunford, C., Bannigan, K., and Wales, L. (2013). Measuring Activity and Participation Outcomes for Children and Youth with Acquired Brain Injury: An Occupational Therapy Perspective. British *Journal of Occupational Therapy*, 76 (2), 67–76. DOI: 10.4276/030802213X13603244419158

Durocher, E., Gibson, B. E., and Rappolt, S. (2014). Occupational Justice: A Conceptual Review. *Journal of Occupational Science*, 21 (4), 418–430.

Gallacher, L., and Gallagher, M. (2008). Methodological Immaturity in Childhood Research? Thinking Through 'Participatory Methods. *Childhood*, 15 (4), 499–516. DOI: 10.1177/0907568208091672

Gibson, J. (1977). The Theory of Affordances. In R. Shaw and J. Bransford (eds), *Perceiving, acting and knowing: Toward an ecological psychology*, pp. 67–82. London: Lawrence Erlbaum Associates.

Grandin, T., and Scariano, M. (1986). *Emergence: labeled autistic*. Novato, CA: Arean Press.

Haight, W. L., and Miller, P. (1993). *Pretending at home: early development in a sociocultural context*. New York: State University of New York Press.

Hammersley, M., and Atkinson, P. (2007). *Ethnography: principles in practice* (3rd ed.). London: Routledge.

Harding, J., Harding, K., Jamieson, P., Mullally, M., Politi, C., Wong-Sing, E., Petrenchik, T. M. (2009). Children with Disabilities' Perceptions of Activity

Participation and Environments: A Pilot Study. *Canadian Journal of Occupational Therapy*, 76 (3), 133–144.

Heft, H. (1988). Affordances of Children's Environments: A Functional Approach to Environmental Description. *Children's Environments Quarterly*, 5 (3), 29–37.

Hocking, C. (2009). The Challenge of Occupation: Describing the Things People Do. *Journal of Occupational Science*, 16 (3), 140–150.

Humphry, R. (2002). Young Children's Occupations: Explicating Dynamics of Developmental Processes. *American Journal of Occupational Therapy*, 56, 171–179.

Humphry, R. (2005). Model of processes transforming occupations: Exploring societal and social influences. *Journal of Occupational Science*, 12 (1), 36–44.

Humphry, R. (2009). Occupation and Development: A Contextual Perspective. In E. Crepeau, E. Cohn and B. Schell (eds), *Willard and Spackman's occupational therapy* (11th ed.), pp. 22–32. London: Wolters Kluwar/Lippincott Williams and Wilkins.

Humphry, R., and Wakeford, L. (2006). An Occupation-Centred Discussion of Development and Implications for Practice. *American Journal of Occupational Therapy*, 60 (3), 258–267.

Jonsson, H. (2007). *Participation- a central concept in health that should be problematised*. Paper presented at the European Network of Teachers in Higher Education Annual Conference, UCC, Cork, Ireland.

Kellegrew, D. (2000). Constructing Daily Routines: A Qualitative Examination of Mothers with Young Children with Disabilities. *The American Journal of Occupational Therapy*, 54 (3), 252–259.

Kilkelly, U., Lynch, H., O'Connell, A., Moore, A., and Field, S. (2016). *Children and the Outdoors: Contact with the Outdoors and Natural Heritage among Children aged 6 to 12: Current Trends, Benefits, Barriers and Research Requirements*. Heritage Council. Retrieved From: <http://www.heritagecouncil.ie/content/files/children_%20outdoors_commissioned_report_26mb.pdf>.

King, G., Law, M., Petrenchik, T., and Hurley, P. (2013). Psychosocial Determinants of Out of School Activity Participation for Children with and without Physical Disabilities. *Physical and Occupational Therapy in Paediatrics*, 1–21. DOI:10.3109/01942638.2013.791915.

Knoblauch, H., and Tuma, R. (2011). Videography: An Interpretative Approach to Video-Recorded Micro-Social Interaction. In E. Margolis and L. Pauwels (eds), *The SAGE handbook of visual research methods*, pp. 414–430. London, UK: SAGE Publications Ltd.

Knox, S. (2008). Development and Current Use of the Revised Knox Preschool Play Scale. In L. D. Parham and L. Fazio (eds), *Play in occupational therapy for children* (2nd ed.), pp. 55–70. St Louis, MO: Mosby Elsevier.

Law, M., Petrenchik, T., King, G., and Hurley, P. (2007). Perceived Environmental Barriers to Recreational, Community, and School Participation for Children and Youth with Physical Disabilities. *Archives of Physical Medicine and Rehabilitation*, 88 (12), 1636–1642.

Lundy, L., and McEvoy, L. (2012). Children's Rights and Research Processes: Assisting Children to (In) formed Views. *Childhood*, 19 (1), 129–144.

Lynch, H. (2009). Patterns of Activity of Irish Children aged Five to Eight Years: City Living in Ireland Today. *Journal of Occupational Science*, 16 (1), 44–49.

Lynch, H. (2010). *The emergence of occupation: infant-environment transactions in the home.* Paper presented at the Redefining Boundaries and Bridges in Occupational Science, London, Ontario, London, Ontario.

Lynch, H. (2012). *Infant places, spaces and objects: exploring the physical in learning environments for infants under two.* Unpublished PhD thesis. School of Social Science and Law. Dublin Institute of Technology.

Lynch, H., Hayes, N., and Ryan, S. (2015). Exploring Socio-Cultural Influences that Impact on Infant Play Occupations in Irish Home Environments. *Journal of Occupational Science.* DOI: 10.1080/14427591.2015.1080181

Lynch, H., and Moore, A. (2016). Play as an Occupation in Occupational Therapy. *British Journal of Occupational Therapy*, 79 (9), 519–520. DOI: 10.1177/0308022616664540

Lynch, H., and Stanley, M. (2017). Beyond Words: Using Qualitative Video Methods for Researching Occupation with Children. *OTJR: Occupation, Participation & Health*, 1–11. DOI: 10.1177/1539449217718504

Lynch, R., and Lynch, H. (2013). Exploring Children's Decisions to Participate in Occupational Therapy Research. *Irish Journal of Occupational Therapy*, 40 (1), 22–30.

Mason, J. (2002). *Qualitative research* (2nd edn). London: Sage Publications.

Minkoff, Y., and Riley, J. (2011). Perspectives of Time-Use: Exploring the Use of Drawings, Interviews, and Rating-Scales with Children aged 6–7 years. *Journal of Occupational Science*, 18 (4), 306–321. doi:10.1080/14427591.2011.586323

Nagy, E. (2011). The Newborn Infant: A Missing Stage in Developmental Psychology. *Infant and Child Development*, 20, 3–19.

Orban, K., Edberg, A., Thorngren-Jerneck, K., Onnerfalt, J., and Erlandsson, L. (2013). Changes in Parent's Time-Use and its Relationship to Child Obesity. *Physical and Occupational Therapy in Pediatrics*, 1–18.

Parham, L. D. (1996). Perspectives on play. In R. Zemke and F. Clark (eds), *Occupational science: the evolving discipline*, pp. 71–80. Philadelphia, PA: F. A. Davis.

Pellegrini, A., Kato, K., Blatchford, P., and Baines, E. (2002). A Short-Term Longitudinal Study of Children's Playground Games across the First Year of School: Implications for Social Competence and Adjustment to School. *American Educational Research Journal*, 39 (4), 991–1019.

Pellegrini, A., and Smith, P. (1998). 'Physical Activity Play: The Nature and Function of a Neglected Aspect of Play', *Child Development*, 69 (3), 577–598.

Pereira, E., laCour, K., Jonsson, H., and Hemmingsson, H. (2010). 'The Participation Experience of Children with Disabilities in Portuguese Mainstream Schools', *British Journal of Occupational Therapy*, 73 (12), 598–606. DOI: 10.4276/030802210X12918167234244.

Phelan, S., and Kinsella, E. A. (2014). 'Occupation and Identity: Perspectives of Children with Disabilities and their Parents. *Journal of Occupational Science*, 21 (3), 334–356.

Pierce, D. (2000). Maternal Management of Home as a Developmental Play Space for Infants and Toddlers. *American Journal of Occupational Therapy*, 54 (3), 290–299.

Pierce, D. (2001). Untangling Occupation from Activity. *American Journal of Occupational Therapy*, 55 (2), 138–146.

Pink, S. (2013). *Doing visual ethnography* (3rd ed.). London: Sage Publications.

Poulsen, A. A., Ziviani, J. M., and Cuskelly, M. (2007). Perceived Freedom in Leisure and Physical Co-ordination Ability: Impact on Out-of-School Activity Participation and Life Satisfaction. *Child: Care, Health and Development*, 33 (4), 432–440.

Primeau, L. (1998). Orchestration of Work and Play within Families. *American Journal of Occupational Therapy*, 52, 188–195.

Ratcliff, D. (2003). Video Methods in Qualitative Research. In P. Camic, J. Rhodes and L. Yardley (eds), *Qualitative research in psychology: expanding perspectives in methodology and design*, pp. 113–130. Washington, DC: American Psychological Corporation.

Ray-Kaeser, S., and Lynch, H. (2016). Play in Occupational Therapy. In S. Besio, V. Stancheva-Popkostadinova and D. Bulgarelli (eds), *Play development and children with disabilities*, pp. 155–165. Berlin: De Gruyter.

Reilly, M. (1974). *Play as exploratory learning*. Beverly Hills, CA: Sage Publications.

Rogoff, B. (2003). *The cultural nature of human development*. Oxford: Oxford University Press.

Rogoff, B., Mistry, J., Goncu, A., and Mosier, C. (1993). Guided Participation in Cultural Activity by Toddlers and Caregivers. *Monographs of the Society for Research in Child Development*, 58 (8), 1–182.

Skard, G., and Bundy, A. (2008). Test of Playfulness. In L. D. Parham and L. Fazio (eds), *Play in occupational therapy for children*, pp. 71–93. St Louis, MO: Mosby Elsevier.

Spitzer, S. (2001). *No words necessary: an ethnography of daily activities with children who don't talk*. Doctoral dissertation. University of Southern California. Los Angeles.

Spitzer, S. (2003a). Using Participant Observation to Study the Meaning of Occupations of Young Children with Autism and Other Developmental Disabilities. *American Journal of Occupational Therapy*, 57 (1), 66–76.

Spitzer, S. (2003b). With and Without Words: Exploring Occupation in Relation to Young Children with Autism. *Journal of Occupational Science*, 10 (2), 67–79.

Spitzer, S. (2004). Common and Uncommon Daily Activities in Individuals with Autism: Challenges and Opportunities for Supporting Occupation. In H. Miller-Kuhaneck (ed.), *Autism: a comprehensive occupational therapy approach* (2nd ed.) pp. 83–106. Bethesda, MD: AOTA.

Stephenson, A. (2002). Opening up the Outdoors: Exploring the Relationship Between the Indoor and Outdoor Environments of a Centre. *European Early Childhood Education Research Journal*, 10 (1), 29–38.

Sutton-Smith, B. (1986). *Toys as culture*. New York: Gardner.

Trevarthen, C. (2011). What is it Like to be a Person Who Knows Nothing? Defining the Active Intersubjective Mind of a Newborn Human Being. *Infant and Child Development*, 20 (1), 119–135.

United Nations (1989). *UN Convention on the rights of the child (UNCRC)*. Geneva: United Nations.

United Nations (2006). *UN convention on the rights of persons with disabilities*. New York: United Nations.

Waller, T. (2007). The Trampoline Tree and the Swamp Monster with 18 Head's: Outdoor Play in the Foundation Stage and Foundation Phase. *Education 3–13*, 35 (4), 393–407.

Wilcock, A. (1998). Doing, Being, Becoming. *Canadian Journal of Occupational Therapy*, 65, 248–257.

Williams, D. (1992). *Nobody nowhere: The extraordinary autobiography of an autistic*. New York: Times Books.

Wood, W., Towers, L., and Malchow, J. (2000). Environment, Time-Use, and Adaptedness in Prosimians: Implications for Discerning Behaviour that is Occupational in Nature. *Journal of Occupational Science*, 7 (1), 5–18.

World Health Organization (2007). *International classification of function, disability and health for children and youth (ICF-CY)*. Geneva: WHO.

Zemke, R., and Clark, F. (1996). Preface. In R. Zemke and F. Clark (eds), *Occupational science: the evolving discipline*, pp vii-xviii. Philadelphia, PA: F. A. Davis.

11   Universal Design for social inclusion:
      Playgrounds for all

Children with disabilities benefit from play, and their right to equal participation in play is enshrined by the Convention on the Rights of the Child
(UNCRC) (United Nations 1989) and the Convention on the Rights of
Persons with Disabilities (UNCRPD) (United Nations 2007). However,
their right to play and participate in play with other children is often
restricted in community playspaces and playgrounds because of physical
barriers and social exclusion. Frequently, spaces and structures set up for children's outdoor play are not accessible to children with disabilities. The result
is lack of interaction between children with and without disabilities, which
reinforces attitudinal barriers and stigmatization. This chapter presents a
background to designing for play, based on research with children with disabilities, landscape architects and other disciplines. Barriers and enablers are
identified in designing, planning and providing for play. Implementation of
a Universal Design approach is proposed as a key solution for making equal
access to participation in play for children with disabilities a reality. In this
chapter the children referred to are between six and twelve years of age and
the term children with disabilities is used to accentuate the person (child)
first, then mention their disability. This is a person-first approach that is
guided by the principle that a person is not defined by his or her condition.

Right to play and participation

All children (including children with disabilities) benefit from play. Play is
established as a fundamental characteristic of childhood and is the primary
drive for learning and development in children. Although many cultures

have different perspectives of the role of play in childhood (Bornstein, Haynes, Pascual, Painter and Galperin 1999; Bazyk, Stalnaker, Llerena, Ekelman and Bazyk 2003) the evidence for the importance of play in health, well-being and development is strong (Ginsburg 2007; Gill 2014). This raises the question then: what about children who struggle to play, due to physical, sensory, cognitive or emotional impairments? How can communities enable social inclusion through play for all children irrespective of ability?

Internationally this issue has been a central part of the United Nations work on children's rights through establishing the 54 articles of the UNCRC (United Nations [UN] 1989). Of particular relevance in relation to play and children with disabilities are articles 12, 23 and 31, which address the need for children to have a voice in things that concern them, to be supported to have a full and independent life, and to have a right to play, Furthermore, in relation to article 31, the UN states that children should have a voice in how playspaces are designed and policy for play in their communities (UN 2013). Through these international policies on children's rights, new roles for children are proposed that include voice and participation in development of policy, planning and legislation on play and playspaces.

However, among health professions, the issue of participation has also been explored by the World Health organization in recent years through the lens of social inclusion. When the World Health Organization (WHO) introduced the International Classification of Function, Disability and Health (ICF) (2001) and the ICF- Children and Youth (ICF-CY) (2007), stakeholders who work to enable play for children began to focus not just on impairments and remediation approaches in therapy provision, but extended the focus of concern to the activity and participation in the environment. According to the ICF-CY, participation is defined as involvement in life situations, including being autonomous to some extent or being able to control your own life. Therefore, in this chapter children's participation is considered from both a UNCRC and an ICF perspective, to capture participation as an issue of voice and action that is fundamental to social inclusion. This approach is based on the understanding that children's engagement in life includes expression through doing as well as through voice (Lynch 2018).

Participation: contexts for play

Researching participation has become more prevalent in relation to children with disabilities, with emerging evidence that barriers to participation are varied, and include physical, and attitudinal as well as societal barriers (Anaby et al. 2013). Furthermore, researchers exploring impact of interventions that address contextual issues rather than impairment, have shown that the outcomes are equally effective (Law et al. 2011). There is now an emerging interest in studying the physical environment as an equal contributor to enabling participation. This opens up many interesting areas for further research, and from the authors' perspective, it strengthens the argument for attending to the physical environment and how it can be designed to maximize and support play for all children.

Outdoor playspaces and playgrounds are the primary sites for outdoor play for many children, especially in recent years when the range and scope of free play outdoors has become more restricted in many countries. For example, across the Netherlands, Australia, UK and Germany, studies have reported the evolving restrictions on children for accessing outdoor play (Karsten 2005; Malone 2007; England Marketing 2009; Blinkert and Weaver 2015). Researchers have noted that public spaces are not designed with children in mind, and consequently children are becoming more invisible in community spaces. In Ireland, it has been noted that this results in primary sites for outdoor play being the back garden at home, the green area in a housing estate, the school yard or the local playground (Fanning 2010). So, from a societal and community perspective, these outdoor playspaces are important sites for social inclusion and participation.

Yet to date few researchers have studied playgrounds with regard to children with disabilities, and children have rarely been included as research participants in such research (Barron et al. 2017). Those who have studied playgrounds have identified multiple barriers to play and social inclusion. For example, in some settings in the UK, special equipment was provided in playgrounds that frequently segregated children with physical disabilities from others, thus exacerbating social exclusion and marginalization (Dunn and Moore 2005). In contrast, Bourke (2014) found that in Australia, design was often considered *after* a playground is built rather than as part of the overall planning for inclusion. Furthermore, in a scoping study of evidence of playground accessibility and usability, Moore and Lynch (2016) found that children are rarely included in the designing of playgrounds, that few guidelines of good practice exist and that there is a need for advocating for play at a societal, policy and local community level. In Sweden, the first author found that children with disabilities are frequently excluded from local playground and that municipalities rarely have adequate knowledge about playground design (Prellwitz and Tamm 1999). Overall, it is evident that when a lack of policy and guidelines exist, decisions can be made that result in even more barriers to participation. In community playgrounds, the lack of knowledge on how to design for social inclusion seems to only compound the segregation between children with and without disabilities, which serves to boost attitudinal barriers even more.

This chapter considers the implementation of the rights for children by exploring the barriers and facilitators for inclusion of children with disabilities in playgrounds and other outdoor play spaces, through explaining the journey of the first author in her quest to search for answers to the question: *how do we ensure playgrounds can be sites for social inclusion for all children?* (Prellwitz and Tamm 1999; Prellwitz and Skar 2006; Prellwitz and Skar 2007; Prellwitz and Skar 2016).

The first author's reflections from playground research: a story from Sweden

My research into playgrounds began over a decade ago and was inspired by children's comments in a study I did about young children's attitudes towards children using wheelchairs. Coming from a background in occupational therapy, I am trained to assess the home and community environment for accessibility (for example for adults who are wheelchair users), but had not learned any theory or knowledge on play environments or environmental assessments of playgrounds. Yet, I could see this was a serious problem for children with disabilities. This is what I have *seen* when I started looking at playgrounds. In the first picture, there is a kerb by the slide, which blocks any child who has restricted mobility from accessing play opportunities; while in the second picture, the play area is level for access, but filled with gravel which prevents a wheelchair user from being able to get to the play components.

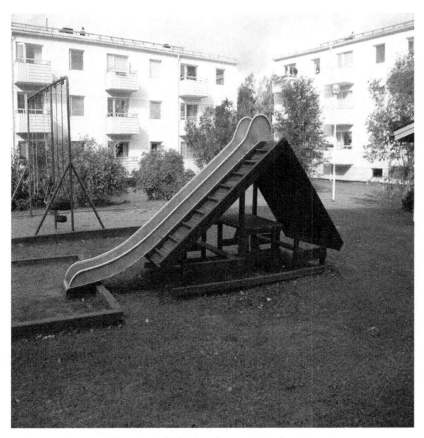

Figure 11.1: Slide placed on a grassy play area

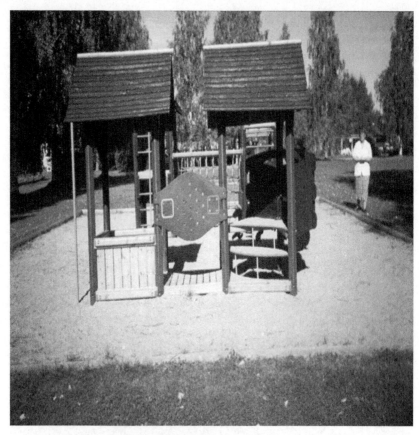

Figure 11.2: Gravel surface underneath the play components

These playgrounds are boring, uninspiring and definitely not accessible. However, this is the way many playgrounds look in Sweden still. According to a survey from 2013 only about 4 per cent of the country's playgrounds are built with the intent of being accessible (Dahlberg et al. 2013).

My reflections on the situation: Playgrounds are important environments where many children play during their childhood. Playgrounds are designed for children, by adults, to be a place where they can perform many different activities. However, playgrounds are not purely physical places they are also a place for children to meet and interact with other children. For children with disabilities playgrounds should be just as important. This is not an issue for Sweden alone. In many countries, few playgrounds are built that are accessible for children with disabilities. In other words, by not having access to playgrounds, a child with a disability can be denied both the opportunity to be in the physical environment and the social environment that exists in a playground. What do children have to say about this?

Beginning my research journey- researching with children: For me it all started with a study called 'If I had a friend in a wheelchair' where I interviewed 48 children without disabilities, between the ages of six and ten years of age from different preschools and schools, in Sweden, about what environmental changes that were needed if a child in a wheelchair were to attend their school. See Table 11.1.

Table 11.1: Characteristics of Participants and Interview Context

Number of participants, boys/ girls (N = 48)	Age	Interview context
8/8 (16)	6	Preschool (small preschool with 30 children in total).
8/8 (16)	8	Early primary school (8 children from a school with approximately 100 children, 8 children from a school with approximately 200 children).
8/8 (16)	10	Early primary school (8 children from a school with approximately 100 children, 8 children from a school with approximately 200 children).

In the study, the children had different solutions to potential problems both indoors and outdoors such as ramps and automatic door openers. However, all of the children regardless of age described that the playground was extremely inaccessible, an unreachable place for a child using a wheelchair. The barriers included snow in the winter, sand in the summer and a high perimeter around the playground that formed an insurmountable obstacle to a wheelchair. This is how a ten-year-old girl put it: 'There are swings and she can't play on them and there is sand and the wheelchair can't go on it. She'll probably have to just sit all the time, so there's no point her going to the playground'.

These obstacles meant that the child using a wheelchair was excluded from any possibility of social participation in games with other children in this environment. The results were something I took note of. In other words, the children in that study were conscious of the physical obstacles that were present in the surrounding environment; obstacles which lead to a child with disabilities becoming isolated from other children who played on the playground. This was contrary to the other results in the same study which showed that the children's attitudes toward including a child with disabilities in different situations were purely positive. They planned to offer help to remove different kinds of obstacle and they made up games that the child with disabilities could take part in. The results from that study indicated no rejection or negative attitudes towards children with disabilities.

In other words, what these children expressed was that children using a wheelchair were excluded from this environment only because of the barriers in the physical environment and not the social. Since play is considered to be a child's primary occupation and play often takes place in playgrounds and since it is often in playgrounds at school and in neighbourhoods that lasting friendships are formed, I realized that playgrounds should be a context that needed to be looked at more in-depth.

The journey continues – researching with children with disabilities: So, I decided to hear from the children themselves who were at risk of exclusion from this environment. I started with school children with restricted mobility by eliciting from them what they had to say about playgrounds at their school. See Table 11.2:

Table 11.2: Characteristics of participants

Child's gender and age	Diagnosis	Assistive device for mobility
Boy 7 yrs.	Spina bifida	Wheelchair (always)
Girl 7 yrs.	Spinal muscular atrophy	Wheelchair (most of the time)
Girl 8 yrs.	Polio	Crutches (mostly)
Boy 9 yrs.	Cerebral palsy	Wheelchair (most of the time)
Girl 9 yrs.	Cerebral palsy	Wheelchair (most of the time)

Child's gender and age	Diagnosis	Assistive device for mobility
Boy 9 yrs.	Spina bifida	Wheelchair (always)
Boy 10 yrs.	Spinal muscular atrophy	Crutches (mostly)
Girl 10 yrs.	Spina bifida	Wheelchair (most of the time)
Boy 12 yrs.	Cerebral palsy	Wheelchair (always)
Girl 12 yrs.	Cerebral palsy	Wheelchair (always)

One girl (aged nine) said: 'My friends are always at the school playground, I can't get there without someone carrying me and that is too embarrassing'.

Another girl (aged eleven) told me: 'I always stay inside during school break, they are too short for me to make it out in time and anyhow there is nowhere to go'.

The outdoor environment received a poor appraisal when I interviewed these children. The breaks for recess or playtime were often too short for the pupils with restricted mobility to get out. Once outside, it was difficult to cope with the physical environment. The playgrounds on the schoolyard were so designed that they were completely inaccessible to anyone using a wheelchair, walking-trolley or crutches, which the children in the study used. Also during the winter months (in Sweden) the schoolyard was poorly cleared of snow and therefore inaccessible to these children. In addition, the schoolyard was often crowded with playing children, which was perceived as a threat to the safety of the children with restricted mobility. Many of the children had found other solutions, such as not going out into the schoolyard at all during breaks.

The journey expands – gaining more insight: In my research, I have interviewed children with and without disabilities. The children with disabilities either had a severe visual impairment, a moderate developmental disability or restricted mobility. The responses I received from them are that the playground is a place that all the children are familiar with. I asked them about the playground at their school and the one closest to their home. All the children were able to describe in detail both playgrounds and they also spoke about the changes that had happened to the playgrounds in previous years: some were renovated while others were rebuilt completely. The only difference was that several of the children I spoke with who had some form of disability, had rarely or never been in these playgrounds. The children without any disability described the playground as a place to get away from adults, a place to sit and talk with friends about secrets. These talks could take place sitting on the swings or high up on a climbing frame. The children with a disability expressed this mostly in the form of wishful thinking or something that had happened once or a couple of times but that had been of great importance. A girl (aged eleven) with restricted mobility described it like this: 'I crawled to the swings and then I sat a long time talking with a friend. We didn't play, we just talked. But it only happened once.'

The girl described this episode in detail as if it was a big event for her. All the children told me how much they wanted places where they could be without adults being present. For children without disabilities, the playground was a meeting place. Here they were with their friends, were waiting for their friends or met new friends. They rarely had any adult with them. For children with disabilities, it was a fundamental difference: the playground was not a place to meet or be with friends and they had always an adult with them as this was a prerequisite for being able to play in the playground. One boy (age nine) had a playground that he saw from his bedroom window. He told me: 'My friends are often in the playground, but there, on our playground, there's sand. What I want most of all in all playgrounds is tiles. Then I would be able to enter the playground.' The boy had never been to this playground.

For those children who had mobility restrictions, sand was the main problem to accessing play equipment. Another was that surfaces were too small to manoeuvre the wheelchair. For children with severe visual impairment, the unpainted wood structures that are often found in playgrounds, were a huge problem. The children with a moderate developmental disability described that some of the playground equipment were too small for them and that some were too complicated and that they did not know how they would use them. A boy with a moderate developmental disability showed me a playground near his home where he dared not go because he did not understand how he would use the equipment: 'I do not know where to start.'

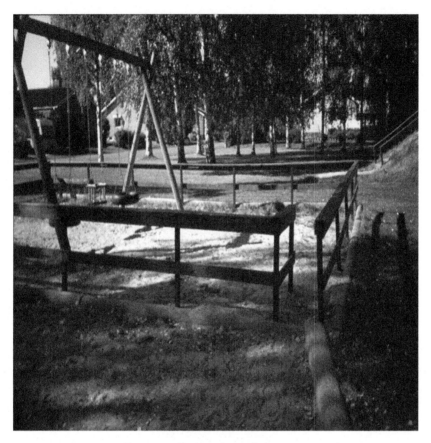

Figure 11.3: Fencing that excludes access

Playground design and the architecture of social participation

The problems identified though the first author's experience highlight the issues faced in playgrounds: these are issues of *socio-spatial inclusion or exclusion* (Yantzi, Young and McKeever 2010). Playground design therefore requires an approach that encompasses 'the architecture of social participation' (Steinfeld and Maisel 2012: 21). Designing for social participation involves a multidimensional approach with expertise needed from varied

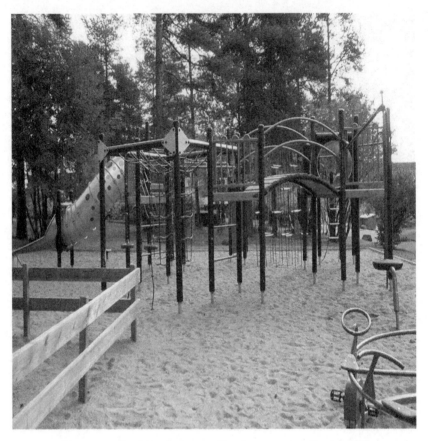

Figure 11.4: Confusing layout resulting in uncertainty for the child

disciplines, from different levels of policy and practice, and from users: for example, landscape architects, urban designers, town planners, municipalities who are responsible for play provision, play officers, occupational therapists, and families and children with and without disabilities. Designing for social participation requires a newer way of thinking: design for all or to give it a specific name: Universal Design (UD) (Goltsman 2011; Steinfeld and Maisel 2012).

The UD concept emerged out of the disability rights movement that aims to strive for equal opportunity and social inclusion, and to eliminate discrimination. It has evolved over time to encompass users' perspectives with a strong advocacy component, yet barriers to inclusion still exist in design and architecture (Steinfeld and Maisel 2012). UD originated in the Center for Universal Design at North Carolina State University, through the work of Mace and Lusher among others (Steinfeld and Maisel 2012), with the primary purpose of eschewing discriminatory design. Many different terms have been used interchangeably to refer to a UD approach: such as accessible design; design for all; inclusive design; barrier-free design. However, this leads to confusion and so UD was adopted by the UNCRPD in 2007 and the Council of Europe (Ginnerup 2009) and is defined as follows:

> Universal design means the design of products, environments, programmes and services to be *usable by all people*, to the greatest extent possible, without the need for adaptation or specialized design. Universal design shall not exclude assistive devices for particular groups of persons with disabilities where this is needed. (UNCRPD 2007: 4)

The intention in the CRPD was to come to some consensus on definitions, to have a cohesive approach in practice and to ensure an international recognition of the importance of a UD approach for all. However, it is important to note that UD is not the same as *accessible design*. According to Steinfeld and Maisel, accessible design 'is intended to benefit only those with disabilities' (Steinfeld and Maisel 2012: 189). Typically, accessible design is closely linked to government legislation and tends to result in the development of a set of *minimum requirements* for design and provision. But designers need to go beyond minimum requirements when designing for play and UD enables this to happen (Sanderson 2014). UD is *more than* an accessible design approach as it adds on principles related to equitable provision for all for example (for example, the same entrance for all, as opposed to having a separate entrance for wheelchair users) (Ginnerup 2009) and is concerned with aesthetic features in design at the same time. UD aims to ensure design is aimed at maximizing usability and minimizing barriers in the physical environment that impede physical, sensory, social, or cognitive interactions. Importantly, UD acknowledges that full usability is not a realistic goal but aims to enable usability to the greatest extent possible. Although many criticize the idealism of UD, others argue that it provides a way to consider individual needs within communities that can improve health and wellbeing outcomes (Steinfeld and Maisel 2012). Interestingly, while it originated as an approach to designing physical spaces and objects, UD has become more evident also in educational approaches and virtual environments.

User's perspective: research evidence on playgrounds from researching with children

When considering a UD approach, it is essential to begin with a user's perspective. Therefore, it is important to explore what is known about playground design from researching with children. Playground research with children, has found that play is significantly influenced by the design of the physical environment. This includes characteristics such as the organization of the playspace, the amount of space per child, and the type of play component (for example, swing) and challenge for the child (Barbour 1999; Min and Lee 2006; Holmes and Procaccino 2009). For example, in Min and Lee's research, the *organization of space* resulted in some playgrounds being more popular for children than others, due to adequate privacy, safety, and freedom to play. *Favourite playground activities* in young children have been identified to include swinging, socialising and sand play (Holmes and Procaccino 2009). In contrast, these activities were not adequate for older children, resulting in a *lack of challenge* being noted, when playgrounds were not designed with older children in mind (Veitch, Bagley, Ball and Salmon 2006). Aside from age-related issues, Prellwitz and Tamm (1999) found that children with disabilities experienced significant barriers to accessing the playground components, through lack of adequate design. So, different play preferences and accessibility features need to be incorporated into the design also. Overall, when playgrounds are designed with a UD approach, equipment is chosen that all children of different ages and abilities can use together. This is highly valued by children with disabilities and their families (Jeanes and Magee 2012) and is established as an important part of providing for the rights of the child (UNCRC 1989). Children's engagement in designing for play is therefore vital to inform better design.

Design is not the only issue however. Play research has also identified that play is significantly influenced by the social environment. In some studies, children expressed their wish to socialize together with other children alongside having opportunities for challenge and fun within the physical space of the playground (for example, Prellwitz and Skar 2007). However, providing accessible settings for play is not enough: there is a need to also consider advocacy to promote attitudinal change in the general public. In their study of four schools in Canada, Yantzi et al. (2010) found that children with disabilities were excluded even in accessible schoolyard playspaces. Although these schools had incorporated some design elements to ensure accessibility, the limitations in design led to social marginalization, and children needed more support from adults to promote social inclusion. This has been explored in other studies where the social environment is also the focus. For example, using a peer model programme in a school setting is one practical and effective method to facilitate social interactions, confidence, and self-esteem for participation in inclusive environments (Harris 2016).

To summarize, from a user's perspective, the challenge is to ensure policy makers, designers, landscape architects, and town planners understand the adoption of UD requires more than simple regulatory change (Steinfeld and Maisel 2012). Playgrounds need to be designed with all the above considerations in mind: to avoid segregation, to aim to design gathering spaces for social play, to include play components for different sizes and abilities of children, to consider space as well as equipment, to aim for challenge in the play affordances. Once solutions are addressed in the physical environment, then social inclusion can be addressed.

Enabling play participation through UD: a framework for practical application when designing playspaces for children

Although UD is acknowledged as a way forward in designing for inclusion, UD is an underexplored concept in relation to playgrounds and playspaces. This final section of the chapter therefore gives attention to how UD might be applied in designing for play, to support social inclusion and participation of all children in our communities.

Designing for play preferences and play styles of a child is important, alongside consideration of age, gender, and size, as these factors influence how a person functions in the environment. In addition, when a child has a disability, a UD approach requires designers to establish what functional limitations might impact users' experience (for example, reliance on walking aids). To address such concerns, an anthropometric approach is adopted (the measurement of characteristics such as weight, size, and functional abilities). It is evident consequently, that when a UD approach is applied to playground design, the playspace *will not* meet the needs of all children at all times, due to these different factors. Instead, UD aims to *maximize* accessibility and usability to the greatest extent possible. The resulting design should therefore provide multiple, varied play opportunities to children, but still result in some play components being too complex or too simple for individual child (see Table 11.3).

Table 11.3: Anne's Play Style and Play Preferences

Anne is a young girl aged six years, who likes to go to her local playground where there is a wooden house with walls, ropes and slopes for climbing up and a slide. It is designed so that there are multiple ways to climb up into the house (accessible use and UD). Anne cannot climb on the climbing wall yet (inaccessible for Anne) but instead she can go up the ramp using a rope to pull herself up. However, Anne chooses to climb up the slide to get to the top (usability)!
On analysis, the play experience of climbing the ramp is not appealing to Anne, and she cannot access the climbing wall, but she finds fun and challenge instead in using the slide in a different way

In this example, the reason for not climbing the ramp might be due to the age of the ability of the child, or indeed her play preference. In many playgrounds, there are play components (a component is a swing or a slide for example) that are beyond the usability of the child, but might be usable in the future as their abilities and motivations for play develop and change over time. So, it is essential that any playground designers[1] operate firstly from an understanding of play, play preferences and play styles in childhood.

---

1   Designers in this case refers to anyone involved in development of community playspaces: Occupational Therapists, Landscape Architects, Engineers, Town Planners.

Once the play context is understood, then UD principles can be applied. One of the most significant contributions from UD is the establishment of seven core principles for operationalising a UD approach. They are as follows: equitable use, flexibility, simple intuitive use, perceptible information, tolerance of error, low physical effort, size and space for approach and use. Below is an attempt to exemplify what the different principles of UD could mean when applied to playgrounds. It is important to remember that UD is about flexibility in how the principles can be applied. It is not about different measurements, therefore one playground built on UD principles should be similar to another.

PRINCIPLE ONE: Equitable Use: The design is useful and marketable to people with diverse abilities and needs: this includes consideration for different sizes.

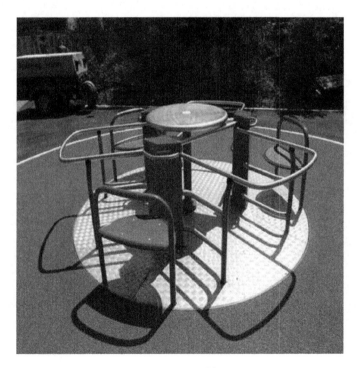

Figure 11.5: Equitable use

Designing for equitable use includes for example, intergenerational play where everybody can use the same route to the play structure. It avoids segregated use, and is designed to appeal to all who wish to use it. The design offers a play environment that provides opportunities for everyone to participate: play components may need to be of different sizes to offer opportunities for children of different sizes also. In this picture, the carousel can be used for children who need to sit, stand or use a wheel chair.

PRINCIPLE TWO: Flexibility in Use: The design accommodates a wide range of individual preferences and abilities and ensures functional comfort.

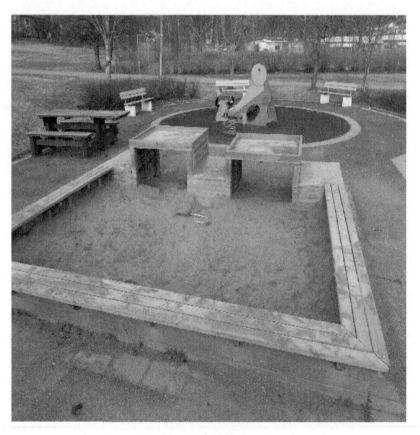

Figure 11.6: Flexibility in use

Designing for flexibility in use includes how the design provides choices and variety of experiences, for example, components at different heights. The design promotes inclusive play by accommodating diverse abilities. This is an example of a sand box that is built with additional sand tables to enable children who have mobility difficulties, to sit beside others, and to play parallel to each other. This example shows multiple ways of doing sand play.

PRINCIPLE THREE: Simple and Intuitive Use: Use of the design is easy to perceive and understand, regardless of the user's experience, knowledge, language skills, or current concentration level.

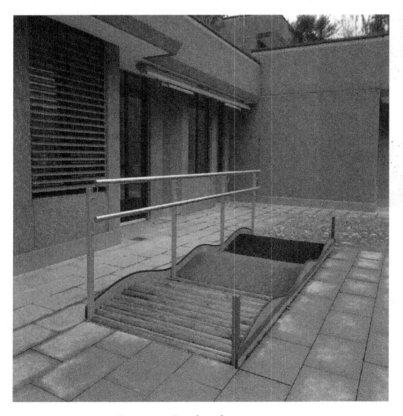

Figure 11.7: Simple and intuitive use

Designing for simple and intuitive use includes adding play structures that are easy to use, with intrinsic play value, while still avoiding unnecessary complexity. The design offers opportunities for discovery and sensory feedback. In this picture, the play structure is easy to figure out, with obvious boundaries and ways to enter and engage in the structure but also includes some risk taking. The function of this play component is clearly laid out. The challenge for play designers is to ensure intuitive use, while still balancing the need for unexpected, creative use.

PRINCIPLE FOUR: Perceptible Information: The design communicates necessary information effectively to the user, regardless of ambient conditions or the user's sensory abilities. It relates to intuitive and unambiguous use.

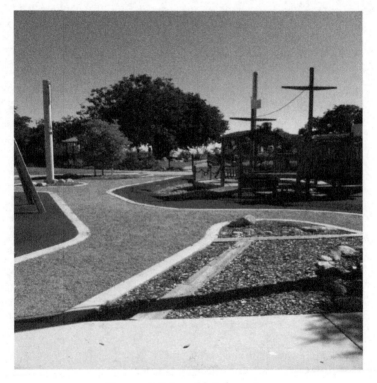

Figure 11.8: Perceptible information

Designing for perceptible information includes for example, colour schemes that mark paths that lead the way to play equipment and it can also signal safety barriers. The design offers a play environment that can be used as independently as possible. In this picture, the colour scheme and different textures on the side of the pathway, give varied forms of cues for where to go.

PRINCIPLE FIVE: Tolerance for Error: The design minimizes hazards and the adverse consequences of accidental or unintended actions.

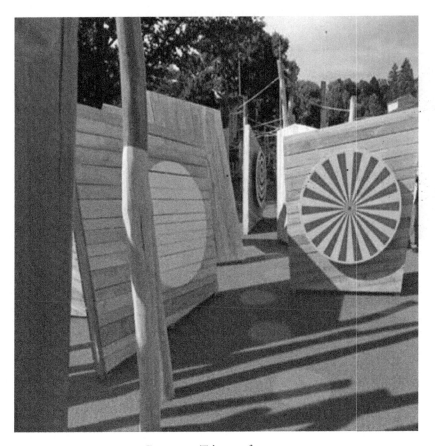

Figure 11.9: Tolerance for error

Designing for tolerance for error in a playground can be done through different levels of challenges and to allow children to interact by taking developmental-related risks. In this picture, the interactive components are arranged spatially removed from heights or slopes that could add potential hazards. In playgrounds, error is part of a rich play experience, play is about trial-and-error. However, in UD for playgrounds, the goal of principle five, is to ensure safety in design, as opposed to removing possibilities for 'error'.

PRINCIPLE SIX: Low Physical Effort: The design can be used efficiently and comfortably and with a minimum of fatigue.

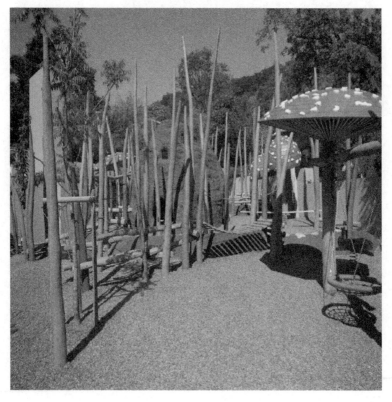

Figure 11.10: Low physical effort

Designing for low physical effort means designing for maximum play activity, for example, including design features that offer a range of opportunities for challenges and social play through the setting. In this picture, the accessible play component is designed with the intent to offer challenges without requiring too much physical effort to be a part of where the play takes place. Children can navigate through varied spaces that encompass shade, height, textures and movement, with ease of use and reasonable force. This means strain is minimized.

PRINCIPLE SEVEN: Size and Space for Approach and Use: Appropriate size and space is provided for approach, reach, manipulation and use regardless of user's body size, posture, or mobility.

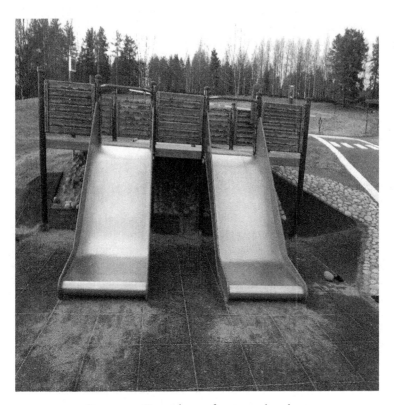

Figure 11.11: Size and space for approach and use

Designing for size and space means ensuring each child is comfortable in play. The design entails that children can approach and use the different components regardless of the child's age or if the child needs assistance. In this picture, the slides are wide enough for a child and an adult to use together if they wish or need to do so.

Finally, once play context and UD principles are considered, a four-phased implementation plan can be conducted (see Table 11.3).

Table 11.3: Outlines a practical application pathway in more detail

A. Environmental analysis: The first steps in designing for play include considering the playability of the space, features of the natural and built environment that meet the needs of the whole child and social/emotional, physical, sensory, cognitive and communication needs. This includes:

1. aiming to provide *sensory-rich* experiences, including among other things, elements of nature within the built environment;
2. varied stimulation for the context/setting- this includes *risk-rich* opportunities, where children can challenge themselves in their play;
3. incorporate varied affordances that provide opportunities for positive experiences of fun and challenge: *social, physical, emotional participation.*

B. Design participation: The next step is to consider design practices that include the users that is, implement design participation strategies, by including users' perspectives in the design development and implementation process from beginning to end (Dunn, Moore and Murray, 2004) and take the users' view seriously (Imrie and Luck, 2014). There is also a need to work in an interdisciplinary way: rehabilitation professionals with their knowledge of functional limitations need to work together with architects and landscape architects (Lid 2014).

C. Establish local or national accessibility regulations: Know the regulatory requirements that apply in your community. Remember that these are more limited than UD, and are usually described as minimum rather than ideal requirements, but that they establish any requirements for example for steps, or graded slopes. In many states, such accessibility regulations exist for general public settings but rarely include specific consideration for playgrounds (Goltsman 2011).

D. Designing from 7 UD principles: Then begin thinking about the 7 principles of UD. The Playcore Association in the USA has worked to establish good practice in applying these principles to playground design and serve to guide the design process. Together with North Carolina State University they have taken the 7 principles and uniquely tailored them to what all children want to feel and experience during outdoor play. According to them no two universally designed play environment projects are alike, but in all play environments, children want to 'Be' and feel fair, included, smart, independent, safe, active, and comfortable during play. [1]

---

1   <http://www.inclusiveplaygrounds.org/me2/overview>

Conclusion

In this chapter, children's participation in play and playspaces was considered as an issue of voice and action: what children tell us and what they show us about their needs. Through researching with children with disability, insights were gained concerning play needs, play preferences, and the physical and social barriers for play, that influence social inclusion. Although there is little evidence to date from the perspective of children with disability, data showed that children value play and need to be included in designing for play. From a child's perspective, it can be deducted that well-designed, risk-rich, fun, inclusive playgrounds are needed.

It is proposed that high-value play opportunities can be created using a UD approach for all children, including those with disabilities. The design approach needs to be one that integrates local community need and is fit for purpose rather than being a 'cookie-cutter' solution (Sanderson 2014: 25). Central to this is ensuring children participate and engage in community planning and have a say in how their play needs are met. Key to successful accessibility, usability and social participation, is designing for diversity, with varied developmentally appropriate play areas and opportunities in the playground. Here are some elements to think about:

- Accessibility to all areas of the playground must be possible, especially where the action is. Even if not everything is accessible or usable to everybody, the possibility of being near the action provides an opportunity to participate. The importance of avoiding an age limit is essential if children with different play preferences and abilities are to be accommodated. This may mean a sixteen-year old playing on a slide that is considered 'age-appropriate' for a five-year old.
- Access onto, through and off equipment should be built for different skill levels and ages. This can involve different ways to successfully use play components through the use of hand-rails, ramps, and transfer platforms for example.
- Integrate accessible play equipment next to equipment that requires greater ability in order to encourage interaction. This speaks to the need to plan the flow and placement of play components within the playspace – the flow needs to be intuitive to the child.

- All play equipment that is raised up should be as accessible as ground-level equipment. This could be provided by ramps, transfer systems or other systems. It is necessary to make sure these systems are integrated in the design so that they are not stigmatizing.
- It is advised to aim to ensure that all children have access to a range of play experiences that include for example swinging, running, sliding, jumping, rotating, climbing, hiding, pulling. Designing for play affordances such as these, will ensure that play opportunities can match play need.
- Make gathering places accessible to promote social interaction.

To conclude, playgrounds are becoming more important to children in many communities as their freedom in outdoor free play becomes more restricted. Hence playgrounds emerge as important sites for consideration in national strategies for social inclusion and participation. For children with disabilities, these sites however are frequently sites of exclusion. Yet there is an abundance of emerging knowledge and experiences that can guide us to design for better play opportunities and promote inclusion. This chapter shares knowledge and experiences of research to date in exploring children's play worlds, and outlines some of the challenges and barriers that exist in providing for play in local communities. This emerging area of research requires significant development: more studies are required to explore different play needs of different children and to identify methods for developing good practice in participatory engagement with children as designers of their playspaces. This is a children's rights issue and one that needs to be taken more seriously by adults. By promoting an increasing commitment to UD, the authors offer a starting point that can guide play providers in the right direction. Promoting participatory design is part of a broader commitment to participation of children in things that matter to them: it is one step in the right direction.

References

Anaby, D., Hand, C., Bradley, L., DiRezze, B., Forhan, M., DiGiacomo, A., and Law, M. (2013). The effect of the environment on participation of children and youth with disabilities: a scoping review. *Disability and Rehabilitation*, 1–10. DOI: 10.3109/09638288.2012.748840.

Barbour, A. C. (1999). The impact of playground design on the play behaviours of children with differing levels of physical competence. *Early Childhood Research Quarterly*, 14 (1), 75–98.

Barron, C., Beckett, A., Coussens, M., Desoete, A., Cannon Jones, N., Lynch, H., ... Fenney Salkeld, D. (2017). *Barriers to play and recreation for children and young people with disabilities*. China: De Gruyter.

Bazyk, S., Stalnaker, D., Llerena, M., Ekelman, B., and Bazyk, J. (2003). Play in Mayan children. *American Journal of Occupational Therapy*, 57 (3), 273–283.

Blinkert, B. and Weaver, E. (2015). Residential environment and types of childhood. *Humanities and Social Sciences*, 3 (5), 159–168. DOI: 0.11648/j.hss.20150305.11

Bornstein, M., Haynes, O., Pascual, L., Painter, K., and Galperin, C. (1999). Play in two societies: pervasiveness of process, specificity of structure. *Child Development*, 70 (2), 317–331.

Bourke, J. (2014). 'No Messing Allowed': The Enactment of Childhood in Urban Public Space from the Perspective of the Child. *Children, Youth and Environments*, 24 (1), 25–52.

Dahlberg, A., Gustafsson, J., Lagercrantz, M., Lindqvist, E., Harish, M., and Aslund, K. (2013). *How are things in 2013? Monitoring of disability policy*. Retrieved from: <www.handisam.se>.

Dunn, K., and Moore, M. (2005). Developing accessible play space in the UK: a social model approach. *Children, Youth and Environments*, 15 (1), 331–354.

Dunn, K., Moore, M., and Murray, P. (2004). *Developing accessible play space: final research report*. London: Department for Communities and Local Government.

England Marketing (2009). *Report to Natural England on childhood and nature: a survey on changing relationships with nature across generations*. Cambridgeshire: Natural England.

Fanning, M. (2010). *Wild Child Poll*. Retrieved from: <http://www.heritagecouncil.ie/content/files/Wild_Child_Poll_quantitative_survey.pdf>.

Gill, T. (2014). *The play return: a review of the wider impact of play initiatives*. Children's Play Policy Forum.

Ginnerup, S. (2009) *Achieving full participation through Universal Design*. Retrieved from: <https://book.coe.int/eur/en/integration-of-people-with-disabilities/4143-achieving-full-participation-through-universal-design.html>.

Ginsburg, K. R. (2007). The importance of play in promoting healthy child development and maintaining strong parent-child bonds. *Pediatrics*, 119 (1), 182–191.

Goltsman, S. (2011). Outdoor play settings: an inclusive approach. In W. F. Preiser and K. Smith (eds), *Universal Design Handbook*, 2nd edn, pp. 22.21–22.10. London: McGraw Hill.

Harris, K. (2016). Supporting executive function skills in early childhood: Using a peer buddy approach for community confidence, and citizenship. *Journal of Education and Training*, 3 (1), 158–175. DOI: 10.5296/jet.v3i1.8837.

Holmes, R., and Procaccino, J. (2009). Preschool children's outdoor play area preferences. *Early Child Development and Care,* 179 (8), 1103–1112.

Imrie, R., and Luck, R. (2014). Designing inclusive environments: rehabilitating the body and the relevance of universal design. *Disability and Rehabilitation,* 36 (16), 1315–1319. DOI: 10.3109/09638288.2014.936191

Jeanes, R., and Magee, J. (2012). Can we play on the swings and roundabouts?': creating inclusive playspaces for disabled young people and their families. *Leisure Studies,* 31 (2), 193–210. DOI: 10.1080/02614367.2011.589864.

Karsten, L. (2005). It all used to be better? Different generations on continuity and change in urban children's daily use of space. *Children's Geographies,* 3 (3), 275–290.

Law, M., Darrah, J., Pollock, N., Wilson, B., Russell, D., Walter, S., Galuppi, B. (2011). Focus on function: a cluster, randomized controlled trial comparing child-versus context-focused interventions for young children with cerebral palsy. *Developmental Medicine and Child Neurology,* 53, 621–629. DOI: 10.1111/j.1469-8749.2011.03962.x

Lid, I. (2014). Universal design and disability: An interdisciplinary perspective. *Disability and Rehabilitation,* 36 (16), 1344–1349. DOI: 0.3109/09638288.2014.931472.

Lynch, H. (2018). Beyond voice: Researching through doing. In M. Twomey and C. Carroll (eds), *Seen and heard: Exploring participation, engagement and voice for children with disabilities.* Oxford: Peter Lang.

Malone, K. (2007). The bubble-wrap generation: children growing up in walled gardens. *Environmental Education Research,* 13 (4), 513–527.

Min, B., and Lee, J. (2006). Children's neighborhood place as a psychological and behavioural domain'. *Journal of Environmental Psychology,* 26, 51–71.

Moore, A., and Lynch, H. (2016). Accessibility and usability of playground environments for children under 12: A scoping review. *Scandinavian Journal of Occupational Therapy,* 22, 331–344.

Prellwitz, M., and Skar, L. (2006). How children with restricted mobility perceive the accessibility and usability of their home environment. *Occupational Therapy International,* 13 (4), 193–206.

Prellwitz, M., and Skar, L. (2007). Usability of playgrounds for children with different abilities. *Occupational Therapy International,* 14 (3), 144–155.

Prellwitz, M., and Skar, L. (2016). Are playgrounds a case of occupational injustice? Experiences of parents of children with disabilities. *Children, Youth and Environment,* 26 (2), 28–42.

Prellwitz, M., and Tamm, M. (1999). Attitudes of key persons to accessibility problems in playgrounds for children with restricted mobility: a study in a medium-sized municipality in Northern Sweden. *Scandinavian Journal of Occupational Therapy,* 6, 166–173.

Sanderson, K. (2014). Getting to universal design for the public playspace. *OT Now*, 16 (5), 24–25.

Steinfeld, E., and Maisel, J. (2012). *Universal Design: Creating inclusive environments.* Hoboken, NJ: John Wiley and Sons, Inc.

United Nations (1989). *UN Convention on the Rights of the Child (UNCRC)*. Geneva: United Nations

United Nations (2006). *UN Convention on the Rights of Persons with Disabilities.* New York, NJ: United Nations.

Veitch, J., Bagley, S., Ball, K., and Salmon, J. (2006). Where do children usually play? A qualitative study of parents' perceptions of influences on children's active free play. *Health and Place,* 12, 383–393.

World Health Organization (2007). *International Classification of Function, Disability and Health for Children and Youth (ICF-CY)*. Geneva: WHO.

Yantzi, N., Young, N., and McKeever, P. (2010). The suitability of school playgrounds for physically disabled children. *Children's Geographies,* 8 (1), 65–78. DOI: 10.1080/14733281003650984

12 Seen and heard: The voice of children with speech and developmental language disorders

Introduction

We often take the ability to talk for granted. It is only when children have difficulties with talking that we appreciate the fundamental role that communication plays in enabling them to participate in their daily lives. For example, children form and negotiate relationships with parents, siblings, peers, teachers, and others using speech, language, and communication skills. Literacy skills, both decoding and reading comprehension, and numeracy skills are underpinned by speech and language abilities. To set the scene for this chapter, imagine a young boy called John who is eight years old. John lives with his parents, his two older siblings and his beloved pet dog Ellie. When John was two and a half years old his mother noticed that he was slow to talk. She referred him to the local health centre and he has been in receipt of services since he was three years old. Although he has made progress his speech is still unclear. John's family can understand what he says most of the time but others outside of the family context find it difficult to understand him without knowing the context. He has had several experiences of communication breakdown with his peers. Although John's language difficulties are less visible, they manifest in a number of ways. For example, he gets mixed up when following directions in the classroom and play-ground. His behaviour is often misinterpreted as a behavioural difficulty. Sometimes he cannot think of the words he needs to explain things. He uses strategies to compensate such as circumlocution and use of gestures. He can find it difficult to tell a story coherently and his grammatical skills are less developed than expected for his age. He attends a local mainstream school and he is generally happy there. His teachers noticed that he was not reaching academic targets. He is now in receipt of learning support, which is a pull-out service, where he receives one-to-one teaching for four hours a week in addition to classroom tuition. He has one close friend who he hangs around with in the school-yard. He has been bullied. His peers have called him 'stupid' and 'dumb' and have told him that he can't talk properly. He is becoming increasingly aware of his difficulties and has lashed out at peers. He has a reputation for being 'difficult' in the school. Outside of school, John gets on well with his sister but not with his brother. John enjoys helping his father with jobs around the farm. He also enjoys spending time with his grandmother, who lives nearby, and his pet dog. He loves sports and is a Manchester United supporter. John desperately wants to be picked for the local football team but so far has been on the reserve list.

This vignette provides a context for this chapter which will focus on children like John, who are often seen but not heard, and do not have a voice. Much of our knowledge and understanding of childhood speech and developmental language disorders comes from research which has been underpinned by positivist paradigms, with a focus on measurement of linguistic and cognitive variables. This research has enhanced our knowledge and understanding of processes underpinning speech and developmental language disorders as well as evidence in relation to assessment and intervention. However, the voice of children, like John, is sparse in the literature. Therefore, little is known about living with speech and developmental language disorders from the perspectives of children themselves. There are many potential reasons for the absence of children's voice. Firstly, some claim that listening to the voice of children is one of the most neglected areas of child developmental research (Greig, Taylor, and MacKay 2007). Secondly, children, and indeed adults, with speech and developmental disorders may be excluded from research because of assumptions that they could not participate in data collection activities such as interviews. However, in recent years there has been a shift in thinking with researchers now placing greater emphasis on children as social and cultural actors who have views to express (Woodhead and Faulkner 2000). This chapter will focus on two topics. Firstly, it will discuss arguments for giving voice to children with speech and developmental language disorders. Secondly, it will focus on methods that can be used to enable children with speech and developmental language disorders to participate in research so that we can gain insights into their worlds.

Children with speech and developmental language disorders have a voice

Childhood speech and developmental language disorders are relatively common. In a recent population-based study 7,267 four-five-year-old children were screened and it was estimated that the prevalence of language disorder of unknown origin, like John's, was estimated to be 7.58 per cent (Norbury et al. 2016). Furthermore, these researchers found that children with language disorders presented with more social, emotional and behavioural problems relative to their peers and 88 per cent did not make academic progress expected for their age. This means that two children in a class of 30 are likely to have developmental language disorders. Much of the research on childhood speech and developmental language disorders comes from the fields of medicine, psychology, speech-language pathology, and linguistics. The focus of this research has primarily been deficit-focused and has undoubtedly enhanced our understanding of the processes underpinning speech and developmental language disorders. This research has also provided evidence in relation to assessment, diagnosis and interventions for children with speech and developmental language disorders. There is also research which suggests that some children will not grow out of these disorders and there can be long-term adverse linguistic, academic, and psychosocial outcomes (Snowling, Bishop, Stothard, Chipchase, and Kaplan 2006; Stothard, Snowling, Bishop, Chipchase, and Kaplan 1998). Therefore, it is even more important that we understand what it is like to grow up living with a speech and developmental language disorder from the perspectives of the children themselves. Through listening to the voice of these children we can learn about ways in which they can be supported at different stages of development across the lifespan. However, up until recently, the voice of children with speech and developmental language disorders has been notably sparse in the literature.

However, the landscape is changing and there are now strong arguments for listening to the voice of children. According to Article 12 of the United Nations Convention on the Rights of the Child UNCRC (United Nations, 1989) children have the right to express their views on all matters affecting their lives, in accordance with their age and maturity. This right means that children should be given a chance to express their wishes, feelings and needs about aspects of their lives that affect them, such as education and health. Lundy (2007) reminds us that a second right in Article 12 of the UNCRC is the right to be heard and given due weight in accordance with the child's age and maturity. Therefore, it is important that listening to the views of children does not become a superficial tick-box exercise. Those who elicit children's views have a responsibility to act upon these views as appropriate (Thomas and Percy-Smith 2010). Article 12 of the UNCRC was ratified in Ireland in 1992 and formed the basis for the Irish National Children's Strategy (Department of Health and Children 2000). This strategy was a significant policy commitment to children and young people (Pinkerton 2004). The vision for the Irish National Children's Strategy is

> [an] Ireland where all children are respected as young citizens with a valued contribution to make and a voice of their own; where all children are cherished and supported by family and the wider society; where they enjoy a fulfilling childhood and realise their potential. (Department of Health and Children 2000: 10)

The Irish National Children's Strategy advocates that 'systematic mechanisms [are put] in place for obtaining and ensuring respect for children's views' (Department of Health and Children 2000: 28). However, the reality is that children are not routinely asked for their views and there is debate about whether children's voices really influence policy because their views are rarely included in the final decision-making (Percy-Smith 2011). Indeed, it is argued that the implementation of Article 12, especially with regard to younger children, has been problematic because it depends on the 'cooperation of adults, who may not be committed to or who may have a vested interest in not complying with it (Lundy, 2007) or who simply may not be used to recognising children, especially younger children, as competent meaning-makers in their own lives' (Lundy, McEvoy, and Byrne 2011, : 716).

Lundy (2007) argues that there are four key concepts that underpin successful implementation of Article 12 of the UNCRC and they are: 'space- children must be given the opportunity to express a view; voice— children must be facilitated to express their views; audience—the view must be listened to; and influence—the view must be acted upon as appropriate' (Lundy 2007: 933). Truly listening to children can be challenging and brings with it a responsibility to be reflexive. For example, it is important that practitioners and researchers remain open to understanding children's point of view and agendas, rather than being driven by problem-oriented adult agendas (Christensen 2004; Davis and Edwards 2004; Gallagher 2008; Morrow and Richards 1996). This was exemplified in research carried out by Miskelly and Roulstone (2011). These researchers were challenged to re-frame their research questions, which focused on the difficulties of young people with communication impairments, because the young people wanted to be represented on their own terms.

A second driver for listening to the voice of children is the way in which childhood is conceptualized. Many psychological theories on child development have been concerned with child variables and outcomes rather than with children themselves (Greene 2006; James and James 2008). When we adopt the ontological position that children are social agents and experiencers of their own worlds, we have a duty to listen directly to children's own perspectives (Christensen 2004; Greene and Hill 2005; Grover 2004; James 2001; Tisdall, Davis, and Gallagher 2009). This position also requires practitioners and researchers to work with children in ways that respect their particular competence (Thomas and O'Kane 2000) and to recognize them as competent reporters of their own experiences (Dockett and Perry 2007; France, Bendelow, and Williams 2000; Goodenough, Williamson, Kent, and Ashcroft 2003; Greene 2006; Prout 2002). Along with the trend to listen to the perspectives of children is the belief that 'as educators, researchers and adults, we have much to learn about children and children's experiences from children' (Dockett and Perry 2007: 48).

However, children with speech and developmental language disorders may be disadvantaged in two ways in relation to having their voice heard. Firstly, they may be excluded because they are children and secondly because they have communication difficulties. Some researchers argue that people with communication difficulties may be excluded and marginalized because of the nature of their difficulties and assumptions that they would not be able to engage in research (Lloyd, Gatherer, and Kalsy, 2006; Rabiee, Sloper, and Beresford 2005). However, it is important that these assumptions are challenged and that it is recognized that children with speech and developmental language disorders also have a right to have their voice heard. There is an emerging body of research in the field of speech-language pathology which conceptualizes children as social actors and has listened to the voice to children with speech and language disorders like John (Coad and Hambly 2011; Lyons and Roulstone 2017; Markham, van Laar, Gibbard, and Dean 2009; McLeod, Graham, and Barr 2013; McLeod, McCormack, McAllister, Harrison, and Holliday 2011; Merrick and Roulstone 2011; Roulstone and Lindsay 2012). Moreover, researchers have found innovative ways of successfully engaging with children and young people with complex communication needs (Carroll and Sixsmith 2016; Rabiee et al. 2005; Wickenden 2010). Although research in this field is in its early stages, these studies are beginning to provide us with glimpses into the lives of children with a range of speech, language and communication disorders because we are hearing first-hand accounts of children's experiences. Listening to children's experiences can inform research and practice. For example, we can learn about aspects of children's lives that are going well, things they would like to change, their strengths as well as their deficits, and about aspects of interventions they find helpful and unhelpful. Through consultations with children we can explore better ways of supporting children with speech and developmental language disorders.

Methods to listen to the voice to children with speech and developmental language disorders

Lundy (2007) reminds us that children may require help to express their views. This point is even more important when we want to engage with children speech and developmental language disorders. The onus is on researchers and practitioners to design methodologies which can be used to meaningfully engage children with speech and developmental language disorders. This requires a mind-shift with regard to acknowledging children's competence and finding innovative and respectful ways of facilitating children's engagement in meaningful ways. This section will outline some of methodological considerations when carrying out research with children with speech and developmental language disorders.

There are a range of methods that can be used to listen to children's voice and these can be adapted to facilitate children with speech and language disorders. One of these methods is interviews which can be construed along a continuum from structured to unstructured (Greig et al. 2007). There are advantages and disadvantages to interviews as data collection methods for both adult and child participants. There is some evidence that interviews can be used with children with speech and language disorders particularly when combined with other methods such as brainstorms, mindmaps, as well as sensitive and skilful questioning techniques (Kelly 2007; Watson, Abbott, and Townsley 2006). Other visual methods such as drawings have been used with typically developing children (Driessnack 2006) and young children with communication disability (Holliday, Harrison, and McLeod 2009; McLeod et al. 2011). Some researchers argue that visual methods can be a useful method of engaging children especially when used in combination with other methods (Christensen and James 2000).

When considering interviews, it is important that they are conceptualized as interactional encounters whereby accounts of experiences are co-constructed between the adult researcher and child participant (DeFina and Georgakopoulou 2008, 2012; Dockett and Perry 2007; Mishler 1986). Christensen (2004) suggests that researchers and practitioners carefully consider what children are asked to do in terms of whether the activities are reflective of children's experiences, interests and everyday activities. When conducting research with children with speech and developmental language disorders it is important that researchers are open, sensitive and flexible because each child will have individual needs and interests (Begley 2000; Brewster 2004). It is important to recognize that linguistic and cognitive factors may affect the interview process (Dockrell 2004; Dockrell and Lindsay 2011). For example, Tompkins and Farrar (2011) reported

that children with specific language impairment have difficulty reporting autobiographical memories without scaffolding from their mothers.
Therefore, when talking to children about past experiences it may be useful
to involve others (for example, parents, grandparents, and siblings) who can
provide this scaffolding and the use of visual supports, like photo albums,
may help children to recall past experiences. Other strategies that can be
used in the data collection phase are topic extensions and repeating the
child's sentence with an expectant intonation (Grove 2005). The use of
active listening skills is important and can make it safer for the child to
talk about difficult experiences (Mossige, Jensen, Gulbrandsen, Reichelt,
and Tjersland 2005). It is also important that researchers and practitioners
are aware of strategies that may hinder children's voice such as the adult
inadvertently switching topic, over-use of closed or specific questions, and
lack of tolerance for silences. In addition, some researchers caution against
repeating questions in exactly the same way because children may change
their responses, thinking that the first answer was not the desired response
(Coad and Lewis 2004; Docherty and Sandelowski 1999; Greig et al. 2007;
Irwin and Johnson 2005; Westcott and Littleton 2005).

Drawing on a piece of research conducted by the author with children
with speech and developmental language disorders, aged nine to twelve
years old, it was evident that the children were able to participate in the
research process (Lyons and Roulstone 2017). Children with speech and
developmental language disorders are a heterogeneous group. Therefore,
researchers need a toolkit and a range of supportive strategies which can be
tailored according to each child's interests, temperament, and speech and
language abilities. For example, it took longer for some children to trust the
researcher and trust was built over multiple interviews in locations which
were chosen by the children (that is, home and school settings, bowling
activity, playground). The nature of the co-construction in the interviews
was different for each child. For example, when asked questions some
children talked for extended turns with little input from the researcher.
In other cases children produced short utterances and the researcher had a
more active role in the co-construction of narratives. The use of strategies
such as drawing, prompts, changing the activity, photo-albums, games,
tours of areas of interest to them (for example, their gardens), playing with

their pets, or changing the setting of the interview, ensured that all children were given space and opportunities to express themselves. In the author's experience drawing was not liked by all of the children. Some children were self-conscious about their drawings and therefore researchers cannot make assumptions that all children will enjoy drawing (Gallagher 2009). Single use cameras were also useful for some children to generate discussion about things of interest to them. For example, one of the children took photographs of her dog, another child took photographs of his new bin which he was very proud of, and another took photographs of a family trip to a festival. This method can shift power to the children because they may take photographs of things of interest to them that can then be used to generate conversation. In the author's experience a range of methods and techniques are required so that all children are given opportunities to express their views.

However, engagement with children is not without its challenges. The author experienced the tensions of balancing the agendas of the children with that of the researcher. This was the case with one child in particular who wanted to lead and control the agenda. A flexible topic guide was designed to leave space to foreground the children's agendas (Greig et al. 2007). Although formal discourse analysis approaches were not used, the researcher learned to listen carefully and tune into what was happening in the interactions in the interviews to explore how the agenda was being negotiated (DeFina, 2009; Tanggaard 2009).

> Listening better requires the researcher or evaluator to be reflexive and reflective in decoding the encounter. (Lewis 2011: 20)

Through reflexivity, the researcher realized that one of the children may have controlled the agenda in order to keep the researcher at a distance and negotiate more fun activities. The researcher checked to see whether or not the child wanted to continue to participate in the research. The child wanted to participate and appeared to enjoy the one-to-one attention and the games. In this case, the researcher conceded power to the child and did not push her own agenda because she made judgement that the child was deliberately keeping the researcher at a distance. Gallacher and Gallagher (2008) describe power struggles whereby children found ways of using the researcher's presence to their own advantage, such as play partners. These actions can be conceptualized as children exercising agency. Some argue that power can be viewed as a negotiated process (Emond 2006; Hill, Davis, Prout, and Tisdall 2004). It is important that researchers are mindful of power differentials and that they do not exert their own power. Valentine (2011) argues that agency can be conceptualized not as a space where children can act autonomously but where the child can reproduce and/or disrupt social norms. Therefore, it is important that researchers are reflexive and consider ways in which power is exerted, shared, and negotiated in the research process. This may require adults conceding power in order to foreground children's agendas and this can be easier said than done. Morris (2003) cautions researchers not to react to their feelings of disempowerment by trying to take more control. Being truly child-centred is not without its challenges. Christensen (2004) urged researchers and practitioners to retrain their attention so that they do not dominate conversation, something that adults may be accustomed to doing in adult-child interactions. It is important to remain open to children's agendas in order to understand children's lives from their own perspectives.

Conclusion

In summary, children with speech and developmental language disorders, like John, have a voice and have the right to have their voice heard. Compliance with Article 12 of the UNCRC presents many challenges. Children are not routinely given opportunities to express their views on matters that concern them and their views may be sought but not acted upon (Lundy 2007). There are strong arguments for including children's views on matters that affect their lives. Listening to children can provide them with a sense of control over their lives and respect for their dignity and worth. Some models of good practice have been developed which engage children and young people in meaningful ways in the education system (Yamashita and Davies 2010).

One of the goals of speech and language therapy is to empower people to make changes to make their lives better in some way (Bunning 2004). Therefore, children and young people attending services, like speech and language therapy, should be given opportunities to be actively involved in decision-making in the therapy process for example, decisions about attending therapy, goal-setting, exploring what and why they want to learn. Indeed, a toolkit has been developed to facilitate children with speech, language and communication disorders in decision-making (Roulstone, Harding, and Morgan 2016). However, engaging with children may present challenges and fears for adults. For example, if given a choice it is entirely possible that a child may choose not to attend services. Baines (2008) argues that children's decision-making may be influenced by short-term advantages rather than long-term gain and suggests that children are encouraged to take responsibility for decisions initially in areas where the consequences of choosing unwisely are less severe or are short-term rather than long-term. Furthermore, Lundy (2007) reminds us that children should be asked whether or not they wish to be part of the decision-making process. Article 12 is a right not a duty.

It is important that speech and developmental language disorders are not be viewed as a barrier to children having a voice. Children, like John, should be both seen and heard. There is evidence that children with speech and developmental language disorders may be at risk in relation to emotional well-being and social exclusion. Therefore, it is necessary to build in ring-fenced time where children are given opportunities to express their views and concerns. It is important that they are supported to express these views, their views should be listened to, and acted upon as appropriate as suggested in Lundy's (2007) framework. Greene and Hill (2005) remind us that for too long we have assumed that children do not have much of importance to tell us and that adults have a better understanding of what is best for children. It is incumbent on us to listen to the voice of children with speech and developmental language disorders so that we can better understand their everyday experiences and explore better ways of supporting them. Listening to children will enable us to co-design services which meet their needs in their daily lives. We are still in the early stages of this journey but the conversation about listening to the voice of children with speech and developmental language disorders has started and is moving in the right direction.

References

Begley, A. (2000). The Educational Self-perceptions of Children with Down Syndrome. In A. Lewis and G. Lindsay (eds), *Researching Children's Perspectives*. Buckingham: Open University Press.

Brewster, S. (2004). Putting Words into their Mouths? Interviewing People with Learning Disabilities and Little/No Speech. *British Journal of Learning Disabilities*, 32, 166–169.

Bunning, K. (2004). *Speech and Language Therapy Interventions: Frameworks and Processes*. London: Whurr Publisher.

Carroll, C., and Sixsmith, J. (2016). Exploring the Facilitation of Young Children with Disabilities in Research about their Early Intervention Service. *Child Language Teaching and Therapy*, 32 (3), 313–325.

Christensen, P. (2004). Children's Participation in Ethnographic Research: Issues of Power and Representation. *Children and Society*, 18 (2), 165.

Christensen, P., and James, A. (2000). Childhood Diversity and Commonality: Some Methodological Insights. In P. Christensen and A. James (eds), *Research with Children – Perspectives and Practices,* pp. 160–178. London: Routledge Falmer.

Coad, J., and Hambly, H. (2011). Listening to Children with Speech, Language and Communication Needs through Arts-based Methods. In S. Roulstone and S. McLeod (eds), *Listening to Children and Young People with Speech, Language and Communication needs*, pp. 131–141. Croyden: J and R Press.

Coad, J., and Lewis, A. (2004). Engaging Children and Young People in Research – Literature Review for the National Evaluation of Children's Funds (NECF). Retrieved from <http://www.ne-cf.org>.

Davis, J., and Edwards, R. (2004). Setting the Agenda: Social Inclusion, Children and Young People. *Children and Society*, 18, (2), 97.

DeFina, A. (2009). Narratives in Interview – The case of accounts: For an Interactional Approach to Narrative Genres. *Narrative Inquiry*, 19 (2), 233–258.

DeFina, A., and Georgakopoulou, A. (2008). 'Analysing Narratives as Practices'. *Qualitative Research*, 8 (3), 379–387.

DeFina, A., and Georgakopoulou, A. (2012). *Analysing Narrative: Discourse and sociolinguistic Perspectives*. Cambridge: Cambridge University Press.

Department of Health and Children (2000). The National Children's Strategy: Our Children-Their Lives. Retrieved from: <http://childrensdatabase.ie/documents/publications/full_english_version.pdf>.

Docherty, S., and Sandelowski, M. (1999). Interviewing Children. *Research in Nursing and Health*, 22, 177–185.

Dockett, S., and Perry, B. (2007). Trusting Children's Accounts in Research. *Journal of Early Childhood Research*, 5 (1), 47–63.

Dockrell, J. E. (2004). How Can Studies of Memory and Language Enhance the Authenticity, Validity and Reliability of Interviews?. *British Journal of Learning Disabilities*, 32 (4), 161.

Dockrell, J. E., and Lindsay, G. (2011). Cognitive and Linguistic Factors in the Interview Process. In S. Roulstone and S. McLeod (eds), *Listening to Children and Young People with Speech, Language and Communication Needs*, pp. 143–152. Croydon: J and R Press Ltd.

Driessnack, M. (2006). Draw-and-Tell Conversations with Children about Fear. *Qualitative Health Research*, 16 (10), 1414–1435.

Emond, R. (2006). Reflections of a Researcher on the Use of a Child-Centred Approach. *The Irish Journal of Psychology*, 27 (1–2), 97–104.

France, A., Bendelow, G., and Williams, S. (2000). A 'Risky' Business: Researching the Health Beliefs of Children and Young People. In A. Lewis and G. Lindsay (eds), *Researching Children's Perspectives*. Buckingham: Open University Press.

Gallacher, L. A., and Gallagher, M. (2008). Methodological Immaturity in Childhood Research? Thinking Through 'Participatory Methods'. *Childhood*, 15 (4), 499–516.

Gallagher, M. (2008). 'Power is Not an Evil': Rethinking Power in Participatory Methods. *Children's Geographies*, 6 (2), 137–150.

Gallagher, M. (2009). Data Collection and Analysis. In E. K. M. Tisdall, J. Davis, and M. Gallagher (eds), *Researching with Children and Young People – Research Design, Methods and Analysis*, pp. 64–88. London: Sage.

Goodenough, T., Williamson, E., Kent, J., and Ashcroft, R. (2003). What Did You Think About That? Researching Children's Perceptions of Participation in a Longitudinal Genetic Epidemiological Study. *Children and Society*, 17, 113–125.

Greene, S., (2006). Child Psychology: Taking Account of Children at Last? *The Irish Journal of Psychology*, 27 (1–2), 8–15.

Greene, S. and Hill, M. (2005). Researching Children's Experience: Methods and Methodological Issues. In S. Greene and D. Hogan (eds), *Researching Children's Experience – Approaches and Methods*. London: Sage Publications.

Greig, A., Taylor, J., and MacKay, T. (2007). *Doing Research with Children* (2nd edn). London: Sage Publications Ltd.

Grove, N. (2005). *Ways into literature: Stories, plays and poems for pupils with SEN*. London: David Fulton Publishers.

Grover, S. (2004). Why Don't They Listen to Us? On Giving Power and Voice to Children Participating in Social Research. *Childhood*, 11 (1), 81–93.

Hill, M., Davis, J., Prout, A., and Tisdall, K. (2004). Moving the Participation Agenda Forward. *Children and Society*, 18 (2), 77.

Holliday, E., Harrison, L., and McLeod, S. (2009). Listening to Children with Communication Impairment Talking Through their Drawings. *Journal of Early Childhood Research*, 7 (3), 244–263.

Irwin, L. G., and Johnson, J. (2005). '.Interviewing Young Children: Explicating our Practices and Dilemmas. *Qualitative Health Research*, 15 (6), 821–831.

James, A. (2001). Ethnography in the Study of Children and Childhood. In P. Atkinson, A. Coffey, S. Delamont, J. Lofland, and L. Lofland (eds), *Handbook of Ethnography*. London: Sage Publications.

James, A., and James, A. (2008). *Key Concepts in Childhood Studies*. London: Sage.

Kelly, B. (2007). Methodological Issues for Qualitative Research with Learning Disabled Children. *International Journal of Social Research Methodology*, 10 (1), 21–35.

Lewis, A. (2011). Silence in the context of 'child voice'. *Children and Society*, 24, 14–23.

Lloyd, V., Gatherer, A., and Kalsy, S. (2006). Conducting Qualitative Interview Research with People with Expressive Language Difficulties. *Qualitative Health Research*, 16 (10), 1386–1404.

Lundy, L. (2007). 'Voice is not enough': Conceptualising Article 12 of the United Nations Convention on the Rights of the Child. *British Educational Research Journal*, 33, 927–942.

Lundy, L., McEvoy, L., and Byrne, B. (2011). 'Working With Young Children as Co-Researchers: An Approach Informed by the United Nations Convention on the Rights of the Child'. *Early Education and Development*, 22 (5), 714–736.

Lyons, R., and Roulstone, S. (2017). Labels, Identity and Narratives in Children with Primary Speech and Language Impairments. *International Journal of Speech-Language Pathology*, 19 (5), 503–518.

McLeod, S., Graham, D., and Barr, J. (2013). 'When He's Around his Brothers. He's Not So Quiet': The Private and Public Worlds of School-Aged Children with Speech Sound Disorder. *Journal of Communication Disorders*, 46, 70–83.

McLeod, S., McCormack, J., McAllister, L., Harrison, L., and Holliday, E. (2011). Listening to 4-to 5-Year Old Children with Speech Impairment Using Drawings, Interviews and Questionnaires. In S. Roulstone and S. McLeod (eds), *Listening to Children and Young People with Speech, Language and Communication Needs*, pp. 179–193. Croydon: J and R Publishers.

Markham, C., van Laar, D., Gibbard, D., and Dean, T. (2009). Children with Speech, Language and Communication Needs: Their Perceptions of their Quality of Life. *International Journal of Language and Communication Disorders*, 44 (5), 748–768.

Merrick, R., and Roulstone, S. (2011). Children's Views of Communication and Speech-Language Pathology. *International Journal of Speech-Language Pathology*, 13 (4), 281–290.

Mishler, E. (1986). The Analysis of Interview-Narratives. In T. R. Sarbin (ed.), *Narrative Psychology – the Storied Nature of Human Conduct*, pp. 233–255. London: Praeger.

Miskelly, C., and Roulstone, S. (2011). Issues and Assumptions of Participatory Research with Children and Young People with Speech, Language and Communication Needs. In S. Roulstone and S. McLeod (eds), *Listening to Children and Young People with Speech, Language and Communication Needs*, pp. 73–85. Albury: J and R Publishers.

Morris, J. (2003). Including All Children: Finding Out About The Experiences of Children with Communication and/or Cognitive Impairments. *Children and Society*, 17, 337–348.

Morrow, V., and Richards, M. (1996). The Ethics of Social Research with Children: An Overview. *Children and Society*, 10, 90–105.

Mossige, S., Jensen, T., Gulbrandsen, W., Reichelt, S., and Tjersland, O. A. (2005). Children's Narratives of Sexual Abuse – What Characterises Them and How Do They Contribute to Meaning-Making?. *Narrative Inquiry*, 15 (2), 377–404.

Norbury, C., Gooch, D., Wray, C., Baird, G., Charman, T., Simonoff, E., ... Pickles, A. (2016). The Impact of Nonverbal Ability on Prevalence and Clinical Presentation of Language Disorder: Evidence from a Population Study. *Journal of Child Psychology and Psychiatry*, 57 (11), 1247–1257.

Percy-Smith, B. (2011). Children's Voice and Perspectives: The Struggle for Recognition, Meaning, and Effectiveness. In S. Roulstone and S. McLeod (3ds.), *Listening to Children and Young People with Speech, Language and Communication Needs*, pp. 41–53. Croydon: J and R Press Ltd.

Pinkerton, J. (2004). Children's Participation in the Policy Process: Some Thoughts in Policy Evaluation Based on the Irish National Children's Strategy. *Children and Society*, 18, 119–130.

Prout, A. (2002). Researching Children as Social Actors: An Introduction to the Children 5–16 Programme. *Children and Society*, 16, 67–76.

Rabiee, P., Sloper, P., and Beresford, B. (2005). Doing Research with Children and Young People Who Do Not Use Speech for Communication. *Children and Society*, 19, 385–396.

Roulstone, S., Harding, S., and Morgan, L. (2016). *Exploring the involvement of children and young people with speech, language and communication needs and their families in decision-making*. Retrieved from: <https://www.thecommuni-cationtrust.org.uk/resources/resources/resources-for practitioners/>.

Roulstone, S., and Lindsay, G. (2012). The Perspectives of Children and Young People Who Have Speech, Language and Communication Needs, and Their Parents. *Better Communication Research Programme*. Retrieved from: <https://www.education.gov.uk/publications/standard/publicationDetail/Page1/DFE-RR247-BCRP7>.

Snowling, M., Bishop, D. V. M., Stothard, S., Chipchase, B., and Kaplan, C. (2006). Psychosocial Outcomes at 15 Years of Children with a Preschool History of Speech-Language Impairment. *Journal of Child Psychology and Psychiatry*, 47 (8), 759–765.

Stothard, S., Snowling, M., Bishop, D. V. M., Chipchase, B., and Kaplan, C. (1998). Language Impaired Preschoolers: A Follow-up into Adolescents. *Journal of Speech, Language, and Hearing Research*, 41, 407–418.

Tanggaard, L. (2009). The Research Interview as a Dialogical Context for the Production of Social Life and Personal Narrative. *Qualitative Inquiry*, 15 (9), 1498–1515.

Thomas, N., and O'Kane, C. (2000). Discovering What Children Think: Connections Between Research and Practice. *British Journal of Social Work*, 30, 819–835.

Thomas, N., and Percy-Smith, B. (2010). Introduction. In B. Percy-Smith and N. Thomas (eds), *A Handbook of Children and Young People's Participation: Perspectives from Theory and Practice*, pp. 1–7. Routledge: London.

Tisdall, E. K. M., Davis, J., and Gallagher, M. (2009). Introduction. In E. K. M. Tisdall, J. Davis, and M. Gallagher (eds), *Researching for Children and Young People- Research Design, Methods and Analysis*, pp. 1–10. London: Sage.

Tompkins, V., and Farrar, M. J. (2011). Mother's Autobiographical Memory and Book Narratives with Children with Specific Language Impairment. *Journal of Communication Disorders*, 44, 1–22.

United Nations (1989). United Nations Convention on the Rights of the Child. Retrieved from: <http://www.unicef.org/crc/>.

Valentine, K. (2011). Accounting for Agency. *Children and Society*, 25, 347–358.

Watson, N., Abbott, D., and Townsley, R. (2006). Listen to Me, Too! Lessons from Involving Children with Complex Healthcare Needs in Research about Multi-agency Services. *Child: Care, Health and Development*, 33 (1), 90–95.

Westcott, H., and Littleton, K. (2005). Exploring Meaning in Interviews with Children. In S. Greene and D. Hogan (eds), *Researching Children's Experience – Approaches and Methods*. London: Sage Publications.

Wickenden, M. (2010). *Teenage Worlds, Different Voices: An Ethnographic Study of Identity and Lifeworlds of Disabled Teenagers Who Use AAC*. Unpublished PhD. University of Sheffield.

Woodhead, M., and Faulkner, D. (2000). Subjects, Objects or Participants: Dilemmas of Psychological Research with Children. In P. Christensen and A. James (eds), *Research with Children: Perspectives and Practices*, pp. 10–39. London: Routledge.

Yamashita, H., and Davies, L. (2010). Students as Professionals: The London Secondary School Council's Action Research Project. In B. Percy-Smith and N. Thomas (eds), *A Handbook of Children and Young People's Participation: Perspectives from Theory and Practice*, pp. 230–244. London: Routledge.

13   Listen to us! The voices of young children with pain

Listening to children

Pain is an integral part of children's (that is, young people under twelve, pre-adolescent) everyday life. Receiving effective pain management is key for developing adaptive responses towards painful situations. As pain is an inherently subjective experience, it is crucial caregivers have a full understanding of how children's pain expressions evolve throughout development, characterized by increased verbalization skills, in order to provide effective pain management (Craig 2009).

How do we access children to gain an understanding of their perspectives in relation to their pain experiences? 'To hear children's voices, a method is required that values subjectivity, enhances empowerment and allows us to enter the respondent's world of meaning and belief' (Coyne et al. 2006:21).

Giving children a voice in their pain experience with integrity and professionalism respects their rights and dignity (Kilkelly and Donnelly 2006). This voice can be given in various ways, but a particularly strong method, both in research and practice, is using qualitative approaches to listen to the child's narrative of pain. The advantage of qualitative methods is that they encourage freedom of expression, thereby giving children a voice and agency (Carter 2004). Their strength rests in leaving participants' perceptions intact, while generating rich, detailed and valid data (Bender and Ewbank 1994). It has also been argued that, when conducting research, qualitative methodologies make it easier to create relaxed and trusting spaces to work in (Hyde and Howlett 2004). Building trust with children is particularly relevant in the clinical context and can be facilitated through adopting qualitative methods of pain assessment, so that the healthcare professional becomes less distanced and passive (Carter 2004). If the methods are flexible enough to take account of differences in age, personalities, context and preferred forms of communication (Coyne et al. 2006), adults can then glimpse the world inhabited by children (Greene and Hill 2005). In this chapter, we will provide some examples of how qualitative methods can be used to assess children's pain by giving them a voice. Before we explain these methods, we will first provide more details on the prevalence of acute and chronic pain among young children, how it impacts on them and the role parents play in these pain experiences.

Prevalence of acute pain experiences in young children

The majority of childhood pain experiences represent acute pain, defined as pain of a relatively brief duration, with a sudden onset and an apparent aetiology such as everyday bumps and scrapes, medical procedures or illness (Cummings, Reid, Finley, McGrath, and Ritchie 1996). Most prevalence studies have focused on school-aged children (nine to thirteen years of age) and adolescents (thirteen to eighteen years of age), revealing an average 3.5 incidence of acute pain per month, with headaches being the most frequently reported and bothersome type of pain (van Dijk, McGrath, Pickett, and Van Den Kerkhof 2006). Moreover, girls tend to report higher levels of pain compared to boys and the overall prevalence of pain has been found to increase with age (Perquin et al. 2000).

Nevertheless, evidence indicating that pain is prevalent among younger children is accumulating. In their observational study of everyday pain in pre-schoolers attending day-care, Fearon and colleagues (1996) observed that young children (three to seven years of age) experience a painful event approximately every three waking hours. Using the Pain Experience Interview, a reliable epidemiological tool to assess the prevalence of pain in children, McGrath and team (2000) found that five to seven year olds reported on average eleven acute trauma or disease pain experiences (for example, cut finger, toothache, chest pain), which varied widely in terms of intensity and affect. As with the school-aged sample, headaches were very common in this age group, with a prevalence of 43.2 per cent (McGrath et al. 2000).

Beyond these everyday acute pain experiences, this age group is also subjected to a large variety of medical interventions that might be painful, such as immunizations and blood draws. In Ireland, for example, the Health Service Executive's (HSE) National immunization Office recommends six vaccinations for babies before the age of fourteen months, two additional vaccinations at five years of age, and a further four vaccinations for children aged twelve years (HSE 2013). Pain resulting from needle-related procedures is usually mild, but can be associated with significant levels of fear (Taddio et al. 2009; Taddio et al. 2012), therefore effective pain management is crucial.

Consequently, early childhood represents a critical developmental stage in the child's life for shaping future pain management skills. In particular, these acute pain experiences in young children provide opportunities for children to gain an understanding of what pain is and how to manage pain. While the field of paediatric pain research has been largely dominated by investigations of how young children deal with medical pain (that is, due to immunizations, blood draws), everyday bumps and falls are more frequent and experienced with varying intensities. Furthermore, medical procedures are quite disconnected from the family's normal environment. Taken together, exploring children's responses to everyday painful events might provide a better insight into development of children's typical pain management skills (Fearon et al. 1999). For instance, Fearon and colleagues (1999) found that coping strategies for these pain experiences gradually developed as children gained in independence; older children relied less on adults to provide help and demonstrated more engagement in protective behaviours such as holding and self-quieting.

It is crucial to gain a better understanding of pain during early childhood, as the nervous system is still developing and therefore highly responsive to noxious stimuli (Schwaller and Fitzgerald 2014). In support of this assumption, stressful events in early childhood (including painful events such as surgery and needle procedures), especially when occurring repeatedly, were found to induce long-lasting changes in pain processing (Schwaller and Fitzgerald 2014) and can be a predisposing factor in developing chronic pain later in life (Burke, Finn, McGuire, and Roche 2016).

Prevalence of chronic pain experiences in young children

While acute pain constitutes children's primary experience of pain, considerable numbers of young children also live with chronic pain, regardless of the aetiology. Chronic pain can be described as continuous pain that lasts longer than it should, that is, three months, or, as frequent recurrent pain with a minimum duration of three months, often without a clear biomedical cause (American Pain Society 2001). The meta-analysis of King and colleagues (2011) reported a prevalence of paediatric chronic pain between 11–38 per cent, with higher prevalence in girls and older children. Headache (8–83 per cent), abdominal pain (4–53 per cent) and musculoskeletal pain (4–40 per cent) were the most frequently reported and investigated types of pain (King et al. 2011). Chronic pain can substantially interfere with children's daily functioning as manifested by impaired sleep patterns, and worse academic, physical, and social functioning (Gauntlett-Gilbert and Eccleston 2007; Konijnenberg et al. 2005; Logan and Scharff 2005; Logan, Simons, Stein, and Chastain 2008; Long, Krishnamurthy and Palermo 2008). Moreover, the experience of chronic pain seems to persist in a considerable proportion of children and adolescents (Perquin et al. 2003) and may be predictive of long-term pain complaints and pain-related disability in adulthood (King et al. 2011). Interestingly, findings by McGrath and colleagues (2000) revealed that chronic or recurrent pain often start in early childhood: recurrent headache on average began around 6.8 years of age, and arthritic pain similarly started on average around 6.4 years.

Importantly, while chronic pain is less common than acute pain in normal developing children the reverse appears to be true for children with a cognitive impairment. Cognitive impairment is generally regarded as having a noticeable and measureable difficulty in remembering, learning new things, concentrating and/or making decisions, all of which influence pain expressions (Hadjistavropoulos et al. 2011). Breau et al. (2003) identified higher rates of pain prevalence in children with a cognitive impairment (aged 3–18) with 35–52 per cent of children experiencing pain at least once a week. Contrary to pain in children without cognitive impairments, the cause of the pain was mainly related to a chronic illness. For example, a new Irish study has found one in fifty children with Down syndrome have juvenile arthritis. This four-year project – undertaken at UCD School of Medicine in partnership with clinicians in Our Lady's Children's Hospital Crumlin and supported by Arthritis Ireland, Down Syndrome Ireland and the National Children's Research Centre – found that children with Down syndrome are 18–21 times more likely to suffer from the debilitating disease than children without Down syndrome (Arthritis Ireland 2017). The pain experienced due to a chronic illness in these children was also more severe in intensity and duration compared to accidental pain or pain related to a medical procedure (Breau et al. 2003). Given the vulnerability of children with cognitive impairments due to their limited verbalization skills, it is important to gain a better understanding of and appropriate assessment of their pain.

PRIME C: Prevalence, impact, and cost of chronic pain among five-to twelve-year-olds living in Ireland

PRIME C, an Irish-wide longitudinal prevalence study, led by Dr O'Higgins, found a surprising 10 per cent of children in Irish Primary Schools self-reported that they had chronic pain. Previous research indicated that pain influences children's daily lives, resulting in absence from school, sleep problems, poor school performance, and problems with social activities (Claar et al. 1999; Dick and Riddell 2010; Hainsworth et al. 2007; Palermo et al. 2009). The PRIME C study characterized the nature, extent, impact and cost of chronic pain among five-to twelve-year-olds. Using cluster-systematic random sampling, primary schools were invited to participate and 3,116 five-to twelve-year-olds completed questionnaires in school classrooms, at three time points, one year apart. Questionnaires used internationally valid psychometric measures to assess a range of quality of life factors and chronic pain indicators among children, with corresponding parental/primary care giver questions, which were completed at home. Data were also gathered on the cost of chronic pain.

Of the children who reported having chronic pain, there was a higher prevalence among girls and older children, similar to other studies among this age group. How pain impacted on them was different depending on the age of the child. Children aged five to eight years with chronic pain were significantly more likely to feel alone and not get along as well with their parents. Children with chronic pain aged nine to twelve were significantly more likely to feel bored, alone, scared, different, and worry about doing schoolwork compared to children without chronic pain. Hence the importance of exploring in more depth how their day-to-day lives were impacted by their pain. This led to the final phase of the study under a Knowledge Exchange and Dissemination grant working participatively with children who have chronic pain and their families (see section on Participative Health Research for more details). On the cost side of PRIME C, childhood chronic pain according to parents/care givers incurred an incremental increase of up to €500 in healthcare costs per year.

One interesting feature of the PRIME-C results, which differed from other studies, was that more of the twelve-year-old boys reported pain than girls of the same age, in particular musculoskeletal pain, affecting their ability to participate fully in sports. The large amount of pain noted by boys in their lower limbs may be due to increased intensity of sports activities combined with a decrease in daily physical activity and higher levels of obesity among this age group (Riddiford-Harland et al. 2015), resulting in overuse injuries. It has been suggested that this is becoming increasingly common, especially during pubescent growth spurts (Launay 2015). This may reflect the increasing difficulty of fitting physical activity into 'the time-challenged, gender-stereotyped, highly-technologized, cyber-filled lives of today's youth' (Berger et al. 2008: 277). This is very pertinent for Irish primary school children where there is a strong affiliation with traditional Gaelic sports such as hurling, camogie and Gaelic football, run under the auspices of the Gaelic Athletic Association (GAA). It is important to high-light that pain in children during sports should not be considered normal, 'It is a warning sign of overtraining, which may require the activity to be modified, reduced or even discontinued' (Launay 2015: 139).

How well children learn to cope with their pain has important health implications. So how were these children coping with their pain? Over 300 children shared their pain stories with researchers during PRIME C data collection. The majority of coping strategies discussed by the children involved reduction in physical activity and distraction, this often involved their withdrawal from interactions with friends, family, physical activities and school, and were reported as having only varying degrees of success in reducing their pain.

This was the first study to explore chronic pain extensively amongst young children in Ireland (O'Higgins et al. 2015). PRIME C results suggested that clinicians should explore all aspects of health-related quality of life (HRQoL) for children with chronic pain, leading to improved out-comes and lower long-term costs. Additionally, and according with previ-ous studies, the results revealed the importance of the social environment in this young age group.

In particular, only 50 per cent of the children reporting chronic pain had parents corroborate that their child had chronic pain. These children were older; had more siblings; were more likely to have seen a GP in the last 12 months; had significantly better self-reported school functioning; and had worse self-reported family functioning. Children with chronic pain who reported not telling their parents about their pain explained that it was due to: fear of not being believed; their worries about medical intervention or not being allowed to participate in activities.

> I feel the muscles in my back are very sore, excruciatingly sore. I don't tell my parents because all they do is sort of tease me about needles and stuff. (Boy, age twelve)

These children reported that their pain experiences were not acknowl-edged by parents

> People don't notice my pain, and my parents ignore it. (Boy, age twelve)

> I told my parents but they just say it will go away. (Boy, age twelve)

A further twenty-seven parents reported a child with chronic pain, where the child did not report the same. These children were more likely to: attend a DEIS (Delivering Equality of Opportunity in Schools) school; have a father who was unemployed; have a medical card; have a parent who suffered from chronic pain; and have a chronic illness according to parental report. Relative to children who reported chronic pain, these children had poorer parent-reported physical, family and social functioning (Durand et al. 2016).

> Most of our daughter's pain secondary to her eczema affects our whole family as she has many nights of not sleeping and crying due to pain keeping others awake as a result. (Mother of girl, aged five)

Those children who did not report chronic pain but whose parents did were reported by parents to have impaired functioning across domains. The few children whose parents confirmed their report of chronic pain appeared to engage in more effective coping strategies.

> She knows she can control the pains by understanding them. Work in progress! (Mother of girl, age nine)

Taken together, these findings suggest a strong discordance between parental and child reporting with respect to chronic pain in this young age group. This discordance has important implications for their pain management, given that children are highly dependent on their parents for help and care, and further stress the need for all caregivers to actively listen to children's perspectives to avoid negating the child's sense of agency.

The role of the caregiver responses and reliance of parental proxy reports

A strong evidence base highlights the important role of the environment, particularly parental responses, in understanding childhood pain. This is particularly true for children with cognitive impairments whom, due to limited verbal capacities, rely heavily on caregivers for appropriately advocating their needs with respect to effective pain management (Solodiuk and Curley 2003). Despite this heavy reliance on caregivers for help and care, evidence reveals a lack in confidence in healthcare professionals to undertake pain assessment in children with cognitive impairments (Carter, Simons, Bray and Arnott 2016; Malviya et al. 2005). The *Social Communication Model of Pain* is a well-recognized theoretical model illustrating the key role of pain expressions in understanding how caregivers respond to a child's pain and how these caregiver responses can in turn impact on the child's pain experiences (Craig 2009).

The Social Communication Model of Pain

The social communication model of pain (SCM), based upon Rosenthal's (1982) model of non-verbal communication, takes into account non-verbal as well as verbal pain communications. Both are key in providing effective pain management attuned the child's needs. The model recognizes three important steps in the process of communicating pain. The first, step A, entails the sufferer's (that is, the child's) internal experience of pain, which is encoded in expressive pain behaviours (step B). The observer (that is, caregiver) needs to decode the child's expressive behaviour in order to draw inferences about their pain (step C). The behavioural responses of the observer, based upon the inferences the observer draw, may, in turn, have an impact upon the child's pain experience (step A) and pain expression (step B; Hadjistavropoulos et al. 2011). Detecting, interpreting and responding to the pain of others can have important implications for the recovery or survival of the person in pain, which is especially relevant in the context of paediatric pain.

Non-verbal behavioural expressions, such as facial pain expressions, crying and protective behaviour, are the main repertoire of young infants to communicate pain (Hadjistavropoulos et al. 2011). With increasing age, non-verbal behaviour gradually expands with other means of communication, such as verbal expression of pain (Craig and Korol 2008). It is important to acknowledge, though, that non-verbal pain expression remain the main form of pain communication amongst children with cognitive impairments. While children with cognitive impairments show large individual differences in their pain expression according to their mobility, developmental level, clinical condition, and verbal abilities (LaChapelle 1999), common pain behaviours seem to fit within the following categories: vocal behaviour, eating/sleeping, social behaviour, facial expressions, activity, body and limbs, and physical signs (McGrath, Rosmus, Canfield, Campbell, and Hennigar 1998).

Of the various possible expressions of pain, facial pain expressions and pain verbalizations have been found to be among the most salient in communicating pain to others. The clarity, intensity and type of pain expression are important for accurate decoding by observers and can impact observers' inferences and related behavioural response (Hadjistavropoulos et al. 2011). For instance, these pain expressions are crucial for observers to make estimations about the child's pain intensity, which in turn is considered an important determinant of caregiving responses such as pain control. Indeed, findings have indicated parent and health care professionals' estimates of child pain influence decisions regarding pain medication; with pain underestimations contributing to lower level of comfort among parents to administer pharmacological analgesics (Maimon, Marques, and Goldman 2007; Pillia-Riddell and Racine 2009). Higher pain estimates, on the other hand, have been linked to more health care usage by children (Janicke, Finney, and Riley 2001). Hence, being attuned to both verbal and non-verbal pain expression by any child is a crucial first step in giving them a voice in their pain management.

The impact of caregiver's pain management responses on the sufferer's pain have been well documented in young children, mainly in the context of procedural pain. Specifically, parental protective responses (for example, reassuring, comforting the child and providing empathic comments) have been associated with more pain and distress experienced by the child (Blount, Devine, Cheng, Simons, and Hayutin 2008; Manimala, Blount, and Cohen 2000; McMurtry, McGrath, Asp, and Chambers 2007; Racine, Riddell, Flora, Taddio, Garfield, and Greenberg 2016). While parental engagement in coping-promoting behaviour (for example, distracting the child, using humour, and commands to engage in deep breathing and relaxation) in response to child pain is associated with less pain and distress and more use of adaptive coping strategies by children (Blount et al. 2008;

Manimala et al. 2000). Despite being related to increased child distress, an observational study on parent's naturalistic behaviour during immunizations (Lisi, Campbell, Pillai Riddell, Garfield and Greenberg 2013) revealed soothing behaviours to be the most frequent behaviour parents engaged in. Furthermore, parental behaviours during vaccinations at pre-school age (four to six-year-olds), have been found to be a stronger predictor of child distress in anticipation of the vaccination than the child's own behaviour during previous vaccinations (Racine et al. 2016). While the exact mechanisms underlying these bidirectional influences between child and parent remain unclear (for example, do higher levels of child distress induce more parental protective behaviour or vice versa), these findings highlight the importance of considering childhood pain experiences as social events. Not only have parents a significant impact on their child's pain, due to on-going development of verbal and cognitive abilities across childhood, parents are often used as proxies for their child's pain experience.

Parent/caregiver reports as a proxy for child pain experiences

While self-report of pain is considered the gold standard for pain assessment, this might not be feasible for pre- or non-verbal children, such as children with a cognitive impairment. Consequently, parental or caregivers report of their child's pain is gathered to gain an in-depth report of the child pain experience. However, the accuracy of caregiver report may be limited, with evidence revealing underestimation is common (Hadjistavropoulos et al. 2011). For instance, focus groups with nurses revealed that discordance between child pain behaviour and parent proxy report is one of the barriers to nurses providing effective pain management (Twycross and Collis 2013). This discordance in reporting might be due to the variety of factors that influence parental proxy reports of pain. Beyond reliance on child pain behaviours, parental reports of their child's pain intensity are also influenced by their own worries about the child's pain, with higher parental worry related to more parental reports of child pain and distress (Caes, Vervoort, Devos, Verlooy, Benoit, and Goubert 2017; Racine et al. 2016). Parental report might be the only way to get an insight into children's pain experience for pre-verbal children, but this proxy reporting is often continued in pre-schoolers (von Baeyer, Jaaniste, Vo, Brunsdon, Lao, and Champion 2017) despite the ability of children as young as three years old to understand and communicate their pain (Jaaniste et al. 2016).

While cognitive developmental requirements for reporting on pain experiences need to be considered, especially when the pain is currently not present (see Janniste, Noel, and von Baeyer 2016 for a detailed overview), it might be more appropriate to rely on child self-report where possible (von Baeyer 2014). To support this self-report in younger ages, we need to be more creative in finding appropriate ways to give the child a voice.

How can young children share their experiences?

Adapted self-report scales

The use of the well-validated Faces Pain Scale – Revised (Hicks, von Baeyer, Spafford, van Korlaar, and Goodenough 2001) for children aged five years and older to report on their pain intensity might not be suitable for pre-schoolers due to the tendency of selecting only the first or last item of scales (von Baeyer et al. 2017). Consequently, based upon a systematic review of self-report measures of pain used pre-schoolers, von Baeyer and colleagues (2017) concluded that there is limited validation of existing self-report tools for use in pre-schoolers and recommended a two-step approach with simplified scales (e.g. reduced response options) in this age group. This two-step approach entails first asking the child a binary yes-no question on whether they are in pain, followed by a three-point scale conveying mild, moderate or severe pain in case the answer to the first question is 'yes' (von Baeyer, Chambers, Forsyth, Eisen, and Parker 2013; von Baeyer et al. 2017). Mixed results have been found to date with this simplified, two-step approach. While it significantly improved pain reports in three and four year olds for hypothetical pain (von Baeyer et al. 2013), recent validation efforts within a clinical context was only successful in providing evidence for validity in four year olds undergoing a venepuncture, not for three year olds (Emmott et al. 2017). Further research is needed to establish the most suitable self-report technique for pain in pre-schoolers. For instance, combining the binary yes-no question with observational pain assessment might be a more reliable pain assessment in verbal children younger than three years (Emmott et al. 2017).

Observational assessment

For preverbal children and children with cognitive impairments, the gold standard is observational assessments such as the The Face, Legs, Activity, Cry, and Consolobility (FLACC; Voepel-Lewis, Merkel, Tait, Trzcinka and Malviya 2002). The FLACC is a reliable, valid, and clinically useful tool, providing a comprehensive pain score on a scale from 0–10 based on 5 pain behaviours typically observed in children with cognitive impairments: facial pain expressions, legs activity, general activity level, crying, and difficulty in comforting or consoling the child (Voepel-Lewis et al., 2002). Each of these behaviours are scored on a scale from 0–2 according to their intensity and added up to create a score ranging from 0–10 that is translatable to the traditionally used numeric rating scale (NRS) for pain intensity (Voepel-Lewis et al. 2002). The FLACC has also recently been revised to account for the individual differences in how children with cognitive impairments express their pain (rFLACC). The rFLACC harnesses parents' unique knowledge about their child by allowing them to add specific pain behaviours unique to their child to each section of the coding scheme. For instance, this individualization revealed that for some children with cognitive impairments, a lack of expression, crying or responsiveness are key indicators of pain (Malviya et al. 2006). Despite representing the child's voice indirectly, this development of the rFLACC reflects and recognizes the need to give agency to children independently of their verbal capacities.

Participative Health Research

Going beyond the sole reliance on pain intensity, creative options exist to gain more in-depth perspective of the child's pain and impact on daily life by using participatory paradigms. Deeper insights into children's views and experiences can give adults better understandings of the reality for children, rather than ideas tempered by memories of childhood, when we rely on proxy adult reports (O'Higgins and Nic Gabhainn 2010). Participative Health Research (PHR) is a particularly useful way to understand the health and wellbeing of children, in the present tense. It does this by providing children with opportunities to show their unique point of view and competencies, and to use their perspectives and experiences to shape the research topics, research methods, and the interpretation and reporting of the findings (Gibbs et al. 2017). PHR with children is a rights-based approach, consistent with the United Nations Convention on the Rights of the Child (1989) (Lundy and McEvoy 2012), in Ireland's the National Children's Strategy (2000) and the National Strategy on Children and Young Peoples' Participation Decision Making 2015–2020 (2015). PHR acknowledges children as capable social actors who have their own views and agency while supporting safe spaces for children's participation and is inclusive of different levels of communication skills (Gibbs et al. 2017). It creates conditions for children's empowerment, encouraging their contributions on issues that are relevant to their own lives, as well as their community (Kellett 2010).

Essentially, PHR seeks to undermine power relations in the production of knowledge (Nieuwenhuys 2004). Empowerment, by dissolving the power hierarchy, involves engaging participants in the research process in order to maximize equity. It differs from power balance in that it can be seen as 'the end result of participative practices where each participant has control and/or influence over the issues of concern to them' (Barry1996:2). The possibility of empowerment for those involved is one of the key elements of participatory research approaches (Bowd et al. 2010). However, researchers need to acknowledge they may not actually 'know what would be empowering for others' (Gore 1992: 63). Cross did investigate longer-term consequences as the process unfolded over time and provided evidence that the ways in which children felt participatory research processes to be empowering, and the extent to which they engaged with them, were shaped by the power constraints which children continue to experience (and of which some are aware) within their own lives (Cross 2009). Researchers' argument that children are competent as research participants (Alderson 1995; Alderson and Morrow 2004) works once one accepts that children's competence is different from, and not necessarily of lesser value, than that of adults (Kellett 2005). Empowerment is possible if researchers make the effort to communicate and accept participants as equals; as the experts in their own lives.

Hence, the choice of method of representation during the Knowledge Exchange and Dissemination phase of the longitudinal cohort study of the prevalence, impact and cost of chronic pain among five to twelve year olds living in Ireland (PRIME C) was considered carefully in order to enhance the communication between children and the adult researcher. An important point is that children cannot be reduced to a 'homogenized group of others' (Schafer and Yarwood 2008: 123); age being a significant factor in their differences, experience and maturity being another. Methods need to be both appropriate and acceptable to the group of children involved (Hill 1997); 'even methods that are defined as participatory can be disempowering and excluding for respondents if used with the wrong group, in the wrong situation or the wrong way' (Boyden and Ennew, 1997: 83).

Knowledge Exchange and Dissemination phase of PRIME-C as an example of PHR

The value of adding PHR as a further layer to the PRIME-C study became clear as the children shared their pain stories, which made us aware that not only were children not telling adults about their pain but, when they did tell their teachers, the reaction from staff in the primary schools was not necessarily the best. For example, children reported that they were told to drink water and/or put their head down on their desks, or wait away from their classmates for someone to take them home, so isolating and differentiating them from their peers.

These findings stimulated the researchers to work together with the children to explore how best to create an intervention for teachers to raise awareness of paediatric chronic pain and possibly more effective management strategies. A first step in this approach was to invite 15 children (aged 5–11; 13 girls and 2 boys) who live with chronic pain due Juvenile Idiopathic Arthritis and their families to a PHR workshop. The workshop turned into a picnic on a sunny Saturday afternoon in Dublin; chosen as a central location. In this way, we overcame one of the challenges of working with children out of the school setting, that is, securing parental consent and acquiescence to transport their children to an event. The PHR workshop involved asking our young participants individually to share their perceptions on issues that affect them on a daily basis either with drawings or words on pieces of coloured paper, without any input or direction of the researchers. This first step is crucial, as from past experience and with a commitment to work with 'the experts' (that is, the children living with chronic pain), researchers' and adult ideas may well be different from the lived reality. Working in two small groups, the children collated all their ideas into themes by playing a variation of the snap card game (all the individual ideas were dealt out by the youngest member of each group face up – to increase saturation with all the ideas from the other children – thus piles of similar issues generated and each pile labelled by the children). They all discussed and chose the most important area that they then explored in more detail as: *being part of school life*. With that issue in the centre, they developed a 'Web of Ideas' about how best to support children with chronic pain to participate more fully in primary school life (See figure 13.1). Throughout the activity, all decisions were fully controlled by the children, with minimal direction or input from the researcher.

The ideas identified by the children became the basis of an awareness raising exercise lead by the children. The children on our PHR picnic decided to make videos to illustrate how chronic pain impacts on them and some ideas on how to improve their ability to 'be part of school'. Using their parents' phones, they went to work. This process is still on-going, with work currently focused on finalizing this educational and awareness-raising video for teachers and primary schools. We plan to release the video on YouTube for all the families involved in the project and a wider audience including the thirty-nine schools involved in the PRIME-C study.

Using the video as a starting point, we will then work with primary schools, principals and teachers, to create guidelines on how to proactively best support children who live with chronic pain to participate, as fully as possible, in primary school life. The guidelines will then be circulated to all primary school principals with the expectation that each school will adopt and adapt them to suit their own community context. It is known that

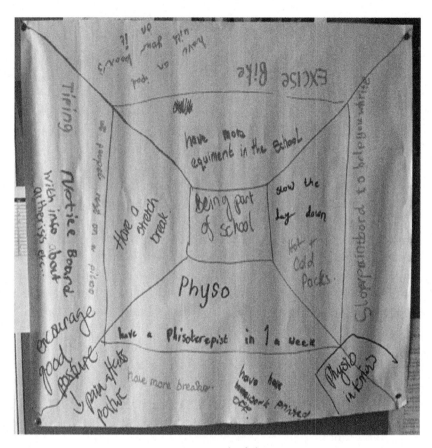

Figure 13.1: Web of ideas

80 per cent of academic achievement is due to the teacher-child interaction (Thackore 2016). If children with chronic pain can remain engaged within the learning environment with the support of their primary teachers, then their potential to thrive and fully participate in post primary school will be enhanced.

While these examples on PHR reflect the usability of listening to children's' narratives within a research context, this technique has also been proven valuable in accepting children as active agents within their clinical pain management. Carter (2004), provided an excellent overview of how to use this narrative approach in clinical settings.

Creative techniques

Other ways of creatively involving children using arts-based techniques have been developed and evaluated. While the application of these approaches is limited in the context of pain, they show promise in offering children a voice, especially non-verbal children (Carter and Ford 2013). Such techniques accommodate to children's skills, capacities, experiences, and interests and include photo-elicitation, poems, performances, collages, as well as drawings. An example of using photographs on a large scale was during the development of Child Indicators of Wellbeing. Children across Ireland identified indicators of their own wellbeing. Using disposable cameras, children were asked to take pictures of '*What makes you well*' and '*What keeps you well*'? Other groups of children then categorized the photographs and a final group of children created a schema of these themes. This process created Ireland's Child Wellbeing Indicators and highlighted how important pets are in many children's lives (Sixsmith, Nic Gabhainn, Fleming and O'Higgins 2007). The main aim of these techniques is to expand the way children express themselves, while appreciating that not everything has to be channelled through words. All these techniques tend to reduce the power imbalance between children and caregivers/researchers by supporting the child's agency (Carter and Ford 2013).

Examples of applying this to the context of pain can include making a collage of worst pain events or drawing your worst headache on a postcard and address this postcard to someone important to the child. These techniques are in their infancy and need further exploration with respect to their reliability for both research and clinical purposes; Carter and Ford (2013) provide an overview of practical tips concerning these creative techniques.

Conclusion

In conclusion, within this chapter we aimed at providing an overview of the prevalence of both acute and chronic pain in young children, from birth up to twelve years of age, as well as highlighting the importance of supporting and listening to the voices to these young children. While children are highly dependent on their parents for help and care, and parental responses to pain influence the child experiences, gaining the child's own perspective is of crucial importance for effective pain management. Discordance between parent proxy and child self-report might pose a difficulty for healthcare professionals, but are important to further explore in more detail as they can reflect an important underlying issue (e.g. high parental proxy reports might reflect heightened levels of parental worries).

Furthermore, continued development and implementation of creative techniques, beyond the reliance on self-reports, are pivotal to gain a better insight of young children's pain and are of importance to empower young children and children with a cognitive impairment to share their experiences. Using creative methodologies to listen to children are particularly appropriate in this young age group as it matches with their usual ways of communication (that is, drawings, pictures) while their verbal skills continue to develop and improve (Caes and Jordan 2017).

Gaining a better understanding of pain experiences in young children by giving them a voice will also facilitate the development of more age-appropriate tools to assist these children in learning adaptive ways to cope with pain. This is of importance as learning adaptive pain management techniques early on in life, might promote resilience when faced with pain and thereby prevent continued disability, due to pain, in later childhood, adolescence and even adulthood.

References

Alderson, P. (1995). *Listening to children. Children, ethics and social research*. Ilford: Barnardos.

Alderson, P., and Morrow, V. (2004). *Ethics, Social Research and Consulting with Children and Young People* (2nd edn). London: Barnardos.

American Pain Society (2001). *Pediatric chronic pain*. Glenview: American Pain Society.

Arthritis Ireland (2017). *Twice as many children with Down syndrome have arthritis than previous estimates*. Retrieved from: <http://www.arthritisireland.ie/go/research/down_s_arthritis_research>.

Barry, M. (1996). The empowering process: Leading from behind? *Youth and Policy*, 54, 1–12.

Bender, D. E., and Ewbank, D. (1994). The focus group as a tool for health research: Issues in design and analysis. *Health Transition Review*, 4 (1), 26–76.

Berger, I. E., O'Reilly, N., Parent, M. M., Séguin, B., and Hernandez, T. (2008). Determinants of Sport Participation among Canadian Adolescents. *Sport Management Review*, 11, 277–307.

Blount, R. L., Devine K. A., Cheng, P. S., Simons, L. E., and Hayutin, L. (2008). The impact of adult behaviors and vocalizations on infant distress during immunizations. *Journal of Pediatric Psychology*, 33(10), 1163–1174.

Boyden, J., and Ennew, J. (eds) (1997). *Children in focus: A manual for participatory research with children*. Stockholm: Radda Barnen.

Burke, N. N., Finn, D. P., McGuire, B. E., and Roche, M. (2017). Psychological stress in early life as a predisposing factor for the development of chronic pain: Clinical and preclinical evidence and neurobiological mechanisms. *Journal of neuroscience research*, 95 (6), 1257–1270.

Caes, L., and Jordan, A. (2017). The pain of youth. *The Psychologist*, 30, 24–27.

Caes, L., Vervoort, T., Devos, P., Verlooy, J., Benoit, Y., and Goubert, L. (2017). Health care professional and parents' level of distress and sympathy influence their estimation of child pain during a painful medical procedure. *Pain Medicine*, 18 (2), 275–282.

Carter, B. (2004). Pain Narratives and Narrative Practitioners: A Way of Working 'In-Relation' With Children Experiencing Pain. *Journal of Nursing Management*, 12 (3), 210–216.

Carter, B., and Ford, K. (2013). Researching children's health experiences: The place for participatory, child-centered, arts-based approaches. *Research in Nursing & Health*, 36, 95–107.

Carter, B., Simons, J., Bray, L., and Arnott, J. (2016). Navigating uncertainty: health professionals' knowledge, skill, and confidence in assessing and managing pain in children with profound cognitive impairment. *Pain Research and Management*, 2016 (1), 1–7.

Claar, R. L., Walker, L. S., and Smith, C. A. (1999). Functional disability in adolescents and young adults with symptoms of irritable bowel syndrome: the role of academic, social, and athletic competence. *Journal of Pediatric Psychology*. 24 (3), 271–80.

Coyne, I., Hayes, E., Gallagher, P., and Regan, G. (2006). *Giving Children a Voice: Investigation of children's experiences of participation in consultation and decision-making in Irish hospitals*. Dublin: Office of the Minister for Children and Youth Affairs.

Craig, K. D. (2009). The social communication model of pain. *Canadian Psychology/ Psychologie Canadienne*, 50 (1), 22.

Cross, B. (2009). Hearing out children's narrative pathways to adulthood: Young people as interpreters of their own childhoods in diverging working-class Scottish communities. *Childhood*, 16 (3), 335–353.

Cummings, E. A., Reid, G. J., Finley, G. A, McGrath, P. J., and Ritchie, J. A. (1996). Prevalence and source of pain in pediatric inpatients. *Pain*, 68 (1), 25–31.

Dick, B., and Pillai Riddell, R. (2010). Cognitive and school functioning in children and adolescents with chronic pain: A critical review. *Pain Research and Management*, 15 (4), 238–244.

Durand, H., O'Higgins, S., Caes, L., Dwyer, C., Slattery, B., Nic Gabhainn, S., O'Neill, C., Murphy, A., and McGuire, B. E. (under review by PAIN 2016). 'Not Seeing Eye-To-Eye: Differential Reporting of Chronic Pain by Children and Their Parents'. (PRIME-C).

Emmott, A., West, N., Zhou, G., Dunsmuir, D., Montgomery, C. J., Lauder, G. R., and von Baeyer, C. L. (2017). Validity of Simplified Versus Standard Self-Report Measures of Pain Intensity in Preschool-Aged Children Undergoing Venipuncture. *The Journal of Pain*, 18 (5), 564–573.

Fearon, I., McGrath, P. J., and Achat, H. (1996). 'Booboos': the study of everyday pain among young children. *Pain*, 68 (1), 55–62.

Gauntlett-Gilbert, J., and Eccleston, C. (2007). Disability in adolescents with chronic pain: Patterns and predictors across different domains of functioning. *Pain*, 131, 132–141.

Gibbs, L., Marinkovic, K., Black, A. L., Gladstone, B. M., Dedding, C., Dadich, A., O'Higgins, S., Abma, T., Casley, M., Cartmel, J., and Acharya, L. (under review). Kids in Action – Participatory Health Research with Children. In M. Wright and K. Kongats (eds), *Participatory Health Research. International Perspectives*: Springer.

Gore, J. (1992). What we can do for you! What can 'we' do for 'you'?: Struggling over empowerment in critical and feminist pedagogy. In C. Luke and J. Gore (eds), *Feminism and critical pedagogy*, pp. 54–73. London: Routledge.

Greene, S., and Hill, M. (2005). Researching Children's Experience: Methods and Methodological Issues. In S. Greene and D. Hogan, (eds), *Researching Children's Experience: Approaches and Methods*, pp. 1–21. London: Sage.

Hainsworth, K., Davies, W., Khan, K., and Weisman, S. (2007). Development and Preliminary Validation of the Child Activity Limitations Questionnaire: Flexible and Efficient Assessment of Pain-Related Functional Disability. *The Journal of Pain*, 8 (9), 746–752.

Hicks, C. L., von Baeyer, C. L., Spafford, P. A., van Korlaar, I., and Goodenough, B. (2001). The Faces Pain Scale–Revised: toward a common metric in pediatric pain measurement. *Pain*, 93 (2), 173–183.

Hill, M. (1997). Participatory research with children. *Child and Family Social Work*, 2 (3), 171–183.

Health Service Executive (2013). Immunisation. *Health Service Executive National Immunisation Office*. Retrieved from: <http://www.hse.ie/eng/health/immunisation/>.

Hyde, A., Howlett, E., Brady, D., and Drennan, J. (2005). The focus group method: Insights from focus group interviews on sexual health with adolescents. *Social Science & Medicine, 61* (12), 2588–2599.

Jaaniste, T., Noel, M., and von Baeyer, C. L. (2016). Young children's ability to report on past, future, and hypothetical pain states: a cognitive-developmental perspective. *Pain, 157* (11), 2399–2409.

Janicke, D. M., Finney, J. W., and Riley, A. W. (2001). Children's Health Care Use A Prospective Investigation of Factors Related to Care-Seeking. *Medical Care, 9* (9), 990–1001.

Kellett, M. (2005). *Children as active researchers: A new research paradigm for the 21st century?*. London: Economic and Social Research Council National Centre for Research Methods.

Kellett, M. (2010). *Rethinking children and research: Attitudes in contemporary society*. London: Continuum International.

Kilkelly, U., and Donnelly, M. (2006). *The Child's Right to be heard in the Healthcare Setting*. Dublin: Office for the Minister of Children and Youth Affairs.

King, S., Chambers, C. T., Huguet, A., MacNevin, R. C., McGrath, P. J., Parker, L., and MacDonald, A. J. (2011). The epidemiology of chronic pain in children and adolescents revisited: A systematic review. *Pain, 152*, 2729–2738.

Konijnenberg, A. Y., Uieterwaal, C. S. P. M., Kimpen, J. L. L., van der Hoeven, J., Buitetlaar, J. K., and de Graeff-Meeder, E. R. (2005). Children with unexplained chronic pain: substantial impairment in everyday life. *Archives of Diseases in Childhood, 90*, 680–688.

LaChapelle, D. L., Hadjistavopoulos, T., and Craig, K. D. (1999). Pain measurement in persons with intellectual disabilities. *The Clinical Journal of Pain, 15*, 13–23.

Launay, F. (2015) Sports-related overuse injuries in children. *Orthopaedics and Traumatology-Surgery and Research, 101*, S139–S147.

Lisi, D., Campbell, L., Riddell, R. P., Garfield, H., and Greenberg, S. (2013). Naturalistic parental pain management during immunizations during the first year of life: Observational norms from the OUCH cohort. *Pain, 154* (8), 1245–1253.

Logan, D. E., and Scharff, L. (2005). Relationships between family and parent characteristics and functional abilities in children with recurrent pain syndromes: an investigation of moderating effects on the pathway from pain to disability. *Journal of Pediatric Psychology, 30* (8), 698–707.

Logan, D. E., Simons, L. E., Stein, M. J., and Chastain, L. (2008). School impairment in adolescents with chronic pain. *The Journal of Pain, 9* (5), 407–416.

Long, A. C., Krishnamurthy, V., and Palermo, T. M. (2008). Sleep disturbances in school-age children with chronic pain. *Journal of Pediatric Psychology*, 33 (3), 258–268.

Lundy, L., and McEvoy, L. (2012). *Childhood, the United Nations convention on the rights of the child and research: What constitutes a 'rights-based' approach?* In M. Freeman (ed.), Law and childhood studies, Vol. 14, pp. 75–91. Oxford: Oxford University Press.

McGrath, P. J., Rosmus, C., Canfield, C., Campbell, M. A., and Hennigar, A. (1998). Behaviours caregivers use to determine pain in non-verbal, cognitively impaired individuals. *Developmental medicine and child neurology*, 40 (5), 340–343.

McGrath, P. A., Speechley, K. N., Seifert, C. E., Biehn, J. T., Cairney, A. E. L., Gorodzinsky, F. P., and Morrissy, J. R. (2000). A survey of children's acute, recurrent, and chronic pain: validation of the pain experience interview. *Pain*, 87 (1), 59–73.

McMurty, C. M., McGrath, P. J., Asp, E., and Chambers, C. T. (2007). Parental reassurance and pediatric procedural pain: a linguistic description. *The Journal of Pain*, 8 (2), 95–101.

Maimon, M. S., Marques, L., and Goldman, R. D. (2007). Parental Administration of Analgesic Medication in Children After a Limb Injury. *Pediatric Emergency Care*, 23 (4), 223–226.

Malviya, S., Voepel-Lewis, T., Merkel, S., and Tait, A. R. (2005). Difficult pain assessment and lack of clinician knowledge are ongoing barriers to effective pain management in children with cognitive impairment. *Acute Pain*, 7 (1), 27–32.

Malviya, S., Voepl-Lewis, T., Burke, C., Merkel, S., and Tait, A. R. (2006). The revised FLACC observational pain tool: improved reliability and validity for pain assessment in children with cognitive impairment. *Pediatric Anesthesia*, 16 (3), 258–265.

Manimala, M. R., Blount R. L., and Cohen, L. (2000). The effects of parental reassurance versus distraction on child distress and coping during immunizations. *Child Health Care*, 29, 161–177.

O'Higgins, S., Doherty, E., NicGahainn, S., Murphy, A., Hogan, M., O' Neill, C., and McGuire, B. E. (2015). The Prevalence, Impact and Cost of Chronic Non-Cancer Pain in Irish Primary School Children (prime-c). Protocol for a longitudinal school-based survey. *BMJ Open*, 5, e007426.

O'Higgins, S., and Nic Gabhainn, S. (2010). Youth Participation in setting the agenda: learning outcomes for sex education in Ireland. *Sex Education,* 10 (4), 367–403.

Palermo, T. M., Wilson, A. C., Peters, M., Lewandowski, A., and Somhegyi, H. (2009). Randomized controlled trial of an Internet-delivered family cognitive–behavioral therapy intervention for children and adolescents with chronic pain. *Pain*, 146 (1), 205–213.

Perquin, C. W., Hazebroek-Kampschreur, A. A. J. M., Hunfeld, J. A. M., Bohnen, A. M., van Suijlekom-Smit, L. W. A., Passchier, J., and van der Wouden, J. C. (2000). Pain in children and adolescents: A common experience. *Pain,* 87, 51–58.

Pillai Riddell, R., and Racine, N. (2009). Assessing pain in infancy: The caregiver context. *Pain Res Manage,* 14 (1), 27–32.

Racine, N. M., Riddell, R. R. P., Flora, D. B., Taddio, A., Garfield, H., and Greenberg, S. (2016). Predicting preschool pain-related anticipatory distress: the relative contribution of longitudinal and concurrent factors. *Pain,* 157 (9), 1918–1932.

Riddiford-Harland, D. L., Steele, J. R., Cliff, D. P., Okely, A. D., Morgan, P. J., Jones, R. A., and Baur, L. A. (2015). Lower activity levels are related to higher plantar pressures in overweight children. *Medicine and Science in Sports and Exercise,* 47 (2), 357–362.

Schafer, N., and Yarwood, R. (2008). Involving young people as researchers: uncovering multiple power relations among youths. *Children's Geographies,* 6 (2), 121–135.

Schwaller, F., and Fitzgerald, M. (2014). The consequences of pain in early life: Injury-induced plasticity in developing pain pathways. *European Journal of Neuroscience,* 39 (3), 344–352.

Sixsmith, J., Nic Gabhainn, S., Fleming, C., and O'Higgins, S. (2007). Children's, parents' and teachers' perceptions of child wellbeing. *Health Education,* 107 (6), 511–523.

Solodiuk, J., and Curley, M. A. (2003). Pain assessment in nonverbal children with severe cognitive impairments: the Individualized Numeric Rating Scale (INRS). *Journal of Pediatric Nursing,* 18 (4), 295–299.

Solodiuk, J. C., Scott-Sutherland, J., Meyers, M., Myette, B., Shusterman, C., Karian, V. E., and Curley, M. A. (2010). Validation of the Individualized Numeric Rating Scale (INRS): a pain assessment tool for nonverbal children with intellectual disability. *Pain,* 150 (2), 231–236.

Taddio, A., Chambers, C. T., Halperin, S. A., Ipp, M., Lockett, D., Rieder, M. J., and Shah, V. (2009). Inadequate pain management during routine childhood immunizations: the nerve of it. *Clinical Therapeutics,* 31, S152–S167.

Taddio, A., Ipp, M., Thivakaran, S., Jamal, A., Parikh, C., Smart, S., and Katz, J. (2012). Survey of the prevalence of immunization non-compliance due to needle fears in children and adults. *Vaccine,* 30 (32), 4807–4812.

Thakore, J. (2016). *Learning Development in Children.* Presentation at St Patrick's Mental Health Founder's Day Conference. November 2016, Dublin.

Twycross, A., and Collis, S. (2013). Nurses' views about the barriers and facilitators to effective management of pediatric pain. *Pain Management Nursing,* 14 (4), e164–e172.

van Dijk, A., McGrath, P. A., Pickett, W., and Van Den Kerkhof, E. G. (2006). Pain prevalence in nine- to 13-year-old school children. *Pain Research and Management,* 11(4), 234–240.

Voepel-Lewis, T., Merkel, S., Tait, A. R., Trzcinka, A., and Malviya, S. (2002). The reliability and validity of the Face, Legs, Activity, Cry, Consolability observational tool as a measure of pain in children with cognitive impairment. *Anesthesia & Analgesia,* 95 (5), 1224–1229.

von Baeyer, C. L. (2014). Self-report: The primary source in assessment after infancy. In P. J. McGrath, B. S. Stevens, S. M. Walker, and W.T Zempsky (eds), *Textbook of Paediatric Pain,* pp. 370–378. Oxford: Oxford University Press.

von Baeyer, C. L., Chambers, C. T., Forsyth, S. J., Eisen, S., and Parker, J. A. (2013). Developmental data supporting simplification of self-report pain scales for preschool-age children. *The Journal of Pain,* 14 (10), 1116–1121.

von Baeyer, C. L., Jaaniste, T., Vo., H. L., Brunsdon, G., Lao, A. H. C., and Champion, G. D. (2017). Systematic review of self-report measures of pain intensity in 3-and 4-year-olds: Bridging a period of rapid cognitive development. *The Journal of Pain,* S1526–5900 (17), 30519–9.

14   Young children's use of private speech in early
        childhood settings: Moving from a deficit
        approach to a rights and agency approach

Speech, language and communication development

Children's speech, language and communication (SLC) develop over time
in the context of relationships and interactions with caregivers and peers
and typically follow an observable sequence, dependent on children's own
genetic inheritance and characteristics and the opportunities afforded to
them to experience and practice communicative interactions with others.
Vygotsky (1978) regarded children as active constructors of their own
knowledge but stressed the role of cultural sign systems. He did not deny
the importance of the child's own spontaneous investigation and everyday experience, especially in the first two years of life, but regarded concepts, language, voluntary attention and memory as mental functions
derived from culture and beginning with interaction between the child
and another person. Moreover, each of these functions appeared twice
in the child's development: first as shared between adult and child (or
social) but secondly within the child (or psychological). Put another way,
Vygotsky (1978) saw the process of development as 'internalizing' social
interactions. What started as a social function became internalized within
the child. This Vygotsky saw as the process by which the development of all
higher mental processes occurred to the extent that language and thought
were inseparable:

> Language is the most powerful tool of any human being. It is undeniably the great-
> est asset we possess. A good grasp of language is synonymous with a sound ability
> to think. In other words language and thought are inseparable. (Vygotsky 1986: 10)

To achieve higher and more abstract concepts and intellectual tools of their community of writing or mathematics, for instance, children need instruction in abstract sign systems. The child has thus a 'zone of proximal development' which he or she can achieve only with the assistance of an adult`. In terms of language development and the role of conceptual tools and knowledge handed on by adults in the same culture, the notion of teaching and social construction is particularly powerful for understanding language acquisition. This view suggests that children need to spend optimum amounts of time interacting with adults and peers in order to promote speech, language and communication (SLC) development and is consistent with Bronfenbrenner's bioecological model. Bronfenbrenner's (1979, 1993) bioecological model acknowledged that children grow and develop in a social and cultural context influenced by the bi-directional interactions and relationships within and between the environments they inhabit. Their learning and development is therefore socially and culturally constructed through interactions and relationships with others in environments where meanings and languages are shared, as summarized by Bronfenbrenner (2001: 6965):

> Over the life course, human development takes place through processes of progressively more complex reciprocal interaction between an active, evolving bio-psychological human organism and the persons, objects, and symbols in its immediate external environments. To be effective the interactions must occur on a fairly regular basis over extended periods of time.

Social and private speech

An important phenomenon that linked language and thinking first identified by Piaget (1959), and reinforced by Vygotsky (1986) was children's use of private speech (or talking aloud to oneself) to help them make meaning from language heard from adult speech. This helped to self-regulate their emotions, keep track of their thoughts and form a bridge between social speech and inner speech. Whilst Piaget (1962) perceived children's private speech to be egocentric, aimed at the self rather than others even when spoken aloud, Vygotksy (1978) saw private speech as externalized thought with a useful purpose. Private speech could be categorized according to whether it was overt or covert and related to a task in hand or was irrelevant to the task the child was engaged in. Children progressed from overt speech to covert speech as they matured. Vygotsky (1978) recognized a developmental role in children's use of private speech which was contingent on both their observation of adult speech and practice of linguistic skills through guided participation with adults (Rogoff 2003). Harris (2000) noted that play is also an important medium in allowing children to deconceptualized language in order to understand abstract concepts in SLC. It enables them to practise their immature speech with peers and through private speech in order to form a bridge between language and thought (Vygotsky 1978). This suggests that although spending time with adults and peers is beneficial, it is also important for children to spend time in solitary periods to rehearse speech alone.

For children with SLCN, extra time may be needed to rehearse speech and internalize conversations in this way as these moments of self-talk and solitary play help children to integrate learning achieved with adults and children's time spent alone to do this should be valued. This raises the question of whether early childhood professionals understand the important role that private speech plays. It also raises the question of how private speech is defined.

Defining private speech

Child and adult speech utterances are typically classified as either social speech or private speech. Social speech is speech addressed to another person as indicated by either a pronoun reference, a gaze to another person, or other signals of social intent, such as physical contact, argumentation, or conversational turn-taking (Diaz 1992; Winsler 1998). Private, or self-directed, speech refers to the audible or visible talk children (and adults) use to communicate with themselves as they go about their daily activities (Berk 1992). While social speech provides a means for communicating with others, private speech provides a tool for thinking, for communicating with the self, and for the self-regulation of behaviour (Berk 1992; Diaz, 1992). Private speech is defined as speech that is not explicitly addressed to another person and thus serves no apparent interpersonal communicative function (Flavell, Beach, and Chinsky 1966). The phenomenon has theoretical significance within both Piaget's and Vygotsky's writings.

A typical approach to drawing the social–private distinction is to classify utterances as social according to characteristics within the communicative interaction such as whether the child involves another person, whether the child shows eye contact with another person, whether their interaction has temporal connection with an earlier conversation or relates to the same topic (Fernyhough and Russell 1997; adapted from Diaz 1992; Furrow 1992; Goudena 1992; Winsler, Carlton, and Barry 2000). Any utterance that does not meet any of these criteria for social speech is classified as private speech. These researchers seem to agree that speech that is not directed to others (peers or adults), does not involve any social rules such as turn taking or reference points is typical of the self-talk that children exhibit during episodes of solitary play.

Speech, language and communication in early childhood settings

This chapter considers findings arising from a mixed-methods policy to practice context study of the acquisition of SLC of young children aged two to five attending early childhood settings in the Early Years Foundation Stage (EYFS) (Department for Education 2017) in one local authority in England (Blackburn and Aubrey 2016). Young children's use of private speech emerged as a key finding from analysis of observation data. The physical and social resources that both promoted and inhibited this aspect of SLC are discussed. The case study approach adopted in the study allowed an in-depth exploration of nine children who had been identified with speech, language and communication needs (SLCN) as defined by Bercow (2008: 13):

> ... encompassing a wide range of difficulties related to all aspects of communication in children, including difficulties with fluency, forming sounds and words, formulating sentences, understanding what others say and using language socially.

Arguably this definition stresses a deficit approach whereby SLCN are perceived from a medical model of being 'within child' rather than being situated within a social model of barriers / promoters within the environment as suggested by Bronfenbrenner. Early childhood professionals have a duty under the statutory framework of the EYFS (Department for Education 2017) to observe, assess and monitor children's SLC in order to provide timely and effective intervention when any delays or deviances are identified. This might also involve referral to other professionals such as Speech and Language Therapists. The nature of adult planning and pedagogy from early childhood professionals (with support from other professionals where necessary) for young children with SLCN and the effect of these on children's communicative interactions is of interest.

Observations

Observations can lie on a continuum from structured to unstructured and from complete participant to non-participant observation (Simons 2009: 55). Observations were carried out by the researcher and were therefore non-participant. Time-sequenced observations were employed to record target children (TC) at specified intervals of time (every two minutes). This method provided numerical data from frequencies of specific interactions and activities in a particular context, which allowed the comparison of children across case study sites. In order to ensure systematic data collection, a structured observation schedule was used. The target child observation schedule developed by Sylva et al. (1980) has been used widely in early childhood research (for example Sylva et al. 2004; Siraj-Blatchford et al. 2002) and allowed the researcher to observe closely an individual child who may (for example) use little language or not appear to relate well to children or adults (Hobart and Frankel 2004). Codes were assigned to denote:

- the task in which the child was engaged (activity);
- what the child was saying/what was said to the child (language);
- what type of educational 'programme' the child was involved in, such as free-play or organized story time (task);
- any non-verbal signs which might indicate the child's social interaction with others (social).

For example, if children were engaged in creative activities such as painting, drawing, chalking, cutting and sticking this was coded as 'ART' and if they were engaged in reading, writing or counting, including attentive looking at books, this was coded as '3Rs'. If children were engaged in activities which combined more than one activity, multiple-coding could be employed, for example, making a book could be coded as 'ART/3Rs'.

Social codes were used to record whether a child was playing alone or with other children and to what extent the play was parallel (playing alongside other children) or associative (playing with other children). Contextual data was also recorded from narrative observations which involved a running record of what was occurring in the early years setting. A digital recorder was used to capture dialogue between target children and adults and target children and peers though it was expected that some children might not have verbal communication skills.

Field notes were analysed thematically and common and discrep-ant themes identified with frequency counts for each theme identified. A sample of 120 minutes of structured observations was analysed for each child in order to determine the amount of time children were involved in different types of social group and communicative interactions. Each struc-tured target-child observation schedule was treated in the same manner for purposes of consistency. The activity record provided social context and environment details. The sections on communication and social records for an observation sample of 120-minutes for each child were analysed in terms of frequencies in order to discover:

- what the social context was for each child and how long children were engaged in particular types of social groups;
- who initiated communicative interactions with whom and how many times in unstructured free-play situations and episodes of joint-attention between adults and children.

For the communication record, a sample of 30 minutes observation comprised 15 minutes of structured adult-led activity and 15 minutes unstructured child-led activity. Analysis of structured activities provided information about how children responded to adults in episodes of joint-attention. Therefore, the observation sample included structured tasks where these episodes were present and unstructured where children were able to choose who they interacted with. Further to this, the observations were analysed qualitatively in order to identify themes, in particular the diverse SLC of children in case study settings, including verbal and non-verbal modalities. For this chapter, only the communication record will be reported on for the purposes of brevity.

Consent was sought firstly from the leaders in early childhood settings and the parents and carers of children who were considered suitable for inclusion in the study. Simple explanations were provided to children that an adult would be watching them because she was interested in how they played. Young children can be quite demonstrative in expressing their views, even if they do not verbally reject a researcher's presence or questions. They can, for example, move away from a person they do not wish to be near (Aubrey et al. 2000), refuse to answer questions, change the topic of conversation or in extreme cases be physically aggressive if they feel particularly unhappy about situations. The decision to adopt an ongoing process of assent whereby the child's acceptance of the researcher within the setting was taken as assent to participate in the research was considered appropriate. Early childhood professionals were considered competent, as secondary caregivers, to make ongoing judgements regarding any unwillingness on the part of children to participate or distress exhibited by children in relation to the researcher's presence, and to allow withdrawal from observations when deemed necessary. For some of the children involved in this study, where speech was not their preferred or main method of communicating with others, this relied on early childhood professionals interpreting children's gestural communication for the researcher.

Participants

A total of nine children between the ages of two years, three months and five years, two months were observed in eleven settings, four providing specialist SLC provision and seven mainstream early childhood settings outlined in Table 14.1.

Table 14.1: Early Childhood Settings Involved in the Study

Type of setting	Area of county	Age at which children can enter the setting	Demographics of families using the setting
Sessional pre-school	City centre (urban)	Two	Mixed (from affluent two-income families to single parent not working and varied cultural backgrounds)
Private day nursery	North-East (semi-rural)	Three months	Predominantly professional both parents working (varied cultural background)
LA maintained nursery provision	South (semi-rural)	Three	High number of vulnerable children with a lot of needs and low SES (varied cultural backgrounds)
Private early years centre	South (rural)	Birth	Mixed (from affluent two-income families to single parent not working and varied cultural backgrounds)

Type of setting	Area of county	Age at which children can enter the setting	Demographics of families using the setting
Childminder	North-East (semi-rural)	Birth	Mixed (from affluent two-income families to single parent not working and varied cultural backgrounds)
Children's Centre	North-East (semi-rural)	Two	Mostly middle income White families
Physical and sensory special school (PS)	North-East (semi-rural)	Two years, six months	Mixed (from affluent two-income families to single parent not working and varied cultural backgrounds)
Communication and interaction special school (CI)	North-West (urban)	Two	Mixed (from affluent two-income families to single parent not working and varied cultural backgrounds)
Language Centre	Middle (urban)	Three	Mixed (from affluent two-income families to single parent not working and varied cultural backgrounds)
Additional settings			
Pre-school	North-East (urban)	Two years, nine months	Mixed (from affluent two-income families to single parent not working and varied cultural backgrounds)
Outreach nursery assessment centre	North-West (urban)	Two years, six months	Mixed (from affluent two-income families to single parent not working and varied cultural backgrounds)

The children were selected by early childhood professionals from nine settings who originally volunteered to be involved in the research study (an initial survey of all early childhood settings in the chosen local authority facilitated this process). Two of the children attending mainstream provision also attended specialist provision. These two children were observed in both their mainstream and specialist settings. Details of child participants are provided in Table 14.2 organized chronologically from the youngest child to the eldest child. Early childhood professionals' descriptions of children's current SLC (at the time of data collection) are also provided from those who originally selected the child to be included in the study.

Table 14.2: Children Observed in Early Childhood Settings

Child	Gender	Age	Home Language(s)	Practitioner description of child's current SLC
1	Male	Two years, three months	English	Delayed speech and difficulty with control of emotions and behaviour. Screams in a shrill voice when he wants something. Exhibits tantrums, immature behaviour, hurts peers by biting or hitting them. Can make some things clear using gesture. Passes out in temper if he cannot have his own way or express his emotions verbally.
2	Male	Three years, five months	English	Some speech, lots of muttering, will come and take adults to objects he wants. Plays alone most of the time but will sometimes interact with peers. Understands most of what is said to him. Attention and listening skills are limited and can be over-excited when hugging and cuddling other children. Has hurt other children in disputes over toys in the past, does not like eye contact and will only eat facing away from others.
3	Male	Three years, five months	Ilocano Tagalog English	Delayed language development (uses single words and babble, pointing and gesture). Is beginning to follow some simple instructions within nursery routine which have been learned over time, but struggles with new concepts. Will play alongside peers but does not interact with them.
4	Female	Four years, one month	English	Speech and language difficulties. Word findings problems and difficulties discriminating between the letter 'S' and 'P'. Difficulty forming sentences. Has recently started to stutter. Good understanding and interaction with adults and peers. Attended both mainstream and specialist settings.

Child	Gender	Age	Home Language(s)	Practitioner description of child's current SLC
5	Male	Four years, two months	English	Delayed speech, babbles a lot and speech is difficult to understand. Has good listening skills, is attentive and joins in with adult-led activities. Interacts well with other children. Has tongue-tie (ankyloglossia).
6	Male	Four years, four months	English	Had no verbal communication skills on joining the mainstream nursery at the age of three. Now he uses mainly verbal communication, but also gestures sometimes, for example will take adult by hand to what he wants. Uses photographs occasionally. Will interact with familiar adults and is content to play alongside peers. Attended both mainstream and specialist settings
7	Female	Four years, four months	English	Delayed language development (probably specific language difficulty). Speech is supported with visual cues. Sometimes substitutes semantically related words or uses gesture and pointing. Sociable, spontaneously communicates through actions, facial expressions and speech. Listening skills are gradually improving. Sometimes needs adult attention to refocus on a task.
8	Male	Five years, one month	English	Communicates using pointing, gesture, facial expression, beginning to sign 'more' and will say 'no' in context. Demonstrates a good understanding of what is being asked of him. Has a short attention span but will maintain interest if the activity is highly motivating, for example painting. Very sociable, enjoys being with the other children but tends to engage in 'rough' play.
9	Male	Five years, two months	Polish English	Communicates mainly through picture exchange using photographs. Has some speech but it is non-functional. Understanding is at a one key word level. Prefers to play alone. Will listen in a 1:1 situation but is inattentive in group situations.

Seven of the children were male and two were female. For three children (child-6, child-8 and child-9), SLCN was associated with overall broader developmental delays associated with a primary diagnosis such as Cerebral Palsy or Autism Spectrum Disorder and their SLCN was therefore secondary to a primary diagnosis. Two of them (child- 8- and child-9) attended specialist SLCN settings, whilst child-6 attended a specialist setting alongside a mainstream setting.

Findings

Observations

COMMUNICATION ANALYSIS: MAINSTREAM SETTINGS

For structured activities, a small group (less than five children) or one-to-one activity was selected for analysis in order to compare activities across settings (not all children participated in large group activities). Due to the wide and varied range of structured adult-led activities, it was not possible to analyse the same activity for all children, therefore activities have been as closely matched as possible in relation to group size and degree of opportunity for adult-child and child-child interactions. In addition, all activities selected could be coded from the Sylva et al. (1980) observation schedule as either 'reading, writing and counting' activities (3Rs) or 'art and music' (AM) and some could also be further coded as 'manipulation of materials and objects' (MAN) and 'movement' (MO) when multi-coding was implemented. This enabled a cross-site comparison.

STRUCTURED ACTIVITIES

Included in structured activities in mainstream settings were: a music activity to help with sound discrimination (child-1), a cooking activity to help with social skills and vocabulary (child-2), craft activities to help with vocabulary and word finding (child-3, child-4 and child-5), a painting activity to help with turn-taking and vocabulary (child-6) and a picture-word game to help with memory and vocabulary (child-7). In all cases a sample of 15 minutes has been analysed.

As shown in Table 14.3, in mainstream settings, A-TC interactions were highest in structured activities for two children (child-3 and child-6).[1] Two children (Child-5 and child-7) initiated the most interactions with adults during structured activities. Two children initiated few interactions (child-1) or none at all (child-3).

Interactions between children were minimal in all settings, although a number of children (child-2, child-4, child-5, and child-6) made comments not directed at others (quiet comments to themselves related to the task, activity or materials in hand) during structured activities, whilst waiting for their turn or when the practitioner was distracted with another child. For example, child-6 repeated the colour of the paint he was using to no-one in particular, saying 'blue', 'it's blue' and child-5 commented on the glue as it dripped from his glue spreader and made his hands sticky, saying 'ah dit, no' whilst flapping his hands in the air. These appeared to be episodes of private speech.

There were many adult initiations in two settings child-3 (26), child-6 (40), whilst the highest number of child initiations were for child-5. A balance between adult and child initiations was experienced by child-2, and child-4.

UNSTRUCTURED

In contrast, when involved in unstructured activities in mainstream settings, children were more likely to initiate interactions with each other and adults, which was not surprising as there was more opportunity for them to do so as shown in Table 14.4.

An interesting finding was the increased episodes of talking aloud to themselves for all children during unstructured activities. Child initiations were higher than adults in most settings apart from child-1. The highest

---

[1]   TC – Target Child; A – Adult; C – One child other than TC; CH – A group of children;

Table 14.3: Frequency of Communicative Interactions in Mainstream Settings: Structured Activity

Setting	Child minding practice	Private early years centre	Pre-school	Pre-school	Children's Centre	Private day nursery	LA Maintained nursery
Time Sample	15-minute observation	15-minute observation	15-minute observation	15-minute observation	15-minute observation	15-minute observation	15-minute observation
Who initiated the interaction	Target Child-1 (Boy)	Target Child-2 (Boy)	Target Child-3 (Boy)	Target Child-4 (Girl)	Target Child-5 (Boy)	Target Child-6 (Boy)	Target Child-7 (Girl)
	Frequency	Frequency	Frequency	Frequency	Frequency	Frequency	Frequency
TC–A	2	3	-	2	4	2	6
TC–C	-	2	-	-	3	-	-
TC–Self	-	2	-	2	2	6	-
C–TC	-	-	-	-	1	-	2
Child initiations	2	7	-	4	10	8	8
A–TC	3	6	26	1	9	40	15
A–TC+CH	5	5	2	6	3	-	2
A–C	1	1	2	-	5	8	4
Adult initiations	9	12	30	7	17	48	21

Table 14.4: Frequency of Communicative Interactions in Mainstream Settings: Unstructured Activity

Setting	Child minding practice	Private early years centre	Pre-school	Pre-school	Children's Centre	Private day nursery	LA Maintained nursery
Sample Time	15-minute observation	15-minute observation	15-minute observation	15-minute observation	15-minute observation	15-minute observation	15-minute observation
Who initiated the interaction	Target Child-1 (Boy)	Target Child-2 (Boy)	Target Child-3 (Boy)	Target Child-4 (Girl)	Target Child-5 (Boy)	Target Child-6 (Boy)	Target Child-7 (Girl)
	Frequency	Frequency	Frequency	Frequency	Frequency	Frequency	Frequency
TC–A	2	5	-	3	6	2	3
TC–C	3	2	5	3	5	6	6
TC–Self	2	5	7	7	4	15	3
C–TC	2	3	-	1	6	1	9
Child initiations	9	15	12	14	21	24	21
A–TC	8	3	4	-	5	6	2
A–TC+CH	2	-	5	-	2	2	3
A–C	1	-	2	-	-	3	2
Adult initiations	11	3	11	-	7	11	7

child initiations were for child-6, although most of these were comments he made to himself. This is illuminated further as follows. The unstructured activity occurred during a fifteen-minute play episode in the outside area of the nursery which comprised a climbing frame with slide, a pergola with seating, a sand-pit and path leading to a tarmacked area where children could ride bikes and scooters. Child-6 spent three minutes standing next to or under the pergola with a toy hammer in solitary play, two minutes riding a three-wheeled scooter, four minutes turn-taking with an adult on the slide and three minutes attempting to retrieve a scooter from another child that he had been playing with before he was engaged with an adult on the slide. There were seven children and two supervising adults.

Adult-child and child-child interactions during this time were recorded. Interactions with peers occurred whilst child-6 was attempting to retrieve a three-wheeled scooter from another child. He twice attempted to take the scooter when the child paused for a rest and twice he crashed his scooter into another child's scooter. He apologized, saying 'sorry H'. His KW on hearing him questioned him by saying 'Sorry H?' Child-6 corrected himself, saying 'Sorry B', then rode off saying to himself 'Sorry H, oh no, babble'. On one occasion he attempted unsuccessfully to draw another child's attention to an object in the distance, and on a further occasion another child pushed child-6 aside in order to descend the slide. He made fifteen comments to himself which occurred whilst pretending to hammer the pergola with a toy hammer. He made comments such as 'oops, oh dear', 'there's going to be trouble', 'oh no'. Although he was aware of peers and could attempt to initiate interactions with him, they appeared to be disinterested. Again, these appeared to represent Vygotsky's concept of private speech and were unobserved and unrecorded by adults in the setting.

Interactions with adults occurred during a turn-taking episode on the slide. The adult took the opportunity to comment on whose turn it was during this time by asking child-6 whose turn it was, pointing at herself when it was her turn, inviting child-6 to do the same when it was his. Also observed were adult-child questions such as 'Whose turn is it now?' and 'yes it's your turn T', and adult-child interventions such as when child-6 was attempting to retrieve a scooter from another child. An adult reminded him that he needed to share and it was not his turn.

Communication analysis: specialist settings

STRUCTURED

In specialist settings structured activities selected for analysis included: a circle activity to help with semantic memory (child-4), a story to help with turn-taking, social interaction and vocabulary (child-6), a painting activity to help with motivation to communicate with others (child-8) and a picture-game to help with functional communication skills and vocabulary (child-9). In all cases, a sample of 15 minutes of observation has been analysed.

Table 14.5 shows that the highest number of TC-A interactions was in the specialist PS school and lowest in the Language Centre and specialist

Table 14.5: Frequency of Communicative Interactions in
Specialist Settings: Structured Activity

Setting	Language Centre	Specialist Nursery Assessment Centre	Specialist Physical and Sensory (PS) Special School	Specialist Communication and Interaction (CI) Special School
Sample Time	15-minute observation	15-minute observation	15-minute observation	15-minute observation
Who initiated the interaction	Target Child-4 (Girl) Verbal	Target Child-6 (Boy) Verbal	Target Child-8 (Boy) Non-verbal	Target Child-9 (Boy) Verbal
	Frequency	Frequency	Frequency	Frequency
TC –A	2	3	7	2
TC –C	-	2	1	-
TC –Self	-	-	-	-
C –TC	-	2	4	-
Child initiations	2	7	12	2
A –TC	2	8	14	10
A–TC + CH	6	3	6	-
A –C	-	3	2	-
Adult initiations	8	14	22	10

Communication and Interaction (CI) school. This appeared to be a consequence of the nature of activities and size of group, as well as the number of adults available to interact with children in the settings. For example, child-6 did not have to wait very long for his turn in activities that involved turn taking as there were only three children present.

The low number of TC –A interactions in the Language Centre and specialist CI school reflected the amount of time it took for child-9 to carry out instructions requested by adults, mainly due to his distraction from background classroom noise and other children, and the large group size for child-4 as well as the number of A –TC+CH questions involved in each interaction.

UNSTRUCTURED

As shown in Table 14.6, for unstructured activities, child-6 initiated the highest number of interactions followed by child-4.

For child-4 there was a more even distribution of interaction amongst children and adults, whereas child-8 only initiated interactions with adults although this was due to his lack of proximity to other children during the activity. Child-9 talked aloud to himself when sitting alone on the bridge to a climbing frame and playing with an 'animal hospital' ambulance. He made comments such as 'I can see you' and 'and some ice-cream' whilst smiling to himself. He also appeared to be singing a nursery rhyme and to be unaware of peers running past him as he did not move to let them past, look at them when they approached him or respond when they collided with him. Adult initiations were highest for child-6 and lowest for child-9. On the whole adults in specialist settings were observed to re-direct children who played alone in episodes of solitary play during unstructured activities in order to engage them in conversation with others. Therefore in specialist settings children had fewer opportunities to engage in private speech either due to the dominance of adult-led activities. The exception to this was child 9.

From analysis of field notes, it emerged that whilst in mainstream settings, children were largely accommodated in group sizes of up to 26 children, in specialist settings, children were organized into groups of 6 – 8 children. Similarly in mainstream settings, activities were planned and provided for children in large groups whilst in specialist settings there

Table 14.6: Frequency of communicative interactions in specialist settings: unstructured activity

Setting	ICAN language centre	Specialist Nursery Assessment Centre	Specialist Physical and Sensory (PS) Special School	Specialist Communication and Interaction (CI) Special School
Sample Time	15-minute observation	15-minute observation	15-minute observation	15-minute observation
Who initiated the interaction	Target Child-4 (Girl) Verbal	Target Child-6 (Boy) Verbal	Target Child-8 (Boy) Pre-linguistic	Target Child-9 (Boy) Verbal
	Frequency	Frequency	Frequency	Frequency
TC–A	3	10	5	-
TC–C	4	3	-	-
TC–Self	2	2	-	7
C–TC	2	2	-	-
Child initiations	11	17	5	7
A–TC	2	10	6	3
A–TC + CH	2	2	1	-
A–C	-	2	1	-
Adult initiations	4	14	8	3

were a higher number small group and one-to-one activities. In addition, there were more structured adult-led activities planned for children in specialist settings than in mainstream settings. This meant that children had fewer opportunities to play alone in specialist settings than mainstream.

Discussion and Conclusion

As mentioned earlier children's SLC develop over time in the context of relationships and interactions with caregivers (such as early childhood professionals) and peers and typically follow an observable sequence, dependent on children's own genetic inheritance and characteristics and the opportunities afforded to them to experience and practice communicative interactions with others. Early childhood professionals have a statutory role to observe, assess and monitor young children's SLC development and report to parents and other professionals when any delays or deviances from so-called norms are identified. This chapter has reported the findings from a policy-to-practice study relating to young children's SLC in early childhood settings in one local authority in England.

This study shows that children who are identified with severe and long term SLCN are more likely to spend prolonged focused time with adults undertaking adult-directed tasks and less likely to initiate communicative interactions with peers or adults during these tasks. Children attending mainstream early childhood settings may have transient delays and difficulties with SLC that may need more exposure to language-rich environments and / or some focused adult intervention. Findings from this study show that these children are more likely to spend time in child-led play activities where there are higher instances of child-initiated communicative interactions.

It was noted by Vygotsky (1978) that children used private speech (or talking aloud to oneself) to help make meaning from language heard from adult speech. Vygotsky argued that the use of private speech was beneficial in helping children to self-regulate their emotions, keep track of their thoughts and form a bridge between social speech and inner speech. Children were observed to use speech in this way more often during unstructured child-led activities than structured adult-led activities and child-6 (who had a severe cognitive delay and Cerebral Palsy) talked aloud to himself more often in his mainstream setting than his specialist setting. For example, he was observed to repeat paraphrases to himself such as 'Oh no!' and 'That's terrible!' usually at transition times when he was engrossed in solitary play and was being asked to do something different. Child-2 appeared to enjoy small-world play, particularly farms and soft toys and had ongoing conversations with them often, repeating particular phrases such as 'The mummy lamb is holding the baby lamb.' whilst holding a soft lamb.

Similarly child-3 was more likely to talk aloud to himself during unstructured child-led activities. Comments made by child-3 to himself included instructions, issued during outside play such as saying 'quick' to himself with no one else within hearing distance, when he wanted to catch up with other boys on their scooters. He also practised words in new contexts on his own. For example, a practitioner had explained to child-3 and two of his peers that the traffic sign they were playing with during outside play meant '*stop!*' (with emphasis and using gesture). Five minutes later he was observed holding the stop sign, holding his hand in the same gesture and saying 'stop!' to no-one in particular (no other children were within hearing distance).

In all observed cases, private speech was used in a social context as target children played alongside but not collaboratively with other children. Children's self-comments were attended to only by themselves, as if they were rehearsing phrases for later use with others. Children learn from practising what they know and through turning their experience, in this case pre-school experience, into personal meaning.

For children in mainstream settings, moments of solitary play and self-talk were allowed, but not recorded to enter in children's learning journals. By contrast, in specialist settings, children were encouraged to engage in adult-led activities for significant amounts of time which allowed little time for children's self-talk or private speech. This might serve to devalue the important role and contribution of children's private speech to their overall development and suggests that training is needed to inform early childhood professionals about this.

Physical and social resources which appear to promote private speech include the degree of adult-led structured activities planned and the size of groups that children are organized into to undertake activities. Children in this study were more likely to initiate communicative interactions and engage in episodes of private speech during child-led unstructured activities although some would occasionally make comments directed at themselves during adult-led structured activities. These episodes provide an opportunity for early childhood professionals to observe children's language and thought and to record children's progress and achievements in SLC differently, moving from a deficit approach to a more positive perspective.

Children's communicative interactions have been shown to vary according to multiple interactive influences from the physical and social structures inherent in the microcontext of early childhood settings in which they participated (Bronfenbrenner 1979; 1993). Early childhood professionals have the opportunity to provide children with SLCN with opportunities to engage in private speech and for this to be valued as an important aspect of their right to have a voice.

References

Aubrey, C., David, T., Godfrey, R., and Thompson, L. (2000). *Early Childhood Educational Research: Issues in methodology and Ethics.* Oxon: Routledge.

Bercow, J. (2008). *The Bercow Report. A Review of Services for Children and Young People (0–19) with Speech, Language and Communication Needs.* Nottingham: Department of Children, Schools and Families.

Berk, L. E. (1992). Children's private speech: An overview of theory and the status of research. In R. M. Diaz and L. E. Berk (eds), *Private speech: From social interaction to self-regulation*, pp.17–53. Hillsdale, NJ: Erlbaum.

Blackburn, C., and Aubrey, C. (2016). Policy to Practice context to the delays and difficulties in the acquisition of speech language and communication in early years. *International Journal of Early Years Education*, 24 (4), 414–434.

Bronfenbrenner, U. (1979). *The Ecology of Human Development.* Cambridge: Harvard University Press.

Bronfenbrenner, U. (1993). The ecology of cognitive development: Research models and fugitive findings. In R. H. Wozniak and K. W. Fisher (eds), *Development in context: Acting and thinking in specific environments,* pp. 3–44. Hillsdale, NJ: Erlbaum.

Bronfenbrenner, U. (2001). The bioecology theory of human development. In N. J. Smelser and P. B. Baltes (eds), *International encyclopedia of the social and behavioural sciences,* 10, pp. 6963–6970.

Diaz, R. M. (1992). Methodological concerns in the study of private speech. In R. M. Diaz and L. E. Berk (eds), *Private speech: From social interaction to self-regulation,* pp. 55–81. Hillsdale, NJ: Erlbaum.

Department for Education (2017). Statutory Framework for the Early Years Foundation Stage London: DfE. Retrieved from: <https://www.foundationyears.org.uk/files/2017/03/EYFS_STATUTORY_FRAMEWORK_2017.pdf>.

Fernyhough, C., and Russell, J. (1997). Distinguishing one's own voice from those of others: A function for private speech? *International Journal of Behavioral Development,* 20 (4), 651–665.

Flavell, J. H., Beach, D. R., and Chinsky, J. M. (1966). Spontaneous verbal rehearsal in a memory task as a function of age. *Child Development*, 37, 283–299.

Furrow, D. R. (1992). Developmental trends in the differentiation of social and private speech. In R. M. Diaz and L. E. Berk (eds), *Private speech: From social interaction to self-regulation,* pp. 143–158. Hillsdale, NJ: Erlbaum.

Goudena, P. P. (1992). The problem of abbreviation and internalization of private speech. In R. M. Diaz and L. E. Berk (eds), *Private speech: From social interaction to self-regulation*, pp. 215–224. Hillsdale, NJ: Erlbaum.

Harris, P. (2000). *The work of the imagination.* Oxford: Blackwell.

Hobart, C., and Frankel, J. (2004). *A Practical Guide to Child Observation and Assessment* (3rd edn). Cheltenham: Nelson Thornes.

Piaget, J. (1962). *The Language and Thought of the Child* (3rd ed.). London: Routledge and Kegan Paul Ltd.

Rogoff, B. (2003). *The Cultural Nature of Human Development.* Oxford: Oxford University Press.

Simons, H. (2009). *Case Study Research in Practice.* London: Sage Publications Ltd.

Siraj-Blatchford, I., Sylva, K., Muttock S., Gilden, R., and Bell, D. (2002). *Researching Effective Pedagogy in the Early Years*, Department for Education and Skills Research Report 365.

Sylva, K., Roy, C., and Painter, M. (1980). *Child Watching at Playgroup and Nursery School.* London: Grant McIntyre.

Sylva, K., Melhuish, E., Siraj-Blatchford, I., Sammons, P., and Taggart, B. (2004). *Final Report of the Effective Provision of Pre-school Education project.* London: Institute of Education.

Vygotsky, L. (1978). Interaction between learning and development. In M. Cole, V. John-Steiner, S. Scribner and E. Souberman (eds), *Mind in society: The development of higher psychological processes,* pp. 79–91. Cambridge, MA: Harvard University Press.

Winsler, A. (1998). Parent-child interaction and private speech in boys with ADHD. *Applied Developmental Science*, 2, 17–39.

Winsler, A., Carlton, M. P., and Barry, M. J. (2000). Age-related changes in preschool children's systematic use of private speech in a natural setting. *Journal of Child Language*, 27, 665–687.

Winsler, A., Fernyhough, C., McClaren, E. M., and Way, E. (2005). *Private speech coding manual.* Unpublished manuscript. George Mason University, Fairfax, VA, USA. Retrieved from: <http://classweb.gmu.edu/awinsler/Resources/PsCodingManual.pdf>.

15   We are all in this together: Inclusive early childhood education

The importance of the early years

Over the last two decades developments within childhood studies have led to increased recognition of the importance of listening to children's voices and experiences with an emphasis on their rights to participation and expression of their views (Powell et al. 2012). This contemporary view of children as active agents in their learning and development is underpinned by, the almost universally ratified United Nations Convention on the Rights of the Child (UNCRC) (1989). In locating children's rights within a social justice frame Smith (2016) argues that the convention has proved to be a very powerful charter for all children. The convention challenges adults to acknowledge children as competent citizens with rights, even the very youngest children. There are four key principles underpinning the convention and they are captured in Articles 2, 3, 6 and 12. Article 2 makes it clear that the UNCRC is for all children, Article 3 challenges adults to maintain a focus on the best interests of the child while Article 6 notes children's right to life, survival and development. Finally, one of the most influential articles in the convention, Article 12, recognizes children as active participants in society with the right to say what they think about decisions that affect them and have those views heard and respected.

Since the dawn of psychology scholars interested in understanding child development have applied scientific insights and the scientific method to the study of children and child development. This approach led to the rise of developmental psychology as a distinct field of study and research. Meanwhile, educational reformers since the late eighteenth century have identified school and education as a central agent for social reform. Of particular relevance to early childhood education was the work of such educationalists as Pestalozzi (1746–1827) and Froebel (1782–1852) who influentially advocated for the creation of early learning environments that identified the unique significance of early childhood and the powerful role of play and exploration as key features of early learning and development.

Psychological, sociological and educational research continues to highlight the importance of early experiences in the child's immediate present and later life. During the last century such research led to increased investment in the development of early education interventions such as the US Headstart and HighScope initiatives (Zigler and Muenchow 1992; Weikart 2004) and the Irish Early Start programme (Ryan, et al. 1998). More recent initiatives include the UK Sure Start project (NESS, 2012) and the Prevention and Early Intervention initiatives supported by the Irish government (CES, 2014). The belief underlying such interventions is that providing young disadvantaged children with early learning opportunities that are more commonplace for their advantaged peers can create equality between the two groups in terms of child outcomes and later educational experiences. Faith in the benefits of simply providing early pre-school experiences in the absence of more sophisticated understanding of the dynamics of child development and early childhood education and care was, however misplaced and many early intervention projects failed to achieve their ambitious aims. Contemporary research indicates that, to be effective, significant effort must be put into the design and support of early childhood education and care programmes which must be well planned, contextually sensitive, well resourced, professionally provided and of high quality (Dahlberg and Moss 2005; OECD 2006; EC 2014).

The science of early childhood education

Early childhood education[1] is a relatively new strand in educational scholarship and is only recently moving 'from the margins' with early education professionals being accorded recognition for their status and contribution

---

1   The terms early childhood education [ECE] and early childhood education and care [ECEC] are used interchangeably throughout the text to refer to any type (i.e. public,

to educational discourse although in many contexts this recognition continues to be somewhat ambiguous (Woodrow and Newman 2015). This development owes much to the recognition of the importance of quality early childhood experiences for all children in terms of lasting educational, developmental and social benefits in addition to a view of access to quality early childhood education and care as a right for all children.

In reviewing the development of early education as an academic discipline Hujala and Niikko (2009) assert that it emerged as a response to the overly influential discourse of traditional disciplines seen as no longer sufficient to meet the needs of fully understanding the role and potential of early childhood education in a post-modern society. They argue that the science of early childhood education, with its emphasis on a sociocultural and participatory approach, has developed to allow for a better understanding of how early education can contribute effectively within the multi-dimensional, complex and culturally diverse environments of contemporary childhoods.

In unpacking the underlying theoretical foundations informing the science of early childhood education – and its implications for practice – Martin Woodhead (2005) juxtaposes two contrasting discourses for considering children's developmental rights. He characterized the discourse as either focusing on 'individual development' or the developing 'child-in-context' drawing attention to the different ways in which different theoretical viewpoints of child development can influence early educational practice, policy and research. The individual development discourse draws heavily on the work of Piaget and views child development as universal, natural and normative. Such an approach locates a child's development trajectory as largely innate, located within the child. On the other hand, within the child-in-context discourse child development is seen as a culturally bound social process which acknowledges that a child is born into a specific cultural-historical context. This approach owes much to the work of Vygotsky (1978). Within this discourse a child's development is considered to be culturally and contextually constructed.

---

private or voluntary) of provision for young children that is subject to a national regulatory framework.

In their book, *Engaging Children's Minds*, Katz and Chard (1994) pointed out that practice in early childhood education and care settings has drawn heavily on traditional psychological studies of human development, which study the child in isolation from her everyday life. Such studies focus on normative development addressing the question of what most children can and cannot do at a given age or stage. It provides us with a general descriptive guide of what children at particular ages can be expected to achieve and how they can be expected to behave; such descriptions are often called milestones. While useful as a general guide, developmental milestones can become problematic if we depend on them to guide early years practice with groups of young children on a day-to-day basis. Features of normative development fail to take account of the diversity of individual children, the dynamics of development and the importance of context (Hayes et al. 2017). The individual child in any group presents with different capabilities, interests and experiences and brings to the learning environment differing and powerful 'funds of knowledge' (Hedges 2014).

The idea of normative development has been a particularly dominant, and contested, influence in early education in both curriculum development and recommendations for practice. This is most evident in the publication and responses to *Developmentally Appropriate Practice* (DAP) (Bredekamp and Copple 1997). This document presents a variety of early education materials and activities identified as either 'appropriate' or 'inappropriate' for children at different ages and stages of their lives. The description (or as some see it, prescription) of 'developmentally appropriate' here was closely tied to the contribution these materials and activities make to the development of the child towards operational thinking and is based primarily on the Piagetian notion of development as a continuous progress toward adulthood. The DAP approach has been criticized (Dahlberg and Moss 2005; Woodhead, 2006); it has limitations as it suggests that all children develop in a predictable way. While this may appear to be the case over time, at an individual level, on a daily basis, things are far messier and entangled. An overemphasis on milestones or outcomes can result in less attention being given to the dynamic dimension of individual development, and the opportunities that arise in children's day-to- day life that contribute to their learning and development (Hayes and Filipovic 2017).

Hujala and Niikki (2009) conclude that the influence of these discourses impacts on our view of children and the degree to which young children are seen as active participant agents in their own development. Within the individual development discourse the 'educator's task is to support each child's development from one level to another, according to individual needs, to determine developmental needs and assess shortcomings' (p. 24). This discourse informs the common early intervention strategy of developing individualized education programmes for children with disabilities. The child-in-context development discourse on the other hand 'perceives the child to be full of opportunities and a competent social actor in co-operation with adults and other children. The child is respected as an individual and his/her emancipation in the community is supported' (ibid.: 25). Within this frame an inclusionary approach to early education embeds inclusive practice within the daily routine of early education without singling out any particular child as different through recognizing that all children are different.

However, while separating out these two different discourses on child development is helpful in distinguishing the way in which different theoretical approaches can impact on the image of the child and on practice it also tends to polarize them. Such polarisation is unhelpful as human development is an intricate and intertwined process involving both normative and dynamic aspects of development (Hayes et al. 2017). Bronfenbrenner's bioecological model of development (Bronfenbrenner 2005) provides an integrating framework of human development within which to consider different theoretical approaches to individual development-in-context taking account of both the individual in development and the socio-cultural contexts. The bioecological model was designed in recognition of the dynamic complexity of human life and the holistic, integrated and bidirectional nature of development.

Meeting this challenge is central to high quality, inclusive and respectful early educational practice. Concentrating more on dynamic development than on normative expectations calls on us to consider what practice is most beneficial to individual children, at a particular moment, within a particular context. Recognizing development as a dynamic and discontinuous process facilitates a pedagogy which is attuned to the connections, interactions and relationships between children and the wider world and sensitive to social, physical and emotional learning opportunities (Hayes 2013). This has particular resonance in early years practice in settings including children from diverse backgrounds or of differing abilities.

Including all children equally

The distinction between what young children can do and what they should do is especially serious in the early years because most children appear willing, if not eager, to do what is asked of them. Because of this they are willing to attempt to meet even the most unrealistic expectations when encouraged by important adults in their lives. It is for this reason that many authors (Singer 2015; Pramling- Samuelsson and Asplond-Carlsson 2008) have cautioned against adult-led, prescriptive models of early years practice. Such approaches tend to be designed to achieve specific learning outcomes in aspects of social development or skills of literacy or numeracy rather than attending to the process of how children become socialized, literate and numerate. Evidence suggests that it is more important to attend to the process of the present, the dynamics of individual development in everyday practice and the cultivation of generative learning dispositions rather than specific skills. This focus is more effective in the long run because, during the early years, it seems that *how* children learn rather than *what* they learn matters most (Pramling-Samuelsson and Asplond-Carlsson 2008). The concept of learning dispositions within the early educational literature has been influential and emerged directly from the socio-cultural pedagogy underpinning the Te Whariki curriculum (Ministry of Education, 1996). Carr (2001) describes learning dispositions in terms of a child being ready, willing and able to participate in learning activities. She names five domains of learning dispositions: (i) taking an interest; (ii) being involved; (iii) persisting with difficulty or uncertainty; (iv) communicating with others and (v) taking responsibility. Dunn writes that learning dispositions 'are the outcome of repeated 'situated learning strategies' ... based on the skills, knowledge and intent of the learner within the learning context, plus their motivation' (2004:123). Where early education practitioners are too concerned with what a child should be doing or learning at a particular stage, they may not only miss the learning / teaching moments of everyday, but may act to inhibit the child's learning (Hayes et al. 2017). Despite the academic literature supporting this more holistic and socio-cultural approach to understanding development the individual development discourse continues to have a profound influence on practice (Hujala and Niikko 2009; Woodrow and Newman 2015).

Woodhead (2006), recognising that the complexities of childhood are multiple, suggested that one way to move day-to-day early education practice towards a more dynamic, responsive process would be to seek out the perspectives of individual children on their own lives. Viewing children as participants in their early education, he argues, demands that adults work with them within contexts that value their voices and contributions in the here and now, engaging with children and learning from them as well as enhancing their learning opportunities. This pedagogical approach is informed by a belief in the dynamic nature of child development and includes all children as partners in their development and learning, irrespective of individual backgrounds or abilities.

The UNCRC, particularly Article 12 has influenced researchers, practitioners and policy-makers alike. It underpins a great deal of policy writing on children and there is an increasing presence of children's research advisory groups, reference groups and consultation panels in many countries (Horgan et al. 2015; Lundy, McEvoy and Byrne 2011). But recognizing the voice of child in a way that is truly respectful of children's views is not an easy task and demands changes in the way in which adults approach working with children. Lundy (2007), in an article entitled 'Voice is not enough', developed an influential model of child participation. The model was designed to elaborate the key elements required to realize Article 12 in a respectful and meaningful way. She identified the following four elements as crucial:

- space – children must be given safe, inclusive opportunities to form and express their views;

- voice – children must be facilitated to express their views;
- audience – children's views must be listened to;
- influence – children's views must be acted upon.

Operationalizing this model of participation with very young children is challenging. While the elements map almost directly on to the general principles of high quality early education in recognizing children as strong, competent, active agents with a right to be heard (Moss 2006; Hayes 2013; Einarsdottir 2007) respectful partnership has proved more difficult. The conceptualization of the agentic child-developing-in-context (Hayes et al. 2017) provides for a dynamic image of learning and development which requires practitioners to appreciate and respond to the reality that even the very youngest children contribute to the context and content of their own development. This is not to underestimate the dependence of the child or the very powerful, protective role of the adult. It does however, challenge adults to reconsider practice and to take account of the rich and diverse nature of each child when planning early care and education, designing learning environments and providing learning opportunities. Early childhood education scholars recognize the importance and respectfulness of including the voice of the young child in early educational practice. By seeking their perspectives we can gather useful information from children to inform and reform practice and future research. There is however, a significant gap between recognizing young children as active participants in their own learning and development with rights to being meaningfully included in day-to-day practice and actually including them as partners in the creation and realization of an inclusive curriculum in practice. This can be explained in part by the tension that exists in balancing a child's right to both protection and participation (Broström 2005). While protecting children is a genuine concern, too strong an emphasis on protection can actually deny children the right to express their views and may render them silent and invisible on the basis of some anticipated potential risk (Molloy et al. 2012). Simply attending an early childhood setting is not sufficient evidence of participation and inclusion, young children must feel that they belong to the setting community. Meaningful participation requires that all young children are actively engaged in activities and that their contributions are valued. A central element of effective early childhood education is the quality of the relational aspect of practice, which should strive to be both respectful and empowering. The issue of power is particularly relevant in working with young children as there is an inevitable inequality in the power relations due to the substantial differences in competencies and experiences between the adult and the young child. Managing this imbalance requires adults to be attuned, engaged and observant and responsive the children's leads. Einarsdottir (2007), in writing about engaging young children in research, suggests that to minimize the power differential and empower young children adults should pay close attention to children's interests and competencies. They should also be sensitive to children's willingness and ability to participate in activities and respect their wishes should they not wish to participate. Other barriers to including young children in curriculum planning and practice are methodological. When discussing the methodological challenges of including young children in research Einarsdottir, drawing on her work with children aged two to six, concludes that adults must be '... be creative and use methods that fit the circumstances and the children they are working with each time. ... Different children ... have different ways of communicating, and therefore they prefer different methods to express their views. Children at different ages also prefer different methods' (2007: 207). These observations also hold for the day-to-day engagements with young children in early learning environments. In fact the issue of methodologies in working collaboratively with young children has given rise to the development of some very creative and useful research and pedagogical instruments (Clark and Moss 2001; Mahoney and Hayes 2006; Sixsmith et al. 2007; Start Strong 2014).

Inclusive early childhood education

Inclusion is a defining feature of high quality early childhood education reflecting societal attitudes that all children should experience a sense of belonging within their communities and have a right to access educational services. The National Association for the Education of Young Children [NAEYC] write that 'The desired results of inclusive experiences for children with and without disabilities and their families include a sense of belonging and membership, positive social relationships and friendships, and development and learning to reach their full potential (2009: 2).

A number of different models of early education commit to high quality inclusive practice. For instance, HighScope's active learning model of early childhood education and care explicitly provides inclusive experiences for children with and without disabilities. Recognizing that all children benefit when they participate actively in their own learning process and engage in positive and meaningful relationships with supportive adults the HighScope approach provides all children in their settings with opportunities for access, participation, and support (www.highscope.org). The Reggio Emilia approach is an influential example of inclusive practice, which has emerged from Italy (Edwards et al., 1993). It is regarded as the gold standard for quality early educational practice and provision (New 2007; Kaga et al. 2010). The pedagogical approach used in Reggio Emilia settings derives from the work of Loris Malaguzzi who argued that the traditional school approaches disconnected the child from the multiple ways in which to learn and communicate, from the 'hundred languages of children' (Edwards et al., 1993). His ideas have been influential and proven to be a source of innovation and exploration within early childhood for both professionals and researchers alike (French 2007). Reggio pedagogy is fundamentally collaborative with children, parents, teachers and specialists participating in the shared experience of learning. There are five key elements to the Reggio approach: the notion of the teacher as learner; a commitment to long term project work; a recognition of children's multiple languages; the learning environment as a third teacher and parental involvement as a form of civic engagement. These features are embedded in an image of all children as competent, strong, active and participating and closely align to the principles of socio-cultural theory and democratic practice. It also reflects a significant refiguring of the role of the educator with associated impacts on practice. In foregrounding the importance of respectful relationships between the teacher and child and the teacher and parent the Reggio approach is, at its core, inclusive. The values underpinning the Reggio approach centre on the image of the 'rich child' – one rich in possibilities – and include concepts of uncertainty, subjectivity, dialogue and democracy. Reggio practice 'represents a way of living and relating that is open-ended (avoiding closure), open-minded (welcoming the unexpected) and open-hearted (valuing difference)' (Moss 2010:1).

Fortunati (2014), describing another Italian early education model, explicitly addresses the issue of inclusion in respect of children under three years of age noting that the '... image of the child as a rich human being recognizes children as citizens in their own right – competent and curious, sociable and strong, and actively engaged in the creation of experience and in the construction of his or her identity and knowledge' (p.42). In addressing the importance of explicit attention to diversity in early education Parrini (2014) critiques the characterization of certain children as having 'special educational needs' and makes the argument for considering all children in terms of their 'special rights'. She argues that a shift in focus to special rights for all children is a necessary one to activate the shift of focus from protection of rights to promotion of rights and from the treatment of children to the education of children. It expands our thinking from a focus on limitations towards a recognition of possibilities. Reflecting an ecological lens this enabling approach to inclusive early years practice with young children 'offers ordinary operating conditions which are sensitive, attentive and capable of responding to the individuality and uniqueness of each child' (Parrini 2014:81). Within this model, early education is understood and activated as a partnership in the development and education of young children and is not characterized as either a support to families or an intervention for particular children.

Within an Irish context these attitudes are implicit in Aistear, the national curriculum framework (National Council for Curriculum and Assessment (NCCA) 2009) through the integrated strands of wellbeing, belonging and identity, communicating and exploring and thinking. Nurturing equality and diversity is one of the twelve central principles underpinning the framework. Equality is recognized as core to a fair society where everyone can participate equally and achieve their potential and diversity is defined in terms of welcoming and valuing difference as part of life. More specifically, diversity is identified as a central feature in ensuring equity and not about treating all young children the same (NCCA 2009).

Current research from developmental psychology highlights the crucial role of interactions and relationships to positive development and supports Bronfenbrenner's contention that proximal processes, the day-to-day interactions in the lives of children, are the engines of development (Bronfenbrenner and Morris 2006). It confirms that it is not simply the opportunity for interactions but the *nature* and *quality* of the interactive process itself that is important. In particular, evidence foregrounds the value of dynamic, bidirectional social interactions as crucial to early development. Studies suggest that early years programmes which have a strong emphasis, both curricular (content) and pedagogical (practice), on the nurturing of affective development and support for social and emotional learning, positively influence children's overall development (Centre on the Developing Child 2007; Dalli et al. 2011). Positive learning environments are those which are warm and provide secure relationships to facilitate children's exploration, play and learning. This is as true for the child of five months of age as it is for the child of five years. Practitioners who provide for these learning opportunities rather than focusing too closely on the development of specific skills are supporting the development of the fundamental, foundational aspects of learning. Positive and supportive adult/child interactions enhance children's security to explore and experience connectedness to peers and are important to wellbeing and flourishing. Nurturing children's learning as part of a caring educative process requires adults to develop skills of non-intrusive planning and provision of learning environments that support and extend children's own learning and quality interactive opportunities. To those outside early childhood education, including parents and other professionals, the complexity involved in such quality practices may not be immediately obvious. There is a continuing tendency to underestimate the educative role of caring and the importance of quality early education to children's happiness and wellbeing (Fleer 2015; Kickbusch 2012; Wood 2013). Hayes (2008), writing about the contested concept of care proposed a shift in early educational practice towards an explicit nurturing pedagogy. This would necessitate a significant shift in understanding and valuing the role of care in practice, requiring explicit acknowledgement of the critical contribution of the interpersonal and relational aspects of early education. A nurturing pedagogy is the manifestation of an inclusive relational early education approach. It is a different style of practice to that many of us have experienced in our own education. It demands that adults let go of some traditional ideas about the educational relationship between adult and child, learner and teacher, where the adult was regarded as the source of knowledge and children were expected to passively receive this knowledge.

Skills of observation and reflection are central to a nurturing pedagogy. They enhance practice and planning, are manifest in well-managed and yet reasonably flexible practice, and assist in the provision of learning environments that include children as active agents, supporting and extending learning. This allows for planning by the adult for future opportunities that might extend the child's learning taking the child, rather than prescribed curricular content, as the central guide. Furthermore, reflective observation encourages movement away from traditional, organizational/management roles, strengthening the focus on the educational, pedagogical role of the adult. Relationships and interactions are central to a nurturing pedagogy as critical spaces for learning individually and in groups. Early childhood educators who are sensitive, attuned and responsive to children's cues and apply a nurturing pedagogy are better able assess what type of assistance children need, if any, and ensure their responses are accordingly respectful of the child. To create this significant shift to understanding the educative role of care in practice it is necessary to explicitly acknowledge the critical contribution of this interpersonal aspect of early education, to make it visible, to realize it as the practice of the everyday interactions, the proximal processes.

Realizing inclusive early childhood education

Mirroring the shift observed in psychology and early education from a normative, developmental model of learning and development towards a socio-cultural, dynamic one the shift from a medical model towards a social model of disability suggests an acceptance of the multiple factors contributing to the experience of disability (Strnadova and Cumming, 2014). In characterizing a person's disability as arising from the interaction of a combination of personal traits and the surrounding environment the social model challenges mainstream institutions to adapt and accommodate the perceived needs of a particular individual. The model is the basis for the UN Convention on the Rights of Persons with Disabilities (2006). Moving from a model of special education as separate towards integrated mainstream education is challenging and has significant implications for the role and practice of educators (Shevlin et al. 2012).

The value of an inclusive approach to practice in early education is captured in a briefing note to the Irish government from the National Disability Authority (NDA), which points out that, in the majority of advanced countries mainstream early education is becoming the norm for the vast majority of children with disabilities (2014). This involves not only the redirection of resources from segregated services to mainstream early education but a commitment to inclusive practice which focuses on whole-setting involvement in supporting and integrating children rather than the traditional one-to-one support for children identified as present-ing with a special educational need. This reflects the inclusive nature of much early educational provision. Noting that children with special needs may not express themselves in traditional ways Vakil, Freeman and Swim (2003) point out that effective practices recommended for inclusive early learning environments are already embedded within the Reggio Emilia model of early education.

Nonetheless, alongside the core principle of inclusion in contem-porary early education literature the discourse of early intervention as a separate mechanism for overcoming disadvantage or disability continues (Dunn 2004; Department of Children and Youth Affairs (DCYA) 2015) creating a tension between mainstream, inclusive early education practices and targeted early intervention initiatives focusing on the individual child. Reflecting on some of the tensions challenging inclusive practice in New Zealand Dunn (2004) argues that the socio-cultural nature of the early childhood curriculum, Te Whariki (Ministry of Education 1996) is in con-flict with the common practice of prescribing individualized programmes for children with disabilities that underpins certain early intervention practices. She notes that such practices feed into a model of deficit thinking (Dunn and Barry 2004) which has been found among both early childhood professionals and parents. She points out that individualized programmes risk excluding children with disabilities from critical learning opportunities within inclusive early education contexts. In effect, early intervention strategies may be more exclusionary than inclusive. Within socio-cultural pedagogy, typified in the pedagogy of Reggio Emilia (Edwards et al. 1993), the Te Whariki curriculum (Ministry of Education 1996) and implicit in the Irish curriculum framework Aistear (NCCA 2009), priority is given to a strengths-based approach to working in partnership with children, focusing on what they are interested in and can do and locating 'early intervention' within daily routine and practices (Jennings et al. 2012).

In considering the discourse of special education Runswick-Cole and Hodge (2009) argue that the term 'special educational needs' has come to 'sustain and construct exclusionary practices within education' (13). While not going as far as Gernsbacher et al. (2016) who reject the concept of special needs as nothing more than a euphemism they do call for an alternative rights based discourse as a start in shifting the focus of both policy and practice. To strengthen their argument they point to the Reggio Emilia approach, embedded as it is in a child's rights framework, and suggest that it offers scholars a way forward from the limiting conceptualization of 'special educational need' towards the more inclusive consideration of 'educational rights'. Noting in particular the Reggio attention to the 'hundred languages of children' (Edwards et al. 1993) they point to the potential of documenting learning through multiple different media as a mechanism for inclusive practice that respects difference without highlighting deficit. Documenting a child's learning has a number of purposes; it provides a record of an individual child's progress, it provides an opportunity and context for teachers to learn and reflect, collaboratively and individually, on their own practice and it makes learning visible to the child, parents and other professionals. Notably the process of documentation applies to all children and is not used as a specific methodology for children presenting with additional needs thus facilitating individualized planning within an inclusive pedagogical context. An approach, which sees collaborative documentation as a core dimension of early education pedagogy presents many challenges and will require support for reformed practice in early education settings to allow time for documentation review, team meetings, engagement with parents and allied professionals and other shifts away from the more didactic approach of traditional practice (Vakil, Freeman and Swim 2003).

Katz and Chard (1996) were among the first authors to identify the power of documenting learning. They noted that 'Documentation typically includes samples of a child's work at several different stages of completion: photographs showing work in progress; comments written by the teacher or other adults working with the children; transcriptions of children's discussions, comments, and explanations of intentions about the activity; and comments made by parents' (1996: 2). Seitz (2008) suggests that documentation is richer when done in collaboration with other teachers, parents and children and as soon after the experience has been observed as possible.

Extending the general idea of documentation into the field of assessment, to include assessment *of* and *for* learning, Margaret Carr (2001) introduced the idea of 'Learning Stories' as a way of assessing children's learning dispositions. Learning stories are 'structured observations, often quite short, that take a 'narrative' or story approach. They keep the assessment anchored in the situation or action' (Carr 2000: 32). They provide a narrative account of children's experiences and make learning visible for others, guiding an understanding of children's learning and development. They are a narrative, strengths-based, credit-based form of assessment written-up by an intentional adult in partnership with the child. They draw from observations in everyday settings and are designed to provide a cumulative series of qualitative 'snapshots' or written vignettes relating to the child, often containing examples of children's own material or play episodes. They document a child's ability, what a child is able to achieve and draw on the child's own interests and experience to provide a context for reflection and realization of learning. Learning stories may also record the teacher's involvement in situations and some may describe situations where a group of children is involved in the same experience. One of the more powerful aspects of the learning story approach to assessment is the potential for meaningful partnerships with parents and allied professionals. This collaborative dimension provides a space within which to find a common language and strengthen the links between the child's key early learning environments to enhance the continuity in children's learning and development. Such collaborations are particularly relevant for children who have additional needs (Vakil et al. 2003).

While the approach has met with some criticism (Blaiklock 2008) the role of learning stories in documenting learning in an accessible format has been broadly welcomed by early childhood educators, children and parents (Carr et al. 2010; Dunphy 2008; Dunn 2004). They provide a mechanism for making valuable and useful statements about children's learning that is more accessible than usual assessment formats. Once written a learning story can be analysed in a 'short term review' which summarizes what learning has occurred and future action building on this learning can then be recorded (Carr 2001). They encourage feedback between the teacher and child, help identify and celebrate a child's progress and achievements and inform next steps. Documenting learning through the use of learning stories takes skill and an understanding of the underlying socio-cultural and participative principles guiding this rich form of assessment.

Although a powerful instrument for collaborative work learning stories in inclusive early intervention have proved challenging. Without careful attention to the underpinning theoretical basis behind the development and application of learning stories research suggests that there is a tendency towards 'an automatic default to a deficit view of the child when considering the child's educational programme' (Dunn 2004: 127). Dunn (2004) suggests that this may reflect a misunderstanding about socio-cultural curriculum which sees it as somehow skill-less. On the contrary, a holistic approach recognizes that the sum is greater than its parts and there is a responsibility on the educator to identify the component skills to be given special attention for each child, particularly those with additional requirements. The important point, as Cullen (2003) notes is that the educator actually has to identify those component skills 'that would help the child achieve their interest-based goals' (282). Dunn (2004) draws our attention to Cullen's focus on the child's 'interest-based' goals as opposed to pre-determined learning goals. Learning stories are not designed to meet externally dictated goals for children but rather move from children's own manifest interests towards supporting the achievement of positive learning and development. This, Dunn (2004) argues is one of the primary distinctions between a deficit approach and the potential of a truly inclusive approach to early childhood education.

Conclusion

Drawing on contemporary research this chapter identifies key features of quality early education arguing that it is, inherently, inclusive. Quality is evident in settings that are well planned, contextually sensitive, well-resourced and professionally provided. Attention is given to the dynamic dimension of individual development, and the opportunities that arise in children's day-to-day life that contribute to learning and development. The conceptualization of the agentic child-developing-in-context provides for a dynamic image of learning and development requiring practitioners to appreciate and respond to the reality that even the very youngest children contribute to the context and content of their own development. This is not to underestimate the dependence of the child or the protective role of the adult. It does however, challenge adults to take account of the rich and diverse nature of each child when planning and providing early learning opportunities.

Positive early learning environments provide secure relationships which facilitate children's exploration, play and learning and are embedded within a child's rights framework offering educators a way forward from the limiting conceptualization of 'special educational need' towards the more inclusive consideration of 'educational rights'. Central to achieving this in a convincing manner for all children requires identifying a mechanism that makes learning visible in a dynamic and respectful way. The value of documenting learning through multiple different methods, but particularly through learning stories, was proposed as a powerful mechanism for inclusive practice that respects difference without highlighting deficit. Learning stories are designed to evolve from children's own manifest interests towards supporting the achievement of positive learning and development. Inclusion is more than simply providing families with access to an early education setting; it is about celebrating diversity, supporting settings to change, facilitating a reformed pedagogy and positively responding to the possibilities and opportunities that all children bring which enrich the early learning environment. While inclusive early education may be challenging to educators it has the potential to contribute to the dynamic and positive development of all children.

References

Blaiklock, K. E. (2008). A Critique of the Use of learning Stories to Assess the learning Dispositions of Young Children. *New Zealand Research in Early Childhood Education Journal,* 11, 77–87

Bredekamp, S., and Copple, C. (eds) (1997). *Developmentally appropriate practice in early childhood programs.* Washington, DC: National Association for the Education of Young Children.

Bronfenbrenner, U. (ed.) (2005). *Making Human Beings Human: Bioecological Perspectives on Human Development.* London: Sage.

Bronfenbrenner, U., and Morris, P. (2006). The Bioecological Model of Human Development. In R. M. Lerner and W. E. Damon (eds). *Handbook of Child Psychology: Vol 1, Theoretical Models of Human Development,* pp. 793–828. West Sussex: John Wiley and Sons.

Carr, M. (2000). Let me count the ways (to do assessment). Proceedings of *Practice, Policy and Politics Conference,* Victoria University of Wellington, 9–12 July 2000. New Zealand: New Zealand Educational Institute.

Carr, M. (2001). *Assessment in early childhood settings.* London: Paul Chapman Publishing.

Carr, M., Smith, A. B., Duncan, J., Jones, C., Lee, W., and Marshall, K. (2010). *Learning in the Making: Dispositions and Design in Early Education.* Rotterdam: Sense Publications.

Centre for Effective Services (CES) (2014). *Prevention and Early Intervention in children and young people's services: Ten Years of Learning.* Dublin: CES.

Center on the Developing Child (CDC) (2007). *The Science of Early Childhood Development: Closing the Gap Between What We Know and What We Do.* Harvard: CDC. Retrieved from: <http://www.developingchild.harvard.edu>.

Clark, A., and Moss, P. (2001). *Listening to Young Children: The Mosaic Approach.* London: National Children's Bureau.

Cullen, J. (2003). The Challenge of *Te Whariki:* Catalyst for change?. In J. Nuttall (ed.), *Weaving Te Whariki,* pp. 269–296. Wellington: New Zealand Council for Educational Research.

Dahlberg, G., and Moss, P. (2005). *Ethics and politics in early childhood education.* London: RoutledgeFalmer.

Dalli, C., White, E. J., Rockel, J., Duhn, I., Buchanan, E., Davidson, S., Ganly, S., Kus, L., and Wang, B. (2011.) *Quality early childhood education for under two-year-olds: What should it look like? A literature review. Report to the Ministry of Education.* New Zealand: Ministry of Education.

Department of Children and Youth Affairs (DCYA). *Supporting Access to the Early Childhood Care and Education (ECCE) Programme for Children with a Disability.* Retrieved from: <https://www.dcya.gov.ie/documents/publications/20151118ECCEAccessSpecialNeedsReport.pdf>.

Dunphy, E. (2008). *Supporting early learning and development through formative assessment.* Research Paper. Dublin: National Council for Curriculum and Assessment.

Dunn, L. (2004). Developmental Assessment and Learning Stories in Inclusive Early Intervention Programmes: Two Constructs in One Context. *NZ Research in Early Childhood Education,* 7, 119–133.

Dunn, L., and Barry, S. (2004). *The Early Childhood Learning and Assessment Exemplar Project: Inclusive assessment for children with early intervention support. Final report to the Ministry of Education.* Wellington: Ministry of Education.

Edwards, C., Gandini, L., and Forman, G. (eds) (1998). *The hundred languages of children: The Reggio Emilia approach—advanced reflections* (2nd edn). Greenwich, CT: Ablex.

Einarsdottir, J. (2007). Research with children: methodological and ethical challenges. *European Early Childhood Education Research Journal,* 15 (2), 197–211.

European Commission (EC) (2014). *Proposal for key principles of a quality framework for early childhood education and care.* Brussels: EC.

Fleer, M. (2015). *Inclusive pedagogy from a child's perspective. A research in practice series title.* Canberra: Early Childhood Australia.

Fortunati, A. (ed.) (2014). *San Miniato's Approach to the Education of Children: Children's protagonism, family participation and community responsibility toward a curriculum of possibilities.* Pisa: Edizioni ETS.

French, G. (2007). *Children's early learning and development.* Research paper. Dublin, National Council for Curriculum and Assessment.

Gernsbacher, M. A., Raimond, A. R., Balinghasay, M. T., and Boston, J. S. (2016). 'Special Needs' is an ineffective euphemism. *Cognitive Research,* 1 (1), 29.

Hayes, N. (2008). Teaching Matters in early educational practice: The case for a nurturing pedagogy. *Early Education and development,* 19 (3), 430–440.

Hayes, N. (2013). *Early Year practice: Getting it Right from the Start.* Dublin: Gukl and Macmillan.

Hayes, N., and Filipović, K. (2017). Nurturing the 'buds of development': changing the narrative from learning outcomes to learning opportunities in early childhood pedagogy. *International Journal of Early Years Education,* DOI: 10.1080/09669760.2017.1341303.

Hayes N., O'Toole, L., and Halpenny, A. M. (2017). *Introducing Bronfenbrenner: A Guide for Practitioners and Students in Early Years Education.* London: Routledge.

Hedges, H. (2014). Children's Content Learning in Play Provision: Competing Tensions and Future Possibilities. In L. Brooker, M. Blaise and S. Edwards (eds). *The Sage Handbook of Play and Learning in Early Childhood,* pp. 192–203. London: Sage.

Horgan, D., Forde, C., Parkes, A. Martin, S., Mages, L., and O'Connell, A. (2015). *Children and young people's experiences of participating in decision-making at home, in schools and in their communities.* Dublin: DCYA.

Hujala, E., and Niikko, A. (2012). The Science of Early Childhood Education – Core Issues. in M. Veisson, E. Hujala, P. K. Smith and M. Waniganayake (eds), *Global Perspectives in Early Childhood Education: Diversity, Challenges and Possibilities,* pp. 21–33. Frankfurt: Peter Lang.

Jennings, D., Hanline, M. F., and Woods, J. (2012). Using Routine-Based Interventions in Early Childhood Special Education. *Dimensions of Early Childhood,* 40 (2), 13–22.

Kaga, Y., Bennett, J., and Moss, P. (2010). *Caring and Learning Together.* Paris: UNESCO.

Katz, L., and Chard, S. C. (1994). *Engaging Children's Minds: The Project Approach* (2nd edn). Norwood, NJ: Ablex Publishing.

Kickbusch, I. (2012). *Learning for Well-being: A Policy Priority for Children and Youth in Europe. A process for change,* with the collaboration of Jean Gordon and Linda O' Toole. Drafted on behalf of the Learning for Well-being Consortium of Foundations in Europe. Brussels: Universal Education Foundation.

Lundy, L. (2007). 'Voice' is not enough: conceptualising Article 12 of the United Nations Convention on the Rights of the Child. *British Educational Research Journal,* 33 (6), 927–942.

Lundy, L., McEvoy, L., and Byrne, B. (2011). Working with young children as co-researchers: an approach informed by the United Nations Convention on the Rights of the Child. *Early Education and Development,* 22 (5), 714–736.

Mahony, K., and Hayes, N. (2006). *In Search of Quality: Multiple Perspectives* Dublin: Centre for Early Childhood Development and Education.

Ministry of Education (1996). *Te Whariki: Early Childhood Curriculum.* Wellington, NZ: Learning Media Ltd.

Molloy, C., Hayes, N., Kearney, J., Glennon Slattery, C., and Corish, C. (2012). Researching young children's perception of food in Irish pre-schools: An ethical dilemma. *Research Ethics,* 8 (3), 155–164.

Moss, P. (2001). The otherness of Reggio. In L. Abbott and C. Nutbrown (eds), *Experiencing Reggio Emilia: Implications for preschool provision,* pp. 125–137. Buckingham: Open University Press.

Moss, P. (2006). *Listening to young children: Beyond rights to ethics. Discussion paper.* Thomas Coram Research Unit: University of London.

National Association for Education of Young Children (NAEYC) (2009). *Position Statement: Developmentally Appropriate Practice in Early Childhood Programs Serving Children from Birth through Age 8.* Washington, DC: National Association for the Education of Young Children.

National Council for Curriculum and Assessment (NCCA) (2009). *Aistear: The Early Childhood Curriculum Framework.* Dublin: National Council for Curriculum and Assessment.

National Disability Authority (2014). *Briefing Paper: Inclusion of children with disabilities in mainstream early childhood care and education. The lessons from research and international practice.* Dublin: National Disability Authority.

National Evaluation of Sure Start Team (2012). *The impact of Sure Start Local programmes on seven year olds and their families.* London: Department for Education.

New, R. (2007). Reggio Emilia as Cultural Activity Theory in Practice. *Theory into Practice,* 46 (1), 5–13.

Organization for Economic Co-Operation and Development (OECD) (2006). *Starting Strong II Early Childhood Education and Care.* Paris: OECD.

Parrini, C. (2014). Recognising Identities to Embrace Diversity: Children with 'special rights' in the nursery. In A. Fortunati (ed), *San Miniato's Approach to the Education of Children: Children's protagonism, family participation and community responsibility toward a curriculum of possibilities,* pp. 78–89. Pisa: Edizioni ETS.

Powell, M. A., Fitzgerald, R., Taylor, N. J., and Graham, A. (2012, March). International Literature Review: *Ethical Issues in Undertaking Research with Children and Young People* (Literature review for the Childwatch International Research Network). Lismore: Southern Cross University, Centre for Children and Young People / Dunedin: University of Otago, Centre for Research on Children and Families.

Pramling Samuelsson, I., and Asplund Carlsson, M. (2008). The Playing Learning Child: Towards a pedagogy of early childhood. *Scandinavian Journal of Educational Research,* 52 (6), 623–641.

Runswick-Cole, K., and Hodge, N. (2009). Needs or rights? A challenge to the discourse of special education. *British Journal of Special Education,* 6 (4), 198–203.

Ryan, S., Ó hUallacháin, S., and Hogan, J. (1998.) *Early Start Preschool Programmes: Final Evaluation Report.* Dublin: Education Research Centre.

Seitz, H. (2008). Power of Documentation in the Early Childhood Classroom. *Young Children,* March, 88–93.

Shevlin, M., Winter, E., and Flynn, P. (2012). Developing inclusive practice: teacher perceptions of opportunities and constraints in the Republic of Ireland. *International Journal of Inclusive Education* 1 – 15.

Singer, E. (2015). Play and playfulness in early childhood education. *Psychology in Russia: State of the Art,* 8 (2), 27–35.

Sixsmith, J., Nic Gabhainn, S., Fleming, C., and O'Higgins, S. (2007). Children's, parents' and teachers' perceptions of child wellbeing. *Health Education,* 107 (6), 511–523.

Smith, A. B. (2016). *Children's Rights: Towards Social Justice.* Talk to Seminar in Wellington, New Zealand, 12 April 2016. Sponsored by Child Well-being Network and Variety.

Start Strong (2014). *If I Had a Magic Wand: Young Children's Visions and Ideas for Early Care and Education Services.* Dublin: Start Strong.

Strnadova, I., and Cumming, T. M. (2014). Editorial: People with Intellectual Disabilities Conducting Research: New Directions for Inclusive Research. *Journal of Applied Research in Intellectual Disabilities,* 27, 1–2.

United Nations (1989). *Convention of the Rights of the Child.* New York: United Nations.

Vakil, S., Freeman, R., and Swim, T. J. (2003). The Reggio Emilia Approach and Inclusive Early Childhood Programs. *Early Childhood Special Education,* 30 (3), 187–192.

Vygotsky, L. (1978). *Mind in Society.* Cambridge, MA: Harvard University Press.

Weikart, D. (2004). *How High/Scope Grew: A Memoir.* Ypsilanti: High/Scope Educational Research Foundation.

Wood, E. (2013,) *Play, learning and the Early Childhood Curriculum* (2nd ed.). London: Sage Publishing.

Woodhead, M. (2005). Early childhood development: A question of rights. *International Journal of Early Childhood,* 37(3), 79–98.

Woodhead, M. (2006). *Changing Perspectives on Early Childhood: Theory, Research and Policy. Paper commissioned for the EFA Global Monitoring Report 2007, Strong foundations: early childhood care and education.* Geneva: UNESCO.

Woodrow, C., and Newman, L. (2015). Recognising, Valuing and Celebrating Practitioner Research in L. Newman and C. Woodrow (eds), *Practitioner Research in Early Childhood: International Issues and Perspectives.* London: Sage Publications.

Zigler, E., and Muenchow, S. (1992). *Head Start: The Inside Story of America's Most Successful Educational Experiment.* New York: Basic Books.

16 Participation, engagement and voice: Where do we go from here?

This final chapter of this book *Seen and Heard* offers some concluding thoughts on participation, engagement and voice and will summarize some of the highlights and innovation in the book, in order to reinforce the main concepts. We shall also explore, through some speculative analysis, key elements described in the various chapters, case studies, and vignettes as examples of innovation. In creating this analysis, we hope that readers will be informed as to how to incorporate these elements into their research, teaching and practice dedicated to researching with children; reinforcing the benefits of a strong rights-based culture. We shall then consider the implications of this book as an example of an academic research-oriented reference text and its potential use in research, pedagogy, practice. In terms of research, pedagogy and practice we will explore its potential use in the career of an advancing researcher, as well as a guide for undergraduate, postgraduate, Master's and Doctoral level teaching and research involving research with children with disabilities. We shall conclude with some ideas on future research and what might happen next in the field of voice.

Adopting a Human Rights approach is fundamental to the design of research and practice that seeks to facilitate the participation, engagement and voice of children with disabilities. Human Rights treaties apply directly to all children's lives. Human Rights were irrevocably violated during two World Wars. The Universal Declaration of Human Rights emanated from such a complete disregard for human existence. Initially considered reactionary to the previous World Wars, the Declaration witnessed for the first time how countries could protect the inalienable rights of their people. This book contributes to the 70th anniversary of the Universal Declaration of Human Rights through the exploration of innovative approaches to researching with children with disabilities from a rights orientation. More recent if not more pertinent to this book, in 1989, the UN General Assembly ratified the United Nations Convention on the Rights of the Child (UNCRC). It is now accepted as the most ratified international human rights treaty ever. Through ratification, it is incumbent on States Parties to implement the Convention's provisions. The UNCRC's participation rights are particularly applicable in this book as Professor Tisdall suggests in Chapter Two, these rights are 'challenging conceptualizations of childhood as merely passive recipients of services and solely vulnerable dependents on their parents, families and communities'. Children have the right to have their views considered in all matters concerning them. More recently, the right to participation was reiterated in the United Nations Convention on the Rights of Persons with Disabilities (UNCRPD) (2006), in Article 7. Children's participation is unequivocally embedded in the human rights agenda internationally.

The ICF-CY serves as a classification system for factors that influence health and wellbeing, but its use in this book demonstrates how researchers investigate the influential factors of child development within a biopsychosocial perspective. Its use is also demonstrates as a conceptual tool and as a universal language to enhance aetiological neutrality, and describe disability and participation in the context of the environment. The ICF-CY also served as a cohesive thread assigning impartiality to the role of participation of children with disabilities in everyday life situations.

This book illustrates a historical and contemporary trajectory of research activity with children to a poststructural, anthropological, and phenomenological [among others] framework including as Dr Watson suggests, research among children. Children are included as collaborators, decision makers, consultants and evaluators. A consensus has been reached by the authors of this book in their sensitive creations of a resistance to the hegemonic view of childhood that characterizes children who have been seen but perhaps not heard. The collective voices in this book confirm a growing expectation that investigation should be with children rather than on or for children. As editors we hope that this book has challenged the subjectification of these children and will encourage researchers and their post graduate students to think about their work from the perspective of the disabled child. It is our hope that researchers will cogitate on this contemporary child's voice, and indeed will ask the question, what would this child say? – as a starting point. Through incorporating the presence and the embodiment of child voice, and the varying interpretations of 'voice', presented in this book where authors explore children's voice from a number of philosophical, methodological and interpretive orientations including psychological, sociological, legal, therapeutic, and educational perspectives, we are now making the assumption that childhood does not limit expression nor disability hinder its freedom. This book engages with readers committed to research with children with disabilities who they acknowledge already have a voice in the home, Early Intervention or education setting.

Highlights from Part I: Legislation, policy and theories

If we recall, in Chapter 1 Professor Kay Tisdall extends notions of participation and voice from a legal and human rights perspective which are situated within a critique of the UNCRC and the UNCRPD in support of children's capacity and competence to participate in research. Professor Tisdall provides us with a theoretical impetus which accounts for a significant 'turn' in the social sciences and related disciplines, to undertaking research with rather than on children acknowledging that children can respond on their own behalf and make meaningful contributions. This chapter heralds new opportunities and challenges that accompany research methods, governance, procedures and ethics. There is a reconsideration of communication and 'voice'; concepts of capacity and competence are embedded in this masterclass and eloquently written chapter.

Many contributors in this volume have incorporated the various strands of the turn that Professor Tisdall refers to. Implementing these strands, our contributors have developed 'participative' and 'creative' methodologies to work directly with children. The authors have provided an intense and extensive focus on ethics; expanding our knowledge of the ways children can be involved in research, from participants to advisers, experts and researchers and they have dedicated their work to a collective research objective – to genuinely and authentically present children's 'voice'. This book explores Professor Tisdall's strands, while cognisant of current challenges and tensions, the contributing authors have creatively developed ideas and concepts based on human rights; recognizing human dignity and valuing all children. This book acknowledges but also meets the challenges Professor Tisdall refers to with regard to the use of participatory methods meeting different children's communication needs when accessing and presenting the voice of the child. Dr Mary Wickenden's chapter draws on global and human rights perspectives, while considering whether and how disabled children's voices can be recognized and heard. This chapter draws on a new sociology of childhood and in the context of a global agenda, challenges concepts of voice, inclusion and participation which are illuminated through multiple research studies involving children who communicate in unusual and unconventional ways. Dr Wickenden presents the challenges of participatory research and encourages readers to consider that all children having the right to be consulted and contributing to society, is not a universal view.

The chapter by Ms Elena Jenkin and colleagues combines theoretical lenses (childhood, disability and postcolonialism) and illuminates how children with a disability in developing country contexts are constructed as underdeveloped, deficient, and incompetent. The authors identify that there is little knowledge of the lives of young children with a disability living in developing countries and their invisibility in children's research exemplifies their marginalization and lack of agency. The authors challenge Western theorizing and develop approaches and methodologies that avert the subjectification of these children. For researchers in developing country contexts, this chapter offers an excellent example of partnership and enablement to engage children in a research project. The authors share innovative methods in the dissemination of research findings by children through the use of film. Dr Karen Watson encourages young children with and without disabilities to share their voice and discourses in her ethnographic research on inclusive Early Years classrooms in Australia. Drawing on a poststructural framework this chapter innovatively explores the idea of researching 'among' children in three 'inclusive' early childhood classrooms. This research-oriented chapter challenges our assumptions and critiques 'adult centric' definitions of participation by listening to children negotiate difference in the classroom; 'taking up or resisting sanctioned circulating discourses' relative to inclusion. How they decide who is included and excluded is particularly innovative and of special interest to the concepts of participation and inclusion of and by children.

Highlights from Part II: Innovative explorations of different forms of voice

The second part of this book presented innovative explorations of voice from hard to reach groups and excelled in approaches to and acknowledgement of what voice is and can be. Professor Melanie Nind's research and methodologically oriented chapter emphasizes the educative value of listening and attending to children with complex disabilities. Professor Nind's chapter presents what she describes as a reciprocal project which she argues begins with the teacher's attitude towards listening and openness to dialogue. At the outset Professor Nind makes a very poignant point and shares the underpinning philosophy to her interactions with learners: 'if it is my job to teach you then I need to be able to reach you'. This chapter focused on educational settings and how listening to voices of children with complex disabilities is important. This chapter recognizes the multiple modalities of communication. Dr Ben Simmons's engaging chapter provides a novel approach to participation and engagement. Using the 'phenomenology of intersubjectivity' to researching with profoundly disabled children as an innovative approach to developing an experiential framework for analysing lived social experiences, this original exploration challenges existing approaches (within the PMLD field), focusing on a philosophical theoretical framework that is applied to profound and complex disability. In his innovative work, Dr Simmons creates new ways of embodying voice; finding alternatives to verbal means. Dr Simmons draws us into the lifeworld of the child with profound and multiple disabilities. Dr Miriam Twomey provides an alternate understanding of voice for nonverbal children. Adopting a phenomenological perspective on ASD and exploring the role of imitation and movement, the author draws attention to the role of movement and being moved in intersubjectivity. Dr Twomey explores movement difficulties for children with ASD and what may present as obstacles to affective engagement and social interaction. Dr Martine M. Smith's chapter highlights the difficulties children who have severe speech impairments and who rely on augmentative and alternative communication experience in order to express themselves. Due to their potential unintelligibility they are vulnerable to being silenced and they may have difficulties in producing communication that others can understand. Dr Smith highlights the potential for miscommunication and misrepresentation of these children's voices in a compelling chapter which lays bare the essentials of communication partnerships. She also reiterates Dr Wickenden's point about the individuality and 'uniqueness' of voice and communication style.

Dr Clare Carroll affirms the concepts of participation through a wider lens, highlighting that through the stages of the research we need to be cognisant of Bronfenbrenner's bio-ecological systems' approach. Dr Carroll's contribution has a pervasive appeal and raises many questions; should we design research projects for one system only? Are gatekeepers representative of other systems outside of our control? Can children's voice visually recorded through a SenseCam tell us something that we do not already know? Is participation dependent on the engagement of all stakeholders?

Highlights from Part III: Disciplinary illustrations and explorations around voice

The third part of this book highlighted disciplinary explorations around voice. Play, outdoor playspaces, unstructured private speech, pain, and identity are also seen as ways of expressing voice. This section also explores contexts of expression and inclusion. Dr Helen Lynch's innovative work adopts a beyond voice stance where she interrogates the importance of 'doing' for the young child and explores a newly developed concept of 'being at play'. This chapter paid much needed attention to Universal Design in outdoor spaces. This innovative work much needed attention on the importance of outdoor play and spaces of all children. Drawing on research by Dr Prellwitz, the voices of children are considered a valuable resource amongst those of landscape artists and researchers in the quest for inclusive spaces and the challenge of designing using a Universal Design lens. Dr Rena Lyons challenges us to include the views of children with speech and developmental language disorders in order to understand how we can support them as they develop. Dr Line Caes and Dr Siobhan O'Higgins acknowledge that including children with cognitive impairment to share their expert view of their pain experience requires creativity and requires researchers to use methods that match the child's way of communicating. Dr Carolyn Blackburn presents findings from her study that explored the policy to practice context of young children's speech, language and communication in early childhood settings. This chapter is of particular interest to research and pedagogy where children's use of private speech as self-regulating became an emergent theme. The author illustrates that unstructured activities that are more prominent in mainstream school settings and that children engage more in episodes of private speech during unstructured child-led activities in mainstream settings. Professor Nóirín Hayes presents the final chapter of this section and theorizes on a universal view of inclusion as context for participation and acknowledgement of the 'child-in-context' where children are not defined by their differences. Successfully challenging normative frameworks within which children find themselves is a good starting point if we are to view participation and inclusion seriously.

Implications for research

Professor Tisdall emphasizes how a human rights framework can support how children with disabilities are perceived by society and also has significant implications for research with children. While research that is

child led and designed to their liking as well as being respectful of children, research must consider the debate on the ethical issues of informed
consent, ownership of research, and the ethical sensitivities when involving children as co-producers or collaborators. Many of the contributors in
this book incorporated stringent and rigorous ethical, consent and assent
procedures in all aspects of the research process – from design, data collection and analysis, to dissemination. Contributors demonstrate how
research that authentically involves children will create better knowledge,
be more ethical and inclusive and will recognize all means of communication. A child's participation in research must respect their human rights
not to mention their right to communicate. It has been highlighted in the
chapters that children with disabilities want to share their views on issues
other than their disability. This book challenges researchers, funders and
ethics committees to be radical in their views relating to children with
communication difficulties while being respectful of the human rights of
all children. In chapters by Nind, Jenkins et al., Simmons, Twomey, Smith
and Carroll, the researchers argue that we must recognize the diversity of
children's voice, in whatever form it takes. This understanding and recognition will support researchers in the development of data collection tools
to enable the participation of all children. With future research in mind
Professor Nind provides a place for the authors to raise questions about
research practice with particular relevance to inclusivity and exclusivity,
children's competence and ethical issues. These questions challenge current thinking and views on research involving children in research and
in particular young children with disabilities. Dr Wickenden argues that
'having a voice' or 'hearing people's voices' can be understood as a powerful trope. Dr Simmons shares his innovative phenomenological framework and the importance of pre-observations to support partnership in
choice of methods. He shares two examples of vignette writing which he
used as a method and shares how he analysed these. Challenging existing
research methods Dr Simmons draws on the lived experience of the child
with PMLD and Dr Twomey shares the importance for researchers and
practitioners and families to be creative, inventive and open-minded in
considering movement as a means of engagement. Dr Twomey challenges
readers to view a person's life as a trajectory rather than a destination and

to focus on timing, tuning in, being responsive to children who may not verbally communicate. Movement and being moved are brought into the foreground with the purpose of engaging readers to be open to engagement at a bodily level with individuals with ASD.

Future potential of children using the puppets and microphone – designing their own research – becoming mini-ethnographers. Dr Clare Carroll encourages viewing children as collaborators – widening the lens of participation. Dr Helen Lynch shares that observing children's play can enable researching children's lives. Dr Lynch's innovative use of videography as a qualitative data collection tool and how using this tool offered a way to analyse occupational behaviour of young infants and to consider play in context is very significant and can be applied to all young children in the determination of affordances. When interpreting children's actions adults need to understand these actions from a child's perspective the researcher needs to share experiences and 'listen' to the child and what the child does ... through play. Dr Prellwitz and Dr Lynch continue the theme of outdoor play and emphasize the importance of collaborative partnership and significance of consultations with children as preparatory to design of the research project. Themes of openness, sensitivity and flexibility during the data collection process are raised in work by many of the authors, for example, Lyons, Smith, Cases and O'Higgins. Dr Lyons calls on researchers to allow data collection activities to reflect the experiences and interests of the children.

Implications for pedagogy

Within early educational settings there are set practices and routines that may not nurture or foster listening to the voice of children. As Professor Nind points out, educational settings vary in their philosophy on inclusivity and listening. Dr Watson explores the role of inclusive Early Years settings and the unwitting knowledge of children and Dr Simmons challenges the field of PMLD with the importance of alternative theoretical

frameworks. Dr Wickenden guides the reader to explore voices as a concept
and explore the meaning of voice. She stresses that we need to understand
how children with disabilities see themselves. We need to explore this
view across their contexts they engage in. Dr Twomey emphasizes the
opportunities that present during the integration programme of a young
child with ASD. Interaction with peers became a daily occurrence. The
School Buddy System contributed greatly to Aaron's socialization and
learning. Dr Smith's chapter exemplifies the need for training on the optimal role of the communication partner. Dr Carroll's chapter emphasizes
on collaboration and participation at all levels is vitally important for the
trainee Speech and Language Therapist as she illustrates her own participatory qualities in collaboration with the stakeholders in her research.
Dr Lyons calls for us to explore openness and use choices in interactions
with children. Professor Hayes emphasizes the role of the child-in-context
and how inclusion in early years needs to accommodate this. Professor
Nind shares how listening and attending to learners with complex needs
can support their learning, mutual pleasure, and a healthy environment.
Dr Blackburn's research illustrates the need for unstructured approaches
and the potential for development of private speech that enhances
self-regulation.

Implications for practice

If we are to consider children's views seriously, as researchers we have a serious responsibility to make this a reality. As Professor Tisdall in Chapter
1 stressed 'participation must be part of young children's everyday lives'.
This book recognizes the agency of children with disabilities and considers
views of children from both Western countries and developing countries.
Jenkins and colleagues outline the importance of partnerships and sharing
of expertise between researchers and community organizations to support research design. Participatory research challenges research practice.
Professor Nind has deftly presented a valued approach to innovative practice

and emphasized a nuanced emphasis on the educative priority. This is followed by the importance of listening for the well-being of learners, which Professor Nind sees as integrally linked to the educational endeavour, followed by the need to listen for research purposes, culminating in the rights of children and disabled persons to be involved in research as in all aspects of the social world. She assumes that the benefits of voice are apparent; providing information for teachers, strengthening partnerships between pupils and teachers, helping with setting priorities and understanding what matters from pupils' perspectives, which creates a listening organization in which pupils feel valued and respected; fostering a sense of belonging and creative thinking. However, Professor Nind reminds us of Fielding's 'recalcitrant realities' where schools are challenged by students' complex disabilities or behaviour that challenges. Using Intensive Interaction as a tool in the educational setting with children with complex disabilities undoubtedly supports the educationalist to listen, attend and observe. In effect this enables the practitioner to really hear the child's voice and enable agency. Furthermore, this way of engaging with children with complex disabilities facilitates the researcher to use a 'multimodal lens' as described by Flewitt (2005) during data collection and data analysis. Dr Smith highlights that using aided communication can create barriers for the person to share their identity and voice and encourages practitioners to be creative, open, flexible and willing in their role as communication partner in the co-construction of interactions. Dr Wickenden recognizes that the 'voice' of the disabled children and adults may be unconventional and of a 'different kind'. She calls on researchers and practitioners to take the stance that all children can join in research. Dr Lyons encourages practitioners to be open to let children's points of view drive the agenda and for children to be actively involved in decision making in the therapy process. Dr Twomey's use of puppetry builds on notions of imitation and movement but also defers to approaches such as Intensive Interaction developed by Nind and Hewett and later used by Caldwell (2006). Dr Smith urges communicative partners, not to discredit choice making possibilities for children with severe communication difficulties. Dr Carroll suggests that not only do we need to continue our development of creativity around research with children but we need to collaborate more with the child and family.

Where do we go from here?

This book raises questions raised as to how innovative practices might be sustained. This brings professional development opportunities to the fore. Within pre-registration courses, for health and social care professionals and with the professionalization of educationalists, understanding the purpose for using multiple modalities to communicate and having opportunities to practice using multimodal communication in their interactions with children, in particular those with complex disabilities, will support their interactions. This learning will also help practitioners to understand and create opportunities to listen to the child's experiences more. Already conversations are taking place about the position of this book in our lives, re-imaginings of voice for different groups, and for groups who before now haven't had a voice. Conversations will continue to be immersed in participation, engagement, agency and voice, what it means and whose voice we need to listen to. We are already planning new sections/parts to our next edition. We hope to look at the life trajectory and the place of voice at different critical moments and transitions in the life of the person who finds communicating difficult. This reflects a key concept from Bakhtin's (1986) polyphony, that our speech is filled with the words of others. Understanding the words of others needs a multitude of voices and the capacity of my words to embody yours, creating a dialogic relationship between two voices:

> The person who understands must not reject the possibility or even abandoning his [sic] already prepared opinions and viewpoints. In the act of understanding a struggle occurs that involves mutual change and enrichment. (Bakhtin 1986: 142)

References

Bakhtin, M. (1986). *Speech Genres and Other Late Essays*. Edited by Caryl Emerson and Michael Holquist. Translated by Vern W. McGee. Austin, TX: University of Texas Press.

Caldwell, P. (2006). *Finding You Finding Me: Using Intensive Interaction to Get in Touch with People Whose Severe Learning Disabilities Are Combined with Autistic Spectrum Disorder.* London and Philadelphia, PA: Jessica Kingsley.

Flewitt, R. (2005). Is Every Child's Voice Heard? Researching the Different Ways 3-year-old Children Communicate and Make Meaning at Home and in a Pre-school Playgroup. *Early Years*, 25 (3), 207–222.

United Nations (1989). *Convention on the Rights of the Child.* New York: United Nations. <http://www.ohchr.org/EN/ProfessionalInterest/Pages/CRC.aspx>.

United Nations (2006). *Convention on the Rights of Persons with Disabilities.* New York: United Nations. <https://www.un.org/development/desa/disabilities/resources/general-assembly/convention-on-the-rights-of-persons-with-disabilities-ares61106.html>

Glossary

Augmentative and alternative communication refers to the use of modalities other than speech to augment or enhance speech that is difficult to understand or to replace speech as a mode of communication, both for expressive purposes and/or to support comprehension or understanding.

Bioecological model is a model of development conceptualized by Urie Bronfenbrenner and his colleagues. Central features include emphasis on relationships and interactions within contexts.

Cognitive impairment is generally regarded as having a noticeable and measurable difficulty in remembering, learning new things, concentrating and/or making decisions.

Complex disabilities is a term used to indicate not just multiple disabilities, but disabilities that interact to compound each other or create a complex profile of challenges. The UK Special Educational Needs Code of Practice: 0–25 years (Dept of Education, Dept of Health 2015) regards children with complex disabilities as those who need integrated or coordinated services from more than one agency.

Developmental delays are delays in meeting developmental milestones, such as sitting, walking, and talking, at the average age specified in standardized development charts.

Developmental language disorder is a term used to describe language difficulties that are unlikely to resolve by five years of age and create obstacles to communication or learning in everyday life. These language problems are not associated with a known condition such as autism spectrum disorder, brain injury, genetic conditions such as Down syndrome and sensorineural hearing loss (Bishop, D. V. M., Snowling, M., Thompson, P. A., Greenhalgh, T., & CATALISE Consortium. (2017). Phase 2 of CATALISE:

a multinational and multidisciplinary Delphi consensus study of problems with language development: Terminology. *Journal of Child Psychology and Psychiatry*, 58(10), 1068–1080).

Developmentally appropriate practice (DAP) is an approach to teaching grounded in the research on how young children develop and learn and in what is known about effective early education.

Dynamic development refers to the day-to-day development of individual children.

Early childhood education [ECE] and early childhood education and care [ECEC] are terms used interchangeably throughout the text to refer to any type (i.e. public, private or voluntary) of provision for young children that is subject to a national regulatory framework.

Impairments refers to problems in body function resulting in barriers to activity participation.

Intellectual disability is defined as a neurodevelopmental disorder with onset in early childhood, which results in functioning deficits in domains of cognitive social, emotional, sensory and motor development.

Intellectual impairment is a term used internationally (especially Australia and USA) and interchangeably with intellectual disability, for impairment occurring from childhood affecting conceptual, social and practical domains such as language, empathy and independence.

Learning Stories are an assessment tool used to document and describe a child's learning process and are also a way of making learning visible.

Neurodevelopmental disorder refers to significant developmental challenges that impact on a child's personal, social, educational or occupational functioning, for example, global developmental delay, intellectual disability, and autism spectrum disorder.

Normative development emphasizes the stages of development that the majority of children of that specific age are expected to achieve.

Nurturing pedagogy is an approach to early educational practice which foregrounds the educative nature of care and the caring nature of education.

Pain-related disability or impaired functioning refers to how pain impacts on everyday activities, including sleep patterns, school, physical, mental, social and family life.

Profound and multiple learning disabilities is the term used in the UK National Health Service when a child has more than one disability, with the most significant being a learning disability. Such a child will also often have a sensory or physical disability, complex health needs, or mental health difficulties. The term is also used by voluntary organizations, such as Mencap and British Institute of Learning Disabilities, who emphasize the uniqueness of each child with PMLD. Profound and multiple learning disabilities (PMLD) is a term used in the UK education system to refer to children with congenital neurological impairments that are said to result in global developmental delay.

Profound and multiple learning difficulties is the term used in the UK Special Educational Needs Code of Practice: 0–25 years (Dept of Education, Dept of Health 2015) for 'children who are likely to have severe and complex learning difficulties as well as a physical disability or sensory impairment'.

Profound intellectual impairment is a term used historically (and still in some circles) in association with an IQ below 20. Used in the book to indicate children with the most profound impairments who are often the most vulnerable because of their restricted autonomy, social exclusion and threats to well-being.

Proximal processes are progressively more complex reciprocal interactions between an active child and the persons, objects and symbols in the immediate environment

Restricted mobility is defined as using a wheelchair, walking-trolley or crutches when moving around,

Severe cognitive delays: children with severe cognitive delays will experience intellectual functioning that is below average compared to peers of the same age and this will exist concurrently with significant problems in adaptive behaviour (how children adapt to environmental demands compared to others of the same age). Children with severe cognitive delays will need additional support to participate in most activities.

Severe visual impairment is defined as a reduction in vision that cannot be corrected by prescription glasses, contact lenses, medicine or surgery (20/200 to 20/400).

Social, emotional and mental health difficulties is the more recent term in the UK replacing 'behavioural, social and emotional difficulties' to indicate children who may manifest withdrawn, isolated, challenging, disruptive or disturbing behaviour reflecting underlying mental health difficulties such as anxiety or depression or labelled conditions such as attention deficit disorder or attachment disorder

Specialist Communication and Interaction School refers to a school that supports children with complex communication and interaction needs.

Specialist Physical and Sensory Special School refers to a school that supports children with complex physical and sensory needs.

Speech disorders/impairments is a general term used to describe problems with speech production. *Speech disorders* may be mild, moderate, or severe, and can affect the child's intelligibility.

Significant communication impairments refers to difficulties in producing communication others can understand.

Acronyms

Augmentative and Alternative Communication (AAC)
Cerebral Palsy (CP)
Communication and Interaction (CI)
Consonant vowel (CV)
Consonant vowel consonant vowel (CVCV)
Delivering Equality of Opportunity in Schools (DEIS)
Department of Children and Youth Affairs (DCYA)
Early childhood education (ECE)
Early childhood education and care (ECEC)
Early Intervention (EI)
Early Years Foundation Stage (EYFS)
Face, Legs, Activity, Cry, and Consolability (FLACC)
Health-related quality of life (HRQoL)
International Classification of Function, Disability, and Health (ICF)
International Classification of Function, Disability, and Health – Children
    and Youth (ICF-CY)
National Association for the Education of Young Children (NAEYC)
National Council for Curriculum and Assessment (NCCA)
National Disability Authority (NDA)
Numeric rating scale (NRS)
Participative Health Research (PHR)
Physical and Sensory (PS)
Process Person Context Time (PPCT)
Profound and multiple learning disabilities (PMLD)
Revised Face, Legs, Activity, Cry, and Consolability (rFLACC)
Routines Based Interview (RBI)
Social communication model of pain (SCM)
Speech and Language Therapists (SLTs)
Speech, Language and Communication (SLC)
Speech Language and Communication Needs (SLCN)

United Nations (UN)
United Nations Convention on the Rights of Persons with Disabilities
    (UNCRPD)
United Nations Convention on the Rights of the Child (UNCRC)
Universal Design (UD)
Vowels (V)
World Health Organization (WHO)

Notes on contributors

CAROLYN BLACKBURN is Senior Research Fellow in the Faculty of Health, Education and Life Sciences at Birmingham City University. She is also a Churchill Early Years Prevention and Intervention Fellow and the Vice Chair of the European Association on Early Childhood Intervention. Her research has focused on family experiences of special educational needs and interdisciplinary practice. Her PhD explored the policy to practice context to young children's speech, language and communication development in the context of family and pre-school experience. More recently she has researched relationship-based early intervention services for children with complex needs, family experiences of premature birth and children's experiences of singing in hospital.

LINE CAES is a lecturer in the Division of Psychology, Faculty of Natural Sciences at the University of Stirling. Her research interests concern the social context of acute and chronic paediatric pain experiences. In particular, her research aims to further our understanding of the bidirectional influence between parents and children during painful experiences and how this influence changes throughout childhood. She is passionate about ensuring that our knowledge on the role of social factors in explaining child pain experiences translates into better treatment opportunities for children with chronic pain. An overview of her publications can be found at <https://www.stir.ac.uk/people/32368>.

ROBERT CAMPAIN is a research fellow at Deakin University, Australia. He has been involved in numerous disability-related projects with both the Victorian disability service provider, Scope, and Deakin University. The focus of his research has been on social inclusion for people with disability involving participatory research methods. His most recent work focuses on personal choice and control relating to individualized funding models in Australia.

CLARE CARROLL is a registered speech and language therapist and a lecturer at the National University of Ireland, Galway. She is part of the teaching team on the pre-registration speech and language therapy course and is Co-Director of the MSc in Childhood Speech, Language and Communication Needs. She has a wealth of clinical experience in the field of early intervention from working in the Irish Health Service and in private practice. She also teaches on the Master's in Education (Early Intervention) at Trinity College Dublin. Her research interests include supporting the engagement and participation of children with disabilities and their families in research and practice. The findings from her PhD on interdisciplinary team-working practices for children with disabilities have been published in *Infants and Young Children*, *Child Language Teaching and Therapy* and the *International Journal of Therapy and Rehabilitation*. She is passionate about services being informed by the people who use them; in particular, understanding what is important to people with communication disabilities. An overview of her publications is available at <http://www.nuigalway.ie/our-research/people/health-sciences/ccarroll/>.

MATTHEW CLARKE is Professor of International Development and Head of the School of Humanities and Social Sciences at Deakin University, Australia. He has worked in the development sector for more than two decades, originally working for a large international non-governmental organization before moving into the tertiary sector. His research has focused on the professional practice of NGOs as well as aid effectiveness, religion and development and humanitarian action. Much of his work focuses on the Pacific.

NÓIRÍN HAYES is Visiting Professor at the School of Education, Trinity College Dublin and Professor Emerita at the Centre for Social and Educational Research, Dublin Institute of Technology. Working within a bio-ecological framework of development and through a child rights lens she researches in early childhood education and care (ECEC) with a particular focus on early learning, curriculum and pedagogy and ECEC policy. She is convener of the Researching Early Childhood Education Collaborative (RECEC) at Trinity and is co-author of *Introducing Bronfenbrenner: A Guide* (2017) and co-editor of *Research and Evaluation in Community, Health and Social Settings* (2018).

ELENA JENKIN has worked alongside children and adults with disabilities, their families and communities in the Pacific and Asia, with a focus on understanding the experiences of inclusion in order to further advance contextually relevant inclusive practice within community and international development and human rights. She is a doctoral candidate at Deakin University, Australia, and a director of Australia Pacific Islands Disability Support (APIDS). She has a diverse disability-focused background, ranging from early intervention and community-based programmes to policy, teaching and research.

HELEN LYNCH is Senior Lecturer in the Department of Occupational Science and Occupational Therapy and a Research Associate of the Institute for Social Sciences at University College Cork. She has been engaged for many years in researching early childhood play environments and the rights of children to play, including children with disabilities. She has authored and presented multiple papers on these topics and has been involved in several research projects, with the Heritage Council, the Centre for Excellence in Universal Design in Ireland and the European Ludi COST Action TD1309. She is a member of Eurochild and the Children's Rights Alliance, Ireland.

RENA LYONS is Senior Lecturer in the Discipline of Speech and Language Therapy at NUI Galway, and previously worked in clinical practice for over fifteen years. Her PhD thesis focused on identity and wellbeing in children with speech and language disorders. Her findings have been published in the *Journal of Speech, Language and Hearing Research* and the *Journal of Communication Disorders*. Her paper 'Labels, identity and narratives in children with primary speech and language impairments' in the *International Journal of Speech-Language Pathology* was awarded the inaugural Taylor and Francis award for Best Paper for 2018. She is co-editing a book with Lindy McAllister entitled *Qualitative Research in Communication Disorders: An Introduction for Students and Clinicians*.

MELANIE NIND is Professor of Education and Director of the Centre for Research in Inclusion at the Southampton Education School, University of Southampton. She is Co-Director of the ESRC National Centre for Research Methods, Editor of the Bloomsbury 'Research Methods for

Education' book series, and Co-Editor of the *International Journal of Research and Method in Education*. She is best known for her work in teaching communication and social connectedness with people of all ages with profound intellectual impairments (*Access to Communication*, 1994/2005). Her current research interests lie in interactive and inclusive pedagogy and research methodology (*What is Inclusive Research?*, 2014 and *Research Methods for Pedagogy*, 2016).

SIOBHAN O'HIGGINS has research interests in adolescents and children with chronic pain, interventions, self-management and transition to adult services, and participative health research methods. Her recent co-authored publications include 'How to conduct mixed methods design' in *How to Conduct Research for Service Improvement*; 'Development of Feeling Better: A web-based pain management programme for children with chronic pain and their parents' in *Frontiers in Public Health*; and 'The prevalence, impact and cost of chronic non-cancer pain in Irish primary school children' in *BMJ Open*.

MARIA PRELLWITZ is Associate Professor in Occupational Therapy at Lulea University of Technology, Sweden. Her research interests have a focus on accessibility and usability in different environments for children with different abilities. Her special interests are the use of Universal Design to support accessibility to playgrounds and how to capture what matters to the children by listening to their own voices. Her most recent publications are 'The state of play in children's occupational therapy' in *British Journal of Occupational Therapy* and 'Are playgrounds a case of occupational injustice?' in *Child, Youth and Environment*.

BEN SIMMONS is Senior Lecturer at the Institute for Education, Bath Spa University, and Co-Director of the university's Centre for Research in Equity, Inclusion and Community. His research focuses on the social and educational inclusion of children with profound and multiple learning disabilities (PMLD). His work in this field has been funded through a British Academy Postdoctoral Fellowship (University of Bristol 2014–2017) and an ESRC PhD Studentship (University of Exeter 2005–2009). His doctoral research was published in 2014 as a co-authored book entitled *The*

PMLD Ambiguity: Articulating the Lifeworlds of Children with Profound and Multiple Learning Disabilities.

MARTINE SMITH is Associate Professor in Speech Language Pathology at Trinity College Dublin. Her research and clinical interests focus on speech, language and communication in children and adults who use augmentative and alternative communication. She has published widely on the language learning contexts of children who use aided communication, with over fifty peer-reviewed articles, one single-author volume, *Literacy and AAC*, and an edited volume, *The Silent Partner: Language and Interaction in Aided Communication*. She is the Principal Investigator in Ireland for the international study 'Becoming an Aided Communicator' and has served as Associate Editor and Editor of *Augmentative and Alternative Communication*.

KAY M. TISDALL is Professor of Childhood Policy at the University of Edinburgh. She has extensive policy and research interests in children's human rights. Her current research includes involving children's participation in contested contact cases (in Scotland and with European partners); monitoring of children's participation in international child protection (with partners in Brazil, Canada, China and South Africa); and children's activism to stop child marriage (with World Vision International and World Vision Bangladesh). She has recent and forthcoming publications in such journals as the *Childhood, Global Studies of Childhood, International Journal of Human Rights* and the *Journal of Social Policy*.

MIRIAM TWOMEY has a background in teaching and research in the field of early intervention, supporting children with Autism Spectrum Disorders and intellectual and neurodevelopmental disorders. She is Assistant Professor in Early Intervention at the Centre for People with Intellectual Disabilities (TCPID) in the School of Education, Trinity College Dublin. She leads the Masters in Education (Early Intervention), which is designed to provide postgraduate level study for those who wish to develop or enhance knowledge and experience working with young children with disabilities and/or Special Educational Needs (SEN) in the 0–6 age group. Her publications include 'Parents, Autism Spectrum Disorders and inner journeys' in the *Journal of Research in Special Educational Needs* (2016) and a co-authored article, 'Gaining access to support for children with special educational needs in the early years in Ireland: parental perspectives', in the *International Journal of Early Years Education* (2017).

KAREN WATSON is Lecturer in Early Childhood Education and Inclusive Education at the School of Education at the University of Newcastle, Australia. Her interest in inclusive practices among children shaped her PhD thesis, in which she examined how young children encounter and negotiate disability and difference in early childhood classrooms, and the role that unquestioned normative discourses play in producing both inclusionary and exclusionary practices. She has published a book entitled *Inside the 'Inclusive' Early Childhood Classroom: The Power of the 'Normal'*, as well as several articles and book chapters that focus on the uninterrupted effects of the normal.

MARY WICKENDEN is a disability researcher. She initially worked as a speech and language therapist, clinically and academically. She subsequently broadened her focus to cultural and social aspects of disability in diverse global contexts, training in medical/social anthropology. She carries out disability-related research, intervention and training projects in South Asia and East/Southern Africa, with a particular interest in using participatory and inclusive research methodologies to explore the lives of disabled adults and children and their families. She works at the Institute for Global Health, University College London and the Institute for Development Studies, University of Sussex.

ERIN WILSON is Associate Professor of Disability and Inclusion at Deakin University, Australia, where she occupies leadership roles in both teaching and research. She is an active researcher in the area of disability-inclusive practice and human rights in both Australian and developing country contexts. She has a special interest in research methods that enable the participation of people with disability as researchers, respondents and in advocating change based on research findings. Her most recent work focuses on issues of capacity building relating to individualized funding models in Australia.

Index